Brain, Mind, and the Structure of Reality

Brain, Mind, and the Structure of Reality

PAUL L. NUNEZ, PhD

Emeritus Professor
Department of Biomedical Engineering
Tulane University
New Orleans, Louisiana

OXFORD
UNIVERSITY PRESS

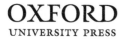

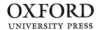

OXFORD
UNIVERSITY PRESS

Oxford University Press, Inc., publishes works that further
Oxford University's objective of excellence
in research, scholarship, and education.

Oxford   New York
Auckland   Cape Town   Dar es Salaam   Hong Kong   Karachi
Kuala Lumpur   Madrid   Melbourne   Mexico City   Nairobi
New Delhi   Shanghai   Taipei   Toronto

With offices in
Argentina   Austria   Brazil   Chile   Czech Republic   France   Greece
Guatemala   Hungary   Italy   Japan   Poland   Portugal   Singapore
South Korea   Switzerland   Thailand   Turkey   Ukraine   Vietnam

Published by Oxford University Press, Inc.
198 Madison Avenue, New York, New York 10016
www.oup.com

First issued as an Oxford University Press paperback, 2012
Oxford is a registered trademark of Oxford University Press

Library of Congress Cataloging-in-Publication Data

Nunez, Paul L.
Brain, mind, and the structure of reality / Paul L. Nunez.
p. ; cm.
Includes bibliographical references and index.
ISBN 978-0-19-534071-6 (hardcover); 978-0-19-991464-7 (paperback)
1. Consciousness.   2. Neuropsychology.   3. Cognitive neuroscience.   I. Title.
[DNLM: 1. Consciousness—physiology.   2. Brain—physiology. WL 705 N972b 2010]
QP411.N855 2010
612.8'2—dc22
2009030940

Cover Photo Credit: The lower part of the book cover was produced from a photograph taken by the Hubble
space telescope. This dying star system is nicknamed "Eskimo" because when viewed through a ground-based
telescope, it looks like a face surrounded by a furry hood. The image reminds us that humans are composed of the
heavy elements "cooked" inside stars by nuclear fusion and later distributed to the wider universe by supernovae;
we are made of star stuff. "The Eskimo Nebula" (NGC 2392). NASA, Andrew Fruchter and the ERO Team [Sylvia
Baggett (STScI), Richard Hook (ST-ECF), Zoltan Levay (STScI)]. Courtesy of the Office of Public Outreach at the
Space Telescope Science Institute (STScI)

9   8   7   6   5   4   3   2   1

Printed in the United States of America
on acid-free paper

Preface

My professional life is largely concerned with the rich dynamic patterns of brain electrical activity, the *shadows of thought* revealed with electroencephalography (EEG or "brain wave") recordings. Such work includes clinical medicine concerned with conditions like epilepsy and coma or the effects of drugs on our mental states. More often I participate in cognitive neuroscience experiments, where relationships between brain activity patterns and different kinds of normal mental states are explored. Like most brain scientists, much of my time is spent in "day science," with its focus on essential experimental or mathematical details. Esoteric reflections on the nature and origins of consciousness are mostly relegated to "night science," the discussions among colleagues after the second round of beers has been consumed. Yet, it was my fascination with consciousness that led to my seduction by brain science from theoretical plasma physics some 30 plus years ago.

To come to the decision to author this, my fourth book, I first had to ask myself if I really had anything substantial to add to the many existing books concerning consciousness. True, as an EEG expert, I could probably paint an enthralling picture of this "window on the working brain." But a number of EEG books already serve this function, so I decided it would be much more fun to opt for a broader view of consciousness. The resulting product integrates ideas from many disparate fields: philosophy, religion, politics, economics, neuroscience, physics, mathematics, and cosmology. With the exception of a few semi technical sections (labeled with asterisks) and some Endnotes material, the presentation level should be readily accessible to motivated college sophomores and many of their friends, parents, and teachers. Readers can simply skip over the more difficult material as desired and still follow the main ideas. Whenever possible, I employ personal and professional experiences and even a little humor to make for an easier read. You may love this book or hate it, but I don't think you will find it to be a clone of any other book.

Three central ideas permeate our discussions. First, consciousness is closely associated with the brain's *nested hierarchical structure,* also the hallmark of complex physical and social systems. This nested hierarchy is believed to enormously enhance brain complexity and scope of behavior, analogous to social networks embedded in cultures. Second, I suggest that any serious scientific study of consciousness must be carried out in the context of a more general study of reality. Thus, the original title *Brain, Mind, and the Emergence of Consciousness* was changed to *Brain, Mind, and the Structure of Reality*. This change led directly to the third idea—more emphasis must be placed on modern physics in consciousness study. One might say that I have been converted from "quantum atheist" to "quantum agnostic." My conversion has little to do with Eastern religions, flaky physics, or Schrödinger's cat; rather it stems from the acknowledged role of *information* in both the brain and physical sciences. I propose a tentative postulate labeled *RQTC*, the conjecture that relativity, quantum mechanics, and thermodynamics *may* somehow play an essential role in the theater of consciousness. I offer no conclusive evidence, only hints of possible connections. Nevertheless, if the study of consciousness indeed boils down to a more general study of reality, the world views provided by modern physics must be seriously considered along with evidence from brain science.

My wife Kirsty is a practical businesswoman; her initial reaction on hearing of my proposed topics was "It sounds like a collection of all the crazy ideas you ever had." But only a few of these "crazy ideas" originate with me; they mostly represent some of the most profound and creative contributions of human minds to philosophy and science. My contribution here is to elaborate on possible connecting links in this nested web of human knowledge, links that are perhaps not widely appreciated, and to discuss what these connections *may* tell us about consciousness.

The first three chapters address the fundamental question, *what do we know about ourselves and our universe and how do we know it?* Complementary models of reality are proposed in the context of our political and economic systems in order to deepen our understanding of *complex systems* including human brains. Appropriate roles for science and religion and graded states of consciousness are considered. I review evidence showing that multiple conscious, unconscious, and semiconscious entities coexist in each human brain. My experiences in poker games and encounter groups are employed to demonstrate contributions from intuition and unconscious processes.

Chapters 4 and 5 describe how brains consist of nested subunits with intricate physical structures, including "non-local" (or "small world") connections that bypass intervening cortical tissue, apparently allowing for much more complex dynamic behavior than would be possible with only "local" interactions. The dominance of non-local connections may be responsible for many of the things that make the human brain "human." Contrary to some popular accounts, the dynamic behaviors associated with higher brain functions are neither simple nor localized in isolated regions. Rather, brains belong to a category called *complex adaptive systems*, which possess the capacity to "learn" from experience and change global behaviors by means of feedback processes. Another hallmark of such complex systems is the presence of intricate *fractal-like* features, where progressively more magnified observations reveal more detailed behavior.

Chapter 6 discusses EEG's *shadows of thought*, revealing a number of newly discovered relationships between mind and brain. A healthy consciousness seems to be associated with a proper "balance" between the functional isolation of brain tissue and global integration; such balance is achieved only in states of high dynamic complexity. Lack of such dynamic balance due to faulty chemical (neurotransmitter) actions may be partly responsible for diseases like schizophrenia and Parkinson's.

Chapter 7 is concerned with dynamic behaviors in cerebral cortex and several analogous physical systems. A proposed conceptual framework embraces the idea of neural networks embedded in global synaptic fields. This approach addresses the so-called *binding problem* of brain science by suggesting top-down resonant interactions between global fields and non overlapping networks. Bottom-up and top-down interactions in complex systems comprise the circular causality of *synergetics*, the science of cooperation. Resonant mechanisms may allow brain subsystems to be functionally isolated in some frequency bands, but at the same time, functionally integrated at other frequencies.

Chapter 8 considers the general limits of scientific knowledge and identifies probability and entropy as important measures of human ignorance; scientific predictions are shown to be severely limited in complex systems. I argue that fundamental limits on computer power may preclude the creation of artificial consciousness, even if natural brains actually do create minds, as assumed by most contemporary scientists.

Chapters 9–11 provide an overview of the strange world views arising from modern observation of the physical universe and the possibility of deep connections between relativity, quantum mechanics, thermodynamics, and consciousness, *the RQTC conjecture*. One hint supporting this idea is that modern physical theories can be cast in the form of fundamental information barriers: relativity, quantum mechanics, and the second law of thermodynamics are all limitations on the speed, quantity, or quality of information transfer.

Chapter 12 takes a highly speculative approach in which the hard problem of consciousness is approached with questions about a category beyond ordinary information, that is, *Ultra-Information*, defined broadly to include ordinary information, unknown physical processes, and consciousness. Thoughts, emotions, self-awareness, memory, and the contents of the unconscious are, by definition, categories of Ultra-Information, whether or not these mental processes also involve ordinary information.

Fractal properties of both brains and physical systems are considered in the context of a thought experiment involving a "brain blueprint." Just how much detail must the blueprint contain in order to construct a conscious entity? Can the blueprint's information hierarchy terminate at classical scales, or are quantum- or even sub-electron-scale descriptions required? Given our limited understanding of both the physical and mental realms, I take seriously the proposition that consciousness may be a fundamental property of the universe. Does the brain create the mind? Or is *Mind* already out there? Read and decide.

The Endnotes contain references, expanded discussion, additional examples, and mathematical background information. Understandably, most readers will skip the mathematics, but they should also appreciate that the Endnote math helps to constrain extreme ideas and facilitates more honest discussion. Readers may take some comfort from the fact that the mathematics is either right or wrong and some readers will know the difference. Think of the mathematics as a safety valve designed to prevent certain kinds of nonsense explosions.

My writing and struggle with difficult concepts have been greatly influenced by cognitive scientist Ed Kelly and by theoretical physicist Lester Ingber; Lester has also made major contributions to theoretical neuroscience. Ed is the major reviewer, having read multiple drafts of the entire book; his comments and criticisms were extensive, insightful, and invaluable. Lester read much of the more technical material and served as an excellent sheriff to enforce physical laws on my ideas. In a book that impinges on so many fields, it should go without saying that the reviewers are not responsible for my mistakes and are unlikely to agree with everything presented. Hey, even my right and left hemispheres failed to achieve full agreement on the controversial material!

It is impossible to credit even a small fraction of the many scientists and philosophers, living and dead, who contributed to the book's conceptual framework; however, I wish to acknowledge comments on specific sections from several experts: Jim Al-Khalili, Todd Feinberg, Walter Freeman, Fred Hornbeck, Alan Gevins, Richard Silberstein, Ramesh Srinivasan, Theresa Vaughan, Brett Wingeier, and Jon Wolpaw. Thanks also to Kirsty, Cindy, Shari, Michelle, Michael, and Lisa for adding joyful complexity to my life.

Contents

Brain, Mind, and the Structure of Reality

Chapter 1

Many Faces of Consciousness

1. A CAN OF WORMS

This is a story about human knowledge and consciousness: the things we know, the things we only think we know, and the things we can perhaps never know. In order to relate our story of the many ingredients of consciousness, we must open a metaphorical can of worms containing many entangled species. Our proverbial worm can holds the scientific worms of neuroscience, physics, engineering, and mathematics as well as the metaphysical worms of philosophy, religion, and ethics. We do not study our worms in the manner of zoologists with their emphasis on anatomy, genetics, or other aspects of worms in isolation. Rather, we ask how the worms are entangled, how they wiggle to and fro and form twisted loops to interact in strange and unexpected ways, forming an exquisite worm society. So dear reader, please be patient as our story undergoes inevitable transitions between multiple fields of knowledge, keeping in mind that the interactions between these normally disparate fields concerns us more than any single field in isolation.

There is another sense in which any serious study of consciousness may employ a worm society. Human minds hold deep-seated beliefs, some shared by nearly all, but many in serious conflict. I will not be timid about calling such beliefs into question whenever the evidence demands it, noting that some strongly held views may be no more than persistent cognitive illusions. The varied phenomena that we humans label "consciousness" span many states and levels of experience and measurement. Misguided views of consciousness, especially those associated with the beginning and end of our lives, can lead to grave consequences. To overcome barriers blocking more realistic views, we must be ready to stomp on any exposed toe, whether it belong to scientist, philosopher, politician, or religious leader.

Human minds have learned quite a bit about consciousness and its relation to brain function over the past century or so: much more than was conceived by Plato and the classical Greek philosophers over two thousand years ago, more than was known in the days of Isaac Newton and his colleague, philosopher John Locke, and more than was understood in the days of eminent psychologist William James near the end of the 19th century. Nevertheless, the phenomenon of consciousness remains the pre-eminent unsolved challenge of our age. Not only do we not have answers, we are unsure of the right questions. This is not to say that consciousness study lies beyond scientific purview. Excellent scientific data are readily available; however, the central theme that permeates our discourse is a delicate balance between knowledge and ignorance: *how much we know, but how little we know of consciousness.*

The two major conflicting views of consciousness are typically labeled *physicalism* and *dualism*.[1] Dualists view the mental and physical realms as distinct and separate conceptions of reality, separate *ontological domains* in philosopher parlance. By contrast, the physicalist view asserts that mental states such as thoughts, feelings, and perceptions are created by brain structure and function. Physicalism says that the brain creates the mind or that the mind *emerges* from brain structure and function. Following the convictions of most modern scientists and philosophers, I mostly adopt a physicalist view, but seriously consider selected aspects of dualism, mainly in later chapters, suggesting that physicalism and dualism are not quite as distinct as normally presented. While generally supporting physicalism, I reject extreme versions of *scientism* that place science at the pinnacle of all forms of knowledge and experience, necessarily taking primacy over ethics, philosophy, religion, and humanistic views of reality. I suggest that no field of knowledge should be insulated from scientific rigor when application of genuine scientific methods is possible. However, our due diligence is required to expose pseudoscientific babble and imposters masquerading as genuine science. No one can say where the limits of science may ultimately lie, but as a practical issue, today's science operates with severe limitations on its ability to reveal the structure of reality, to be examined in several contexts in Chapters 7–12.

2. PEELING THE REALITY ONION

When I return graded exam papers to my students, I am often approached by students uttering the classic line familiar to all science professors: "I understood everything you said in class, but I could not solve the exam problems." My response is to assume my best "guru posture," deepen my voice, and reply: "There are many levels of understanding, my son; your job is to reach for deeper levels." The search for deep truths about consciousness or any other complex subject is analogous to peeling an "infinite onion," a metaphorical vegetable consisting of an infinite number of ignorance layers obscuring central truths. By peeling off more and more ignorance, we approach truths at the core but never really expect to get all the way to the center. Our metaphor follows the true spirit of the scientific method, in which reality is approached as a series of successive approximations; at no time does science claim final accuracy. In the first three chapters, our onion will be linked to several spheres of human activity. What do these disparate knowledge realms have to do with the consciousness challenge? All involve human decision making based on some combination of rational and intuitive mental processes, the latter closely associate with the unconscious. We will sharpen our cognitive knives for more efficient onion peeling, shaking off obvious biases and cognitive illusions by removing outer layers. Only then can we confront the intermediate layers of onion consciousness and its relatives in contemporary science.

My generation's parents typically advised their children to avoid three topics, politics, sex and religion, lest destructive arguments ensue. Discouragement of sexual discourse in Western culture has eased considerably over the past 50 years or so, but the controversial nature of politics and religion remains robust. Why are these topics so controversial? One answer concerns their complexity; I suggest that no one may understand them in any real depth. When no one knows much about something, each of us is free to adopt his favorite position with little danger of being proved wrong. You and I can become instant "experts" with no formal training, indeed, with hardly any effort at all. Choosing a political party or a religion can be a little like choosing a beer or a mate; beauty is in the eye of the beholder. Some libertarians, for example, believe that government power should be severely limited. Even if such views were implemented, we could never really be certain that they were correct, or even if "right" and "wrong" can be defined unambiguously. Any economic or social policy may be good for some and bad for others; identifying the so-called *common good* presents a substantial challenge. Furthermore, history is not a controlled experiment where we have the luxury of changing its parameters so as to evaluate multiple outcomes. In our universe at least, only one history is possible. The religious onion, in particular, has hardly been peeled at all. We are free to form our own conceptual frameworks about the origin of the universe, God, and so forth. Gain a few devoted followers and you have a cult; attract a large number and you have founded a new religion.

Onion layers may be purposely added by those who wish to persuade us with their views, but why do they even care what we believe? Several motives come to mind. If we agree with Smith's position, we reinforce his beliefs and he may find this comforting, especially when his ideas rest on shaky ground. He may feel a compulsion to convert us to his way of thinking. Self-serving human motives also produce very thick onion layers, especially in politics and religion, and despite heroic efforts to remove them, ulterior motives are also no stranger to science. The expression of self-serving opinions in modern societies is commonplace. Revisionist history under both communism and capitalism (think Vietnam war) reminds us of George Orwell's Big Brother dictatorship: "He who controls the present controls the past. He who controls the past controls the future." But, Orwell's famous book *1984* omitted the critical influence of propaganda in democratic societies with its mainstream media influenced by narrow financial interests. Propaganda can have devastating effects when citizens yield to intellectual laziness. Unfortunately, philosopher Bertrand Russell's famous quip, "Most people would rather die than think," often rings true.

As a little warm-up exercise for our explorations into the nature of reality, consider an article published in the *Wall Street Journal* in 1998 claiming that a scientific consensus had been reached on climate change. According to this article, "scientists" had concluded that global warming was *not* caused by human activity. A similar view was more recently provided by conservative columnist Cal Thomas, whose articles appear in more than 500 American newspapers. Here is what he wrote in March, 2009: "New laws and regulations will . . . change our lifestyles and limit our freedoms. . . There is a growing body of opinion that global warming is a fraud perpetrated by liberal politicians and their scientific acolytes who want more control over our lives."[2] Note that neither article was printed on April Fools' Day!

Most of us are not climate experts. How then do we evaluate such issues encompassing critical technical components beyond our expertise, but having profound implications for public policy? With just a little casual reading I come to the following conclusions: (1) Climate research has been ongoing for many years and has further intensified in the past few decades. (2) There is no doubt that human activity has increased atmospheric carbon dioxide, a greenhouse gas, in the past century or so. (3) The greenhouse effect, in which such gas acts to trap heat, is a well-established physical phenomenon. (4) Many government policy changes aimed at reductions in carbon dioxide, especially reductions in wasted energy, are also consistent with good economics and national security. (5) Such policy changes are likely to produce positive financial outcomes for some and negative outcomes for others. Those who perceive themselves as potential economic losers have substantial incentive to obscure any "inconvenient truth."

From these few bits of information, we can conclude that legitimate scientific debates about human-caused global warming are essentially quantitative. Is it a large effect that may threaten our very civilization or is the effect negligible? Unfortunately for humans, past scientific predictions of adverse environmental effects seem to have been substantially understated. When the *Wall Street Journal* article appeared in 1998, a growing body of evidence collected over several decades seemed to support human-induced climate change. There were certainly competent scientists who disagreed at the time, but to claim a scientific consensus *opposing* the existence of human-induced climate change was extremely sloppy journalism, self-delusion, or a deliberate lie. Did the editors act in anticipation of Vice President and climate spokesman Al Gore's 2000 presidential bid? Perhaps not overtly, but as will be argued in Chapter 3, unconscious actions are ever present in human decision making. And what can we make of the article by Cal Thomas? Technical expertise is not required to know that climate science does not rest on the opinions of liberals, conservatives, Al Gore, Dick Cheney, or Donald Duck. Nature does what she does without consulting liberals or anyone else. I cannot say whether Thomas and those of similar ilk are poorly disguised lobbyists for oil companies, simple crackpots, of some combination thereof. As *The Shadow* (from a favorite old radio drama originating in the 1930s) used to say, "Who knows what evil lurks in the hearts of men?"

In the first three chapters, I will move the discussion between several scientific and non scientific issues, the latter including politics, sex, religion, and another controversial field, economics. Economics is an especially appropriate choice in the context of our consciousness study given its traditional link to psychology. The famous 18th century moral philosopher and classical economist Adam Smith described psychological principles underlying human behavior. But during the 20th century, neoclassical economics had largely moved away from psychology, attempting to convert economics to a natural science based on the idea that humans act as rational agents. What? Humans were assumed to be rational; imagine that! By contrast, modern behavioral economics recognizes that humans are, in fact, often irrational; it integrates principles of psychology with neoclassical economic theory. All fields concerned with human beliefs and decision making are related to consciousness; *consciousness study is necessarily a study of the nature of reality.* With this overview in mind, consider my discussions in several disparate areas as more warm-up exercises for the challenges of later chapters.

3. CONSCIOUSNESS VIEWED FROM OUTSIDE

The problem of consciousnesses is uniquely curious. I am conscious, but what about you? We must face the fact that we have no direct experience of any consciousness other than our own. We infer that others share similar kinds of internal experiences mainly because they look, behave, and talk as we do. This similarity encourages the belief that others are aware of their own existence, thoughts, and environment just as we are. Is your experience of the color red the same as mine? If I say the word "red," do you think of red paint, a stop light, a skimpy dress, a wicked communist, or the red shift of cosmology? How do you experience a Rembrandt painting, a Mozart concerto, rap music, a cockroach in your breakfast cereal, or a nude person surprising you in an elevator? What thoughts and emotions are evoked and how do you experience your internal conscious state?

With increased human differences, for example, by not sharing a common language, our understanding of the internal states of others decreases. In extreme cases, we dehumanize others based on differences of language, race, religion, or tribe. Wars with other tribes or nations are easier to justify if we think of their citizens as less human. We typically assume some level of consciousness in humans and higher mammals, providing lower status to lower mammals. But, we have little idea of the internal experiences of animals except by anthropomorphic extension. We certainly have no comprehensive understanding of non human consciousness, whether in dolphins, chimps, dogs, bats, or the future computer intelligence predicted by some.

What can we infer about the internal experiences of a person, animal, or machine with observations limited to external behavior? A clever perspective was developed by neuroscientist Valentino Braitenberg in a little book titled *Vehicles.*[3] The imagined mechanical vehicles are driverless toy cars with simple, easily understood internal structures; however, the interactions between multiple vehicles result in the emergence of complex dynamic behaviors. To a naïve observer who knows nothing of their inner workings, the vehicles appear to exhibit fear, aggression, love, goal-directed behavior, and other human characteristics; they display a "synthetic psychology." Similar ideas were expressed by James Hogan in the science fiction book *Code of the Lifemaker*,[4] in which a race of robots is marooned on Saturn's moon Titan. After several million years, the robots exhibit competition, natural selection, "genetic" variability, and adaptation, apparently a form of life. These works of fiction were evidently inspired by the famous writings on cybernetics by Norbert Wiener in the mid-1900s. They demonstrate one of the central limitations of consciousness studies. Our scientific knowledge is based largely on external observation, but we can be easily fooled when we extrapolate such observations to internal states. In Chapters 5 and 6 we will see that several brain-imaging methods can reveal important correlates of consciousness that are observed inside the brain.

In Chapter 8, I will posit that genuine conscious computers are unlikely to be developed in the foreseeable future, but "con man computers" making false consciousness claims may be close at hand; such claims may be sufficiently credible to persuade many. Consider the famous test proposed by mathematician Alan Turing. Two sealed rooms are occupied, one by a human and the other by a computer. A scientist types questions directed to both rooms on a keyboard and receives answers on a monitor. If after a very large number of answers have been received from both rooms, the scientist cannot tell which room holds the computer, Turing proposed that the computer should be regarded as having "human-level intelligence."

While some have interpreted this experiment as a test for consciousness, I see no compelling reason to equate consciousness with human-level intelligence. The former demands awareness, whereas the latter may not. The implications of Turing-like tests bring us to the intriguing realm of zombies. Our zombies do not rise from the dead and eat the flesh of the living as in horror fiction; rather, these creatures are *philosophical zombies* (*p-zombies*). In the field known as philosophy of mind,[1] p-zombies are hypothetical creatures who lack consciousness but behave otherwise just like normal persons. By this restrictive definition, a perfect p-zombie behaves indistinguishably from a conscious being in all possible tests: Turing tests, psychophysical tests, neurophysiological tests, and all other tests that science is able to devise.

The prominent philosopher Daniel Dennett questions whether p-zombies are possible. Imagine a creature that passes all possible tests, including strident claims like "of course I am conscious, you idiots!" Can we ever say that such a creature is not conscious, that is, a genuine p-zombie? Dennett's choices for the p-zombie are that they are *(1)* metaphysically impossible, *(2)* logically impossible, *(3)* physically impossible, or *(4)* just extremely unlikely to exist. He is skeptical of what he terms the *zombic hunch*, the intuition that there can be a genuine difference between a conscious person and a perfect p-zombie. He suggests that the notion that something fundamentally human is "missing" from the p-zombie may be just one of our persistent cognitive illusions.

In such tests of possible consciousness in computers or zombies, I suggest that the role of the observer is critical. Thus, at this point in our discussion, I engage on a brief detour to consider some general ideas from modern physics. This is not just some gratuitous excursion into *relativity* and *quantum mechanics* based only on the vague idea that these topics are mysterious and consciousness is mysterious, so perhaps there is some connection. There are, in fact, some indications of deeper connections, perhaps not strong evidence, but intriguing hints to be offered in Chapters 9–12. For now, I simply want to use physics as a metaphor to emphasize the critical role of the observer in various *thought experiments.*

The p-zombie and Turing tests cited above are thought experiments, employing imaginary situations and imaginary observers to explore some aspect of reality. The most famous thought experiment led to Einstein's *special theory of relativity.* Einstein imagined physical measurements by two observers, one observer moving at constant velocity with respect to the other. Our intuition about the two observer's separate experiences is correct if their relative velocity is much less than the velocity of light, perhaps seeming to imply that relativistic effects have minimal practical consequences. But, this intuition is wrong. Two well-known predictions of this thought experiment are *time dilation*, the so-called twin paradox, and the famous equivalence of mass and energy $E = mc^2$, derived using only consistent logic and high school algebra. These predictions have been verified in many experiments over the past century, the most dramatic demonstration being the explosion of nuclear weapons. The two fundamental assumptions of special relativity are: *(1)* All physical laws are identical in the two systems, implying that all subjective experiences by identical observers would also be identical. *(2)* The (fixed) speed of light is the fastest speed at which "signals" (*information*) may be transmitted between systems. *An essential aspect of relativity is that natural, not supernatural, observers are required by thought experiments.* The critical role of the observer will surface in several contexts in Chapters 7–12. In Chapter 11, we will see that while ordinary information is limited to light speed, certain other influences are apparently not limited by this barrier. Fundamental limits on ordinary information transfer occur in relativity, quantum mechanics, thermodynamics, and consciousness; we will question whether this implies a connection between physics and consciousness.

Aside from relativity, the other major branch of modern physics is quantum mechanics. In quantum theory, the observer and the system under observation are joined in a new and intimate way that fiercely assaults our worldview based on everyday experience. The implications of quantum mechanics are even more astounding than those of relativity, appearing more akin to witchcraft than science, except for their extensive verification and widespread applications in modern technology. Quantum mechanics places fundamental limits on what we can ever know, limits on the amount of ordinary information we can ever hope to gain from a system. These successful and entirely new ways of thinking may provide some useful hints of new ways of looking at the consciousness challenge. In the philosopher's parlance, modern physics has important *epistemological implications* for consciousness studies. While at this point of our story, I am using the observer's role in modern physics only as a metaphor, the possibility of deeper connections to consciousness will be addressed in Chapters 9–12.

4. A PERSONAL PERSPECTIVE ON CONSCIOUSNESS

The scientific material, interpretations, and opinions in this book are biased by my educational, professional, and other life experiences. This is, of course, true of all books and their authors, but such biases can be obscured by the author's desire to appear objective. In the case of consciousness studies, such illusions of objectivity are unconvincing. For this reason, I choose to reveal my "tribal membership" at the outset. My academic training is selective areas of mathematical physics, engineering, and neuroscience. My professional life has been largely concerned with brain waves (*electroencephalography* or *EEG*) and their relation to other areas of brain science and *complex systems theory*. In Chapters 5 and 6, EEG, fMRI (*functional magnetic resonance imaging*), and PET (*positron emission tomography*) will be cited as useful, if often murky, windows on the working mind, tools for studying brain dynamics and network structures associated with human consciousness. My research work has been divided between mathematical theory and experiments, and between physics and engineering applications in neuroscience. My mother was known as a "spiritual" person by her friends but was not associated with any organized religion. My father was an engineer and businessman. Due to my history of nature and nurture, I am a hybrid product of the esoteric and practical worlds.

Like many species ranging from ants to chimpanzees, we humans tend to join warring tribes, evidently our heritage from natural selection. Modern human tribes develop as *nested hierarchies* with structures analogous to Russian dolls: little dolls within larger dolls within still larger dolls and so forth. Tribal nested hierarchies are demonstrated symbolically in Figure 1–1, in which religious beliefs are separated at the top (outer) level of the hierarchy into atheists, agnostics, organized religions, and all others. The (2nd from the

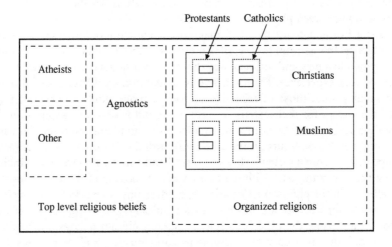

Figure 1–1   A nested hierarchy of religious beliefs.

top) organized religion level consists of Christians, Muslims, Jews, and so forth. The 3rd level consists of subcategories of the major religions: ([Protestants, Catholics, . . .], [Shiites, Sunnis, . . .], and so on). The subcategories of Protestants are 4th level categories (Baptists, Methodists, . . .). Finally, the subcategories of Baptists are 5th level categories (say, born-again Baptists and born-once Baptists). Other tribes often in conflict in modern societies include rich versus poor, conservatives versus liberals, scientists versus religious fundamentalists, and the multiple subcategories of these nested hierarchies. Nested hierarchy is also a critical feature of brain structure and other complex systems. It is also closely related to the important scientific concepts of *fractal structure* and *multiple scales of observation*. In Chapters 4 and 12, I will suggest that nested hierarchies of nerve cells forming dynamic structures may be essential for consciousness to occur.

My "tribe" consists of those who believe in an objective reality (Truth), and that access to parts of this Truth occurs by life experiences, scientific observation, introspection, and logic. My tribe gains knowledge in this manner and tends to be skeptical of self-proclaimed "experts." We believe that Truth is approached by successive approximation, and that one can never be sure that final and complete accuracy has been achieved. My tribal members include scientists, religious persons, agnostics, atheists, and others with differing worldviews from many walks of life. Our religious members differ from the dogmatically religious in making no claim of access to Personal Truths that automatically trump the beliefs of others. Our tribe rejects the idea that any mathematician, philosopher, scientist, rabbi, pope, priest, imam, pastor, Torah, Qurān (Koran), or Bible is immune from criticism. We hold that no single source can claim a monopoly on Truth. Our tribal members may or may not believe in God or gods but eschew notions that some humans have special access or privileged dinner reservations at some Great Table in the sky. Our tribe welcomes a wide range of opinions and complementary models of reality, often resulting in vigorous debate. We recognize that reasonable people often disagree on interpretations of the available evidence. Our tribe has no dues or high barriers to membership, and no particular name. We could be called the John Locke Society, the Albert Einstein Society, The Free Thinkers, The Curious, or many other names. Perhaps some other tribes might label us Satan's Agents or Infidel Evil Doers.

The momentous difference between the typical posture of many gurus, demanding obedience and adherence to a fixed worldview, and a free-thinking member of our tribe is illustrated by Linus Pauling's address in 1954 to university students following the award of his Nobel Prize in chemistry for illuminating the nature of the chemical bond:

> When an old and distinguished person speaks to you, listen to him carefully and with respect, but do not believe him. Never put your trust in anything but your own intellect. Your elder, no matter whether he has gray hair or has lost his hair, no matter whether he is a Nobel Laureate, may be wrong. . . . So you must always be skeptical, always think for yourself.

5. LIGHTING TUNNELS WITH SCIENCE

Science represents our best available tool for studying the structure of reality. Scientists collect data and, based on interpretations of these data, form conceptual frameworks leading to concrete predictions about future events and observations. Young scientists like nothing better than to slaughter the old sacred cows of entrenched ideas, but many of these cows are pretty robust; they can survive for centuries, often outliving the much more populous and flashy bull(s) that inhabit our culture. In Plato's famous allegory, prisoners are chained to the wall of a cave illuminated by fire, unable to turn their heads. The prisoners cannot see the real objects that pass behind them; they see only shadows cast by these objects, the distorted images of reality. When properly applied, science can correct many of these distortions. In order to illustrate the scientific method generally and the science of consciousness in particular, a much larger metaphorical cave is proposed here.

Imagine an enormous labyrinth with hundreds of levels extending for thousands of miles underground. Suppose a human tribe once occupied a few poorly lighted rooms on one level. The room walls opened to dozens of dark tunnels, all leading to multiple branches in many directions. In our fable, some adventurous members of the tribe were compelled to expand their knowledge and ventured several hundred feet or so into the tunnels relying only on light from the room. Others went further, overcoming complete darkness by feeling their way along tunnel walls. Still others were rumored to have ventured still deeper into the tunnels but never returned to tell of their adventures.

Some clever tribal members decided that tunnel explorations were too difficult and dangerous. They stayed put in their comfortable but poorly lighted rooms and claimed to have majestic Visions about vast riches to be found in the tunnels. They formed the Cults, whose members were offered food and sexual favors by tribal leaders in exchange for amazing tales of tunnel wonders. Others, called Cons, aligned themselves with Cult leaders to share their enhanced wealth and power even though many Cons didn't take the Visions seriously. The Cults and Cons combined forces to elect Cons as rulers of the tribe.

One day a box of new artifacts was discovered in the tunnels. The box contained small penlights able to provide effective illumination in the tunnels. Two new groups then developed: the Cautious, who favored only short tunnel trips, and the Curious, who carried out extensive excursions, revealing many new artifacts. It soon became apparent that the Visions of the Cult leaders had failed to predict important aspects of artifacts, and in fact, most of the Visions were just plain wrong. At this point, conflicts escalated between the Cautious and Curious on one side and Cults and Cons on the other. With the assistance of the ruling Cons, the Cults were able to suppress or distort much of the new tunnel information. This censorship was resisted by both the Cautious and Curious, resulting in an ongoing battle for the hearts and minds of the undecided.

Within this nested hierarchy many sub conflicts ensued. Some of the Cults proposed setting fire to tunnels to destroy artifacts that conflicted with Visions but were stopped by the more pragmatic Cons who feared becoming fire victims. The Cautious traded Visions for Introspection, which was more consistent with tunnel knowledge. Some of the Curious called Skeptics denounced Introspection as being poorly disguised Visions. Other Curious known as the Goodcops tentatively accepted Introspection and focused on preserving their alliance with the Cautious, fearing the destructive actions of the Cults–Cons partnership.

Authors of fiction often add a disclaimer to prevent themselves from becoming targets of legal action. Here is mine: *Any similarity to persons living or dead is fully intentional.* In this metaphorical tale, I identify the scientific method with penlights that often fail and provide only minimal illumination rather than powerful light beacons that might be imagined by some. More modest light sources indicate that the actual practice of science requires repeated checking and rechecking of experimental data, followed by extensive analysis and interpretation. Dramatic new discoveries are unlikely to be accepted until repeated in multiple experiments. Furthermore, our metaphorical consciousness tunnels are especially long and treacherous, forming a mammoth sub labyrinth. When the penlight of science fails, as will occur dramatically in Chapter 12, we will attempt to feel our way a little deeper into tunnels with logic and intuition as the only guide. This extra-science approach may provide a poor substitute for a genuine scientific journey. Nevertheless, we shall go as deep as we can.

Experiments in many disparate scientific fields are cited in this book; nearly all fall in the category that I label type 1 experiments as indicated in Figure 1–2. Type 1 experiments are "mature" in the sense of having been successfully repeated so that a clear scientific consensus is achieved. Perform a type 1 experiment and, if you do everything right, outcome A is essentially assured. By contrast, type 2 experiments are more of the "adolescent" ilk; perhaps they have been performed at different laboratories with conflicting results. Or, maybe reported outcomes seem outlandish, even appearing in conflict with accepted physical laws. But most commonly, conflicts arise because *the*

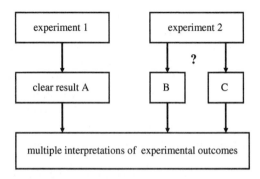

Figure 1–2   Well-established (mature) experiments (1) and adolescent experiments (2).

experimental devil is in the details; small experimental design differences between laboratories sometimes cause unexpected and conflicted outcomes. Type 1 experiments include the EEG work to be described in Chapters 5 and 6, and the quantum studies of Chapters 10 and 11. Type 2 experiments occupy much of the everyday lives of working scientists, but for the most part, I avoid discussion of type 2 studies here and focus on the mature type 1 work. Even though type 1 experimental outcomes are widely accepted, their ontological interpretations often lead to substantial controversy; a worm society limited to type 1 experiments is large enough for one book.

6. COMPLEMENTARY MODELS AND DIFFERENT SCALES OF REALITY

Our journey into consciousness study must consider several interrelated philosophical issues—the nature of reality (*ontology*), the nature of knowledge (*epistemology*), and the fact that reality can have alternate descriptions in different contexts or when viewed by different observers. Diverse models of a single system need not be conflicting; rather, they may constitute *complementary descriptions of reality*. According to the philosophical version of *complementarity*, the views of any two observers (of some system) are complementary if is it is impossible to derive all the observations of one observer from those of the other. Here I employ a so-called *folk philosophy* by picking a few concrete examples. The notion of complementarity was made famous in physics by Niels Bohr as a central part of the Copenhagen interpretation of quantum mechanics, in which electrons, photons, and even small atoms (with today's technology) can behave like either particles or waves, depending on the specific nature of the quantum measurement. I will have more to say about this kind of complementarity in Chapters 10 and 11.

In science, we try to match our models of reality to the scales (levels) at which observations occur. A macroscopic model of an ordinary table is a solid, wooden object with certain shape and strength. But, in the complementary atomic model, the table consists mostly of empty space with atoms held together by electric fields. Still other table models are appropriate for different observational scales; as viewed from afar, the table is just a point in space. The critical issue of scale applies also in economics. Suppose you open a restaurant with capital borrowed from friends. If the restaurant serves good food at reasonable prices, it may be successful; otherwise, it will likely go bankrupt. Some government involvement in your small business may be inconvenient, say, visits by the public health inspector. But government will also provide essential benefits like enforcement of contracts and police protection. Corporate bankruptcy law even limits your risk to capital invested in the restaurant. If it fails, you need not fear debtor's prison; your private wealth will be preserved, and you may even start a new restaurant if willing investors can be found.

Contrast small-scale restaurant capitalism with the large banks that introduced a novel new product called *credit cards* about 50 years ago. Credit cards seemed able to provide banks with enormous profits if only high interest rates could be charged. But, potential profits were constrained by state *usury laws* limiting interest rates. No problem; credit card companies simply lobbied state legislators, located in card-friendly states like Delaware or South Dakota, and issued their cards nationwide. There is now no lawful limit on the interest rate or late charges. The annual interest income of credit card companies is something like $100 billion per year, money that flows directly from the majority of citizens to a banking cabal, enough money to provide 100,000 bankers with regular yearly incomes of $1 million. Nice work if you can get it.

The point here is not whether usury laws or credit cards are good or bad. Rather, the fundamental difference between small- and large-scale capitalism is made quite evident by this example. Small businesses operate within the framework of existing rules, and the success of small- and medium-scale free-market capitalism has been demonstrated over and over in many environments. By contrast, large corporations are often able to change the rules for their benefit and stifle competition. Credit card companies are even free to charge small business exorbitant fees, placing the economic interests of small and large businesses in direct conflict.

In other large-scale examples, oil companies may impede development of alternate energy sources by small companies, and large corporations may absorb competing corporations. United States defense contractors have long operated in an environment of national socialism where contracts are promoted by politicians or government program managers who later accept highly paid positions with the same contractors, the well-documented *revolving door* or *Cheney scheme*. Similarly, the huge banking system bailouts of 2008–2009 might be termed a *Paulson-Summers scheme* after the two treasury secretaries who provided enormous government payoffs to their former Wall Street cronies. In science and engineering, these kinds of processes are called *positive feedback*, or in extreme cases, *runaway positive feedback*, a kind of economic epilepsy. Large-scale corporate wealth and power breeds even more wealth and power; the rich typically get richer in large-scale corporate systems, but revolving door schemes are mostly absent at the scale of small businesses. *Complementary models of corporate reality apply to different scales.* Similarly, we will see in Chapters 7–12 that different scientific principles apply at different scales of operation, in complex physical systems as well as in brains.

7. COMPLEMENTARY MODELS OF POLITICAL-ECONOMIC SYSTEMS

Complementarity is especially useful for studying complex systems, and political- economic systems provide excellent examples. Furthermore, political-economic systems nicely illustrate how propaganda, emotional barriers, and *cognitive dissonance* limit our understanding of complex systems. I like the latter charming label so much that I named my little (brain physics) consulting company *Cognitive Dissonance, LLC*. Cognitive dissonance is the uncomfortable feeling of holding contradictory ideas simultaneously, extensively studied in *social psychology.* Cognitive dissonance can be experienced as guilt, anger, embarrassment, and so forth.

We typically refer to the United States and nations of Western Europe as capitalistic democracies, labels carrying positive connotations. By contrast, the label *socialism* has negative connotations for many, viewed as an evil to be avoided at all costs. The Europeans have a saying, "If you are not a socialist at age 20, you have no heart. If you are still a socialist at age 40, you have no brain." But, most citizens favor state ownership of mass education, state-sponsored military and police functions, public disease control efforts, and so forth. Free markets require government enforcement of contracts; successful democratic systems require education for both rich and poor; soldiers do not normally fight for financial gain; all social classes require police protection, and so on. More controversial, but still favored by most U.S. citizens, are government entitlement programs like Social Security, Medicare, and Medicaid. A bit of cognitive dissonance seems at work here; we like many aspects of government involvement, including many aspects that some call "socialism," provided we religiously avoid this offending label.

Government regulation of private business can be a controversial area. Suppose I start a life or medical insurance company and target only the young and healthy, allowing me to acquire substantial initial capital that, in the absence of government constraints, can be invested in unrelated businesses or simply placed in my offshore bank account. I may have no intention of ever paying claims; my insurance company may be nothing but a scam operation. In order to discourage fraudulent insurance operations of this kind, or even the innocent but risky use of capital, state insurance commissions are empowered to regulate insurance companies, requiring that they meet minimal capital reserve requirements.

Jim, a friend of mine, was once president of a small insurance company in California. The company's owner, a multimillionaire and "pillar of the community," informed Jim that he planned to obtain a private $10 million bank loan using the insurance company's assets as collateral. Jim resisted as such action would violate state insurance law and refused to sign loan documents. Jim thought the issue had been resolved, but some months later he received an urgent call from the bank regarding late payments on a mysterious loan. The owner had forged Jim's signature on loan documents! Jim kept quiet about the crime and retained his well-paid position; fortunately the owner paid off the loan. Several years later, however, the owner was indicted by a grand jury for an unrelated fraud, and the community lost one of its pillars.

The world's financial institutions experienced a major crisis in 2008 partly as a result of the creation of an estimated $65 trillion (that's trillion with a T) in *credit default swaps* (CDS), essentially unregulated, private insurance contracts between individual institutions. The financial game works like this: Suppose I am an investment bank or hedge fund and purchase a package of home mortgages, a *collateralized mortgage-backed security* (CMBS). American International Group (AIG) or some other institution sells me insurance guaranteeing payment if my mortgages default. But, who guarantees that AIG has sufficient capital to pay all the claims if too many mortgages default? Since these bilateral contracts became unregulated in 1999 and AIG has been deemed by federal officials as "too big to fail," the suckers guaranteeing the contracts turn out to be us citizens.[5] But it gets worse. In addition to being unregulated, CDS's are traded in a secondary market where investment banks and hedge funds make leveraged bets on the financial health of their peers. By contrast to the idealized free market encouraging the creation of genuine new wealth, much of the CDC financial activity amounts to gambling in zero sum games. As in all poker games, both big winners and big losers can be expected to emerge from this multitrillion dollar casino. The biggest losers will probably turn out to be the taxpayers, you and I, and most of us didn't even realize we were playing in this game.

Another label that we may avoid is *oligarchy*, a form of government in which most political power rests with a small elite segment of society, distinguished by royalty, family, military power, race, wealth, or religious hegemony. How much power must be concentrated in the hands of the top 0.01% of the citizens before we apply the oligarchy label? This is partly a matter of taste and definition. Most would probably agree on oligarchies like former apartheid South Africa (race), Iran (religious hegemony), Saddam's Iraq (family), China (Communist hegemony), Saudi Arabia (family, wealth), and North Korea (family). More controversial examples may include today's capitalistic societies Russia (wealth), Israel (race, religion), or the United States (wealth).

Is the United States an oligarchy? It may be difficult to quantify the concentration of political power held by different classes, but we can look at how U.S. income is distributed and try to project the relationship of monetary to political power. Here are several typical examples of *daily* incomes in the United States: minimum wage ($50), university professor or engineer ($350), orthopedic surgeon ($1500), Fortune 500 CEO ($50,000), ten-billionaire ($2,000,000). I have cited daily rather than yearly compensation as these convey more dramatically the incredible discrepancies between even highly trained professionals like engineers and surgeons versus an elite class making hundreds of times more. While U.S. taxpayers often complain about the so-called "high salaries" of politicians, the total salary of all 100 U.S. Senate members only equals the typical compensation package of a single CEO of a Fortune 500 company.

About 500 to 1,000 billionaires are U.S. citizens, and the many ways such wealth is used to influence or even dominate public policy are all too obvious. Billionaire Rupert Murdoch is the major stockholder and CEO of *News Corporation*, which publishes more than a 100 newspapers worldwide (including the *Wall Street Journal*) as well as *Fox Broadcasting Company*. Billionaires Harold Simmons, T. Boone Pickens, Sam Wyly, Aubery McClendon, and Sam Fox donated millions to fund the so-called *swift-boat* media attack on John Kerry's war record in the 2004 presidential race, an effort that may well have changed the outcome. "Swift-boating" has now become a generic term for the peddling of propaganda or even outright lies designed to influence elections. Our national TV and radio media apparently have minimal incentive to check the accuracy of such profitable ads.

I don't have direct access to the workings of billionaires or even lesser *plutocrats* with yearly incomes in the $1 million dollar range, but clearly our political-economic system is often dominated by their self-interests and opinions. The news media relies on corporate funding of its commercials, and large corporations are run by the elite. TV's "talking heads" say just about anything they want as long the focus is on sexual misconduct, celebrities in crises, parochial politics, and other issues non threatening to plutocrat status. The plutocrats have many tools at their disposal: propaganda designed to inflame religious and cultural fears, middle-class dread of competition from lower classes, and so forth. Attempts to convey accurate information that could potentially result in serious income reduction or higher taxes on plutocrats are likely to be squashed with misinformation campaigns. Deregularization of the banking industry to allow gambling with taxpayer dollars,[5] the long denial of obvious health hazards of cigarettes, human-caused global warming, transformation of ballistic missile defense into a corporate welfare program,[6] misinformation campaigns leading to the Vietnam and Iraq wars,[7] and media distortions of U.S.-backed military interventions and terrorist campaigns in South and Central America over the past century[8] provide a few prominent examples.

What do my political-economic rants have to do with the central issues of this book? One motivation is to emphasize the importance of complementary models of reality. On one hand, the American political-economic system may be characterized as a Jeffersonian democracy with free markets and a free press. Perhaps equally convincing, however, is an oligarchic model with critical decisions controlled by a small group of plutocrats whose idea of "free markets" often consists of employing financial power (or military power in the third world) to stifle competition and shift the monetary risks of their leveraged bets to the lower and middle classes. A deep understanding of our political-economic system requires consideration of both models to provide the requisite complementarity.

A second motivation for my rants is to point to the critical importance of spatial scale in descriptions of complex dynamic systems. Large and small corporations actually operate under quite different "rules," regardless of what our legal statutes may say. In fact, their interests are often in direct conflict as when the credit card industry dictates fees to small businesses, say, a small restaurant that cannot realistically restrict customers to cash payments. Or, government bailouts of large banks making reckless bets can easily punish small banks that have adopted sound business practices. CEO salaries paid by small businesses are limited by its investors to reasonable ranges determined in a free market. By contrast, the boards of directors of large corporations may be loaded with management's accomplices who are paid, along with the so-called hired "salary consultants," to insure absurdly high management salaries. Were these consultants to make the mistake of recommending more modest management salaries, they would likely be forced to give up salary consultancy and pursue honest work. In my view, the claim by plutocrat apologists and "market fundamentalists" that CEO salaries of $50,000 per day are determined in free markets is a joke.[9]

Finally, I have addressed the issues of self-delusion or propaganda masquerading as knowledge in the context of political and economic systems. In the examples of clear conflicts of interests between small and large businesses cited above, the noisy media advocates of so-called "free markets" should be asked, "free for whom?" As I introduce new ideas originating from disparate scientific fields, we must remember that while scientific methods have been developed to avoid false information, science is, after all, carried out by imperfect human beings. Throughout this book, I will advance similar arguments about complementarity, spatial scale, and human biases in our studies of complex physical systems, brains, and the deep mystery of consciousness itself.

8. THE SCIENTIFIC STUDY OF CONSCIOUSNESS

The important scientific issues of spatial scale and *reductionism* are closely interrelated. One of the hallmarks of modern science is its ability break down complex questions into subsets of simpler questions, often employing mathematics as an essential tool. Such methods typically follow some version of reductionism, the idea that an understanding of a system's constituent parts and their interactions provides a powerful way toward understanding the system as a whole. We must, however, be careful with our language. Philosopher Patricia Churchland[1] has advised that "reductionism" has come in some quarters to indicate a form of insult, sometimes used as a synonym for such diverse sins as atheism, communism, or bourgeois capitalism.

To avoid such peripheral issues, I adopt the terms *weak reductionism* and *strong reductionism*, suggesting a continuous spectrum rather than discrete categories, a continuum of reductionist ideas. The distinction between the weak and strong ends of this reductionist spectrum has much to do with the phrase "nothing more than." Consider any system S composed of interacting elements E as indicated in Figure 1–3. Strong reductionism suggests that system S is nothing more than its elements E and their rules of interaction I. That is, an observer (the eye at the upper right) measures global properties M of the entire system S that may be "explained" in terms of its parts E and the interactions I. In later chapters, I will elaborate on various interpretations of the observer and the word "explain" as used in this context.

In one common example, the elements E are air molecules, and the system S is a room full of air. The "observer" need not be human; it might be a temperature or pressure gauge that records important macroscopic properties of the air mass. A weak reductionist claim is that we can explain temperature M_1 and pressure M_2 in terms of the motion of air molecules; faster molecules result in higher temperatures and pressures if the room boundaries are fixed. A much

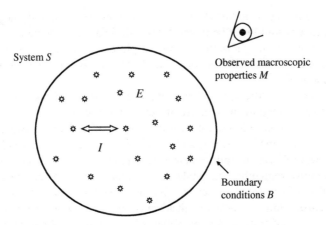

Figure 1–3 Emergence of macroscopic properties M in a system with small-scale elements E and interaction rules I.

stronger reductionist argument is that that our world economic system S is nothing more than the interaction of thousands of microeconomic systems E, and that if we just had perfect knowledge of all the microsystems and their rules of interaction I, we could, "in principle," predict the most important behaviors of the macrosystem M. Dennett has used the term *greedy reductionism* to describe strong scientific reductionism. I am even more critical of strong reductionist views and favor the label *autistic reductionism* to identify what I consider especially vacuous philosophical positions.

In one example of reductionism, some physicists and philosophers (perhaps after being misled by physicists) have claimed that "chemistry is simply applied physics." While it may be argued convincingly that the basic nature of chemical bonds may be understood in the context of quantum mechanics, it is much too big a jump to say that the general field of chemistry may be reduced to physics or that biology may be reduced to chemistry, and so forth, up the hierarchical levels. Such sweeping statements are unsupported by either theory or experiment, as I will outline in Chapter 8.

Much of my objection to strong reductionism has to do with the overused phrase "in principle." Scientists and philosophers generally agree that many complex systems display *emergent properties* that cannot be explained in terms of their constituent parts with today's scientific tools. In other words, such systems cannot yield to reductionist explanations "in practice." One familiar implication of strong reductionism is that all we require are bigger, faster computers to overcome the caveat "in practice." In the economics example, with an imagined "super duper computer," we could then provide perfect predictions of the global economy from knowledge of the microsystems.

Computer simulations of complex systems like global weather and economics can be very illuminating and provide critical practical information.

An important part of my professional life has been directed to such simulations of complex systems. However, I will argue in Chapter 8 that some complex systems S can display emergent properties M that cannot be explained in terms of their constituent parts E and interactions I, even "in principle." We cannot fully solve many important problems at the macro scale even with some imagined "super duper computer." These arguments against strong reductionism are based solely on established science and require no appeal to supernatural phenomena.

When studying complex systems like macroeconomic systems, weather patterns, superconductors, and especially human brains, we should regularly remind ourselves of *how much we know, but how little we know*. A rough idea of complexity and our depth of understanding in several fields of human knowledge is indicated in Figure 1–4. The horizontal axis might be labeled Log[Log (Complexity)] so that some imagined measure of complexity ranges from perhaps 10 to 10^{100}. The double Log operation compresses the scale of the plot to the range 0 to 2. Similarly, the vertical axis might be Log[Log (Understanding)]. These specific numbers don't mean much of anything; I merely suggest large numbers as a communication device to emphasize the enormous differences in complexity and depth of understanding of the fields shown. In Chapters 8–12, I will attempt to illustrate the vast extent of our metaphorical cave or dark labyrinth representing the structure of reality and just how far we are likely to be from anything approaching a comprehensive understanding of consciousness.

Students having struggled to fulfill their mathematics requirements may be aghast at the idea that mathematics is the simplest knowledge category depicted in Figure 1–4. But, in this case, "simple" does not mean "easy," rather, "simple" is the opposite of "complex." Perhaps the most obvious feature that distinguishes the knowledge fields shown at the far left of Figure 1–4 is that once a solution is proposed and considered by those in the field, it is typically judged to be either right or wrong rather quickly. This often occurs whether the solution is

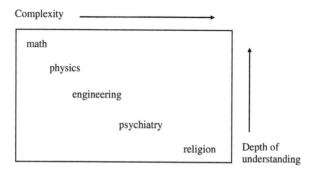

Figure 1–4   Complexity versus depth of understanding in several areas of human endeavor.

proposed by an established guru or an unknown upstart. The mathematics community is quite good at this egalitarian process; the physics community is also pretty effective. By contrast to these "left fields," new ideas proposed in knowledge fields at the right side of Figure 1–4 are much more likely to result in ongoing conflict, with new groups formed at different levels of nested hierarchy as in Figure 1–1. The result is differing schools of economic theory, political philosophy, and especially religion; these schools can represent either competing or complementary models of reality. I will have more to say about such disparate ways of "understanding" in Chapters 8–12.

9. SUMMARY

Our study of consciousness draws upon a broad range of human knowledge from hard science to metaphysics. Many fields overlap and suggest ambiguous or inconsistent answers to our questions. We employ the philosopher's *epistemology*, a field focused on the nature of human knowledge. What do we only think we know, what do we really know, and how do we know it? Science provides an essential tool for answering many such questions and constructing conceptual frameworks supporting consciousness studies. Such frameworks often call for complementary models of reality appropriate at different scales and in different contexts. Political systems, businesses, and financial markets provide familiar examples of complementarity. In the *efficient-market hypothesis*, for example, stock prices already reflect known information about the listed equities. On the other hand, a complementary model might view a stock market as similar to a poker game in which good players and players with inside information take money from the poor and uniformed players.[10]

Self-delusion and propaganda masquerading as knowledge are commonplace in our political and economic systems. Despite heroic efforts to avoid them, such examples of false information are not unknown to science. Today's science is quite limited in its ability to penetrate the behaviors of complex systems, for which human brains provide the pre-eminent examples. Traditional science is often based on reductionism and determinism, but these approaches to knowledge acquisition have serious limitations. Extreme reductionist ideas, for example, that chemistry is just applied physics, biology is just applied chemistry, and so forth up the hierarchical scale, are challenged here and again in Chapters 8–12.

Chapter 2

Ethics, Religion, and the Identity of Self

1. WHEN SCIENCE AND RELIGION COLLIDE

Any journey into the realm of consciousness is likely to tread on sensitive toes, both religious and scientific. Scientific texts typically skirt religious issues, but in the case of consciousness studies, such avoidance may not work very well. Here I will not be shy about the overlap of science and religion; some conflict is unavoidable. Central to the scientific method is the doctrine that knowledge acquisition is a never-ending process based on observation and logic, and no claims of final accuracy can ever be made. Many scientists and non scientists with religious beliefs follow this doctrine to varying degrees; still others appear to reject it entirely. The beliefs of any religion X are likely to seem rigid or even absurd to anyone outside of belief system X, whether religious or not. Religion X is typically based on some combination of sacred text, religious leader, and *faith*. Faith is a willingness to accept doctrine based on peer influences and personal introspection without any need for supporting evidence.

If there is no evidence that something called Y exists and no way to settle the issue, my faith in Y is just a personal choice, and no conflict with science need occur. Maybe I imagine a superior copy of me in another universe that won five Olympic gold metals and two Nobel Prizes. But, why settle for such modest powers? Perhaps I am actually a god; a proposition that apparently cannot be falsified. Discord between science and religion is unnecessary when they operate in separate realms of reality (*ontological domains* in philosopher parlance), but major conflicts can be expected in overlapping realms, as in the formidable challenge of consciousness. Conflicts between science and religion may be viewed as just one level in a nested hierarchy of arguments about the structure of reality. We humans often become stuck in rigid positions or *psychological minima*, borrowing from scientific parlance. This happens with scientists as well as the faithful. To avoid becoming stuck, we must keep reminding the faithful of *how much we know*, and the scientists of *how little we know*.

2. THE WATCHMAKER'S MINIVERSE

The debate between the majority of scientists who accept *evolution by natural selection* and those faithful (including a few scientists) supporting "intelligent design" provides a widely publicized example of science–religion conflicts.

Richard Dawkins, prominent biologist and atheist, has produced several pro-vocative and widely read publications. In *The Blind Watchmaker*[1], Dawkins presents an overview of the theory of evolution by natural selection, the process by which an organism's heritable traits favoring survival become more common in successive generations, while unfavorable traits become less common. Most scientists are comfortable with the following positions.

The theory of evolution is supported by a treasure trove of data from many fields, including genetics, molecular biology, paleontology, comparative anatomy, and biogeography. While some may say, "It's just a theory," in a similar sense, Newton's laws are just theory. Living things are enormously complex, composed of nested hierarchies of sub systems performing specific functions critical to survival. Human understanding of all complex systems, especially living systems, has the gap structure of multidimensional Swiss cheese. When your toilet is flushed, the resulting turbulent flow is understood only in broad outline; many gaps remain. Routine science is able to fill some of the smaller gaps, much like fitting individual pieces in a jigsaw puzzle. Every so often, however, a general principle is discovered that fills gaps in many fields with a single stroke, similar to the sudden recognition of a familiar object covering a large region of our metaphorical jigsaw puzzle. Newton, Darwin, and Einstein closed numerous gaps with single brilliant strokes; the typical Nobel laureate accomplishes much less.

Proponents of "intelligent design" argue that such complexity requires the guiding hand of God. The assumption that an act of God is required to explain processes not yet understood has been labeled the *God-of-the-gaps argument*. Often, the poorly disguised motivation behind *God-of-the-gaps* is proving the existence of God (or some god) to support predetermined religious views. Dawkins and his critics often focus on interpretations of gaps in evolutionary theory and argue whether or not science can be expected to close the gaps. For example, the most fundamental evolutionary gap is the first-life (*biogenesis*) problem, explaining how the first biological molecule capable of replicating itself originated from non biological chemical processes.

For purposes of argument, suppose that the first-life problem remains unsolved for quite some time, say in the year 2050 a large gap remains. How should we interpret this failure? We can list several viewpoints: (*1*) The first-life problem is more difficult than originally thought, but the gap will eventually be filled using standard biochemistry and evolutionary theory. (*2*) While evolu-tionary theory is accurate, new molecular organizational principles are required to explain how the initial conditions of first life came into being. (*3*) Complex processes like life are governed by an as yet to be discovered "information field" that permeates our universe. (*4*) Some unknown super intelligence, call it *Mind*, guides the creation and evolution of life. (*5*) The God of organized religions guides the creation and evolution of life.

My argument addresses several points: First, even if a gap cannot not be closed in the context of Darwin's theory, the jump from (1, Darwin) to (5, God) is large, indeed. Second, explanations 4 and 5 are evidentially not falsifiable, implying that they are unlikely to be subject to scientific study, at least in the foreseeable future. The scientist's job is to assume tentatively explanation (1) and test whether it leads to a solution or an impenetrable barrier. If the latter, he is likely to seek a solution consistent with explanation (2). In this same spirit, the failure of Newton's laws at the level of elementary particles encouraged the development of quantum theory.

Having strongly supported evolution by natural selection, I offer a major caveat. *The Blind Watchmaker* describes Dawkins' simulations to create a synthetic "life form" called Biomorphs on his computer. His purpose is to demonstrate that complex forms may be created by a simple rule for producing stick figures composed of branched lines. His drawing rule was influenced by nine "genes" that determine features like length and angle of branch and number of successive generations. After perhaps 50 or so generations, many Biomorphs looked a bit like living things: bats, foxes, insects, and so forth. His central point is that he didn't plan the animals that evolved; the shapes *emerged* in the absence of his active direction. The simulations demonstrate that complex shapes may emerge from simple one-step processes and no designer is required. By the way, chaotic dynamic systems (Chapter 8) also produce complex structures from the application of simple one-step rules.

Suppose we alter Dawkins' story just a little and assume he has constructed his computer himself and added a natural selection subroutine to the basic evolutionary program. In this case, Dawkins is the god of a *miniverse*; he constructs the genes and the initial Biomorph shapes, the *initial conditions*. He is a powerful god; if he doesn't like his Biomorphs, he can just erase the computer memory and start over. In my little fairy tale, Dawkins as a young child had an unpleasant experience with an aggressive lizard. When big lizard-bird creatures, the Dinomorphs, unexpectedly evolve to prominence in his miniverse, he is not pleased. Rather than destroy his miniverse, he introduces a new subroutine called Meteor that alters natural selection consistent with new Meteor-induced conditions; that is, the environmental *boundary conditions* are changed. The Dinomorphs disappear, and new creatures called Mamomorphs evolve. Dawkins then surveys his miniverse and declares, "It is good." He rests on the 7th day. Dawkins is a powerful god, but not all powerful. He cannot predict nor easily control future evolution of his Biomorphs as evidenced by words from his sacred text, ". . . nothing in my wildest dreams prepared me for what actually emerged. . ."

Dawkins begins his preface to *The Blind Watchmaker* with the claim, "This book is written in the conviction that our own existence once presented the greatest of all mysteries, but that it is a mystery no longer because it is solved." Taken at face value, this is an absurd statement, rivaling fundamentalist voices claiming that the earth is less than 10,000 years old. I don't believe Dawkins really meant what he said. Assume that evolution by natural selection is both 100% complete and accurate. As in our many examples, the mysteries of initial conditions and boundary conditions remain. We don't know why our universe is the way it is. As will be outlined in Chapter 9, we don't know why our universe seems so finely tuned for the production of the observed hierarchy of matter: the elementary particles, atoms, molecular precursors of biological molecules, and ultimately human beings. These are the initial conditions required to get the process of evolution started. The boundary conditions provide the environment in which evolution occurs.

Scientists often assume fixed environmental boundary conditions, punctuated by the random influences of volcanoes, meteors, sunbursts, Earth magnetic field switching, and so forth. But, the assumption of randomness can be interpreted as just an admission of ignorance of causes. The story of Dawkins and his miniverse suggests possible properties of our universe that may be discovered in our future and others that may never be discovered. Perhaps our universe is just one level of an unimaginably large *multiverse*. Maybe our universe just popped out of the multiverse by chance or maybe not. Could so-called empty space be permeated by an "information field," so that in some sense the universe itself is conscious? Or perhaps, the super intelligence that I call *Mind* tinkers with the universe's boundary and initial conditions. My guess is that the true structure of reality may be well beyond our wildest imaginations, but these limitations will not prevent us from continuing our search.

3. THE PROBLEM OF IDENTITY AND PERCEIVED UNITY OF CONSCIOUSNESS

Our internal experiences are normally unified. Imagine that you have a problem causing emotional distress and discuss this problem with a friend on a hot day while driving a car with the windows down. At any particular time, you seem have just one internal experience consisting of your emotional state, the traffic conditions, your friend's demeanor, the conversation, the hot wind in your face, and your memories. There appears to be just one of you inside your brain even though you can identify several distinct experiences. Various interpretations of this apparent unity of consciousness have been debated at least since the time of philosopher Immanuel Kant in the 18th century.

Both William James and Sigmund Freud wrote extensively of the unconscious mind. Freud divided the mind into the conscious mind, the *ego*, and two parts of the unconscious mind: the *Id* associated with primitive desires and the *super ego*, a sort of conscience or internal policeman. The unconscious was meant to account for mental illnesses, especially neurosis. Many of Freud's ideas have been sharply discredited, but the general idea of the unconscious is well supported by modern science.

Marvin Minsky, one of the founders of the field of artificial intelligence, reminds us that every brain has hundreds of parts, each of which evolved to do specific jobs: some recognize faces, others tell muscles to execute actions, some formulate goals and plans, and yet others store memories for later integration with sensory input and subsequent action. Michael Gazzaniga, well known for his work on *split-brain patients* (Section 5) expresses a view consistent with the multipart conscious idea: the mind is not a psychological entity but a sociological entity composed of many mental sub systems, each with the capacity to produce behavior; the sub systems are not necessarily conversant internally.

Many neuroscientists, myself included, have carried out EEG studies suggesting that even moderately complex cognitive tasks involve many interacting brain areas, proverbial constellations of widely distributed and rapidly changing sub systems. The EEG measures dynamic activity from the outer brain layer, the *cerebral cortex*. If we label different cortical areas *A*, *B*, *C*, and so forth, certain tasks are associated with stronger functional connections between, let's say, *A* and *X*, but at the same time weaker connections between *B* and *Z*. Different tasks result in different global patterns of interdependency between cortical sites that can be physically close together or located on opposite sides of the brain. We will consider additional implications of these studies in Chapters 4–6.

Following the pioneering mid 20th century work of psychologist Donald Hebb, we tentatively associate these brain sub systems with *cell assemblies*, groups of neurons that act as unitary systems over some (perhaps very short) time interval. The phrase "cell assembly" is much more accurate than the more common term *neural network*, which implies specific interaction mechanisms and misleading electric circuit analogs. A critical difference is that cell assemblies are not static structures like electric circuits; rather, they continuously form and dissolve, crating ever-changing patterns and sub patterns. Nevertheless, in this book I will often use "network" as shorthand for "cell assembly," consistent with the way neuroscientists often express themselves. In Chapters 6–8, I will argue that distinct cell assemblies need not have distinct locations. Rather, they can overlap both spatially and hierarchically; they can occur in *nested hierarchies*.

Modern brain research is often concerned with the so-called *binding problem*: how different cell assemblies dealing with different aspects of perception (vision, hearing, language, memory, and so forth) can be combined to produce a unified experience. The notion of a unified (or not) consciousness is closely linked to the riddle of personal identity, that is, what properties cause one to remain a single person over time. The following fanciful tale addresses such issues.

4. THE STRANGE CASE OF BILLY BOB O'RILEY

Early in her marriage, Billy Bob's mother Sue had several miscarriages without ever realizing that she had become pregnant. This was not unusual; medical scientists estimate that more than 25% of all conceptions result in spontaneous abortion by the sixth week following the woman's last menstrual period. The most common causes are serious genetic problems with the *embryo*. The risk of miscarriage declines substantially after the embryo reaches the official status of *fetus* in the 8th week.

Sue noticed blood spots when she used the toilet but quickly suppressed any idea that she might have spontaneously aborted a fertilized egg. After all, her priest emphasized that "life begins at the moment of conception," and it just didn't make sense to her to equate a minor blood spot to the death of a child. In Sue's third pregnancy, Billy Bob avoided the fate of his unlucky predecessors and began existence as a successful *zygote*, Sue's egg fertilized by his father's sperm. But several days after conception, the zygote spontaneously divided to form two separate embryos, later to be named Billy and his identical twin Bob.

As Billy and Bob grew to middle age, they retained their identities at birth, at least according to the law and most of their friends. All through their school years, Billy and Bob shared many experiences and outlooks, so much so that their friends often thought of them as the single unit Billy + Bob. However, over the years, most of the cells in their bodies were replaced. In middle age, they lived far apart and had developed many distinct experiences. Many memories were gained and lost, and important aspects of their personalities changed. So much so, that one friend of Billy and Bob from high school initially refused to believe that the middle-aged Bob was the same person he knew in high school. Nevertheless, Billy and Bob each insisted that he was the same person he had always been. But just what was it that made each one the same? Would we ever be able to unmask a clever imposter?

Later in Billy's life, one of his large blood vessels became blocked, thereby cutting off blood supply (and oxygen) to a large portion of his brain. He suffered an *ischemic stroke* and lapsed into a *coma*. After several days, Billy's condition improved somewhat, and he began to show alternating periods of open and closed eyes superficially similar to the normal sleep-waking cycle, a clinical condition called the *vegetative state*. Still later, Billy graduated to the so-called *minimally conscious state* in which he was able to look at and perhaps even recognize some of his visitors and follow simple one-word commands. However, be remained permanently unable to speak and apparently unaware of most of the activity in his hospital room. His doctors and family were able to infer his internal experience only indirectly, by observing his responses and with various medical tests like EEG and fMRI.

5. THE SEPARATION OF BOB'S CONSCIOUSNESS

A more unusual fate was in store for Bob. He had experienced many *complex partial seizures* during his life when he would become confused and unable to respond to those around him for 10 seconds or so. His EEG revealed that he had a mild case of *epilepsy*. Such "absence seizures" are fairly common, occurring at least once in the life of perhaps 5% or 10% of the population, often without the person's knowledge. In Bob's case his absence seizures were only a minor inconvenience. However, following a head injury suffered in an automobile accident, he started having regular *tonic-clonic seizures*. He would first sense an unpleasant smell (aura) that signaled an imminent seizure. He would then lose consciousness, fall to the ground, and convulse violently. For several years, Bob's seizures were kept to a minimum with a succession of anti epilepsy drugs.

However, after a time, all the drugs stopped working, and in desperation, Bob considered brain surgery.

When abnormal electrical activity is confined to a small area of the brain (typically part of the temporal lobe), the event is called a *focal seizure*. Some focal seizures remain isolated, others spread to the whole brain, that is, progress to *generalized seizures*. The location of a seizure focus is typically identified with EEG recorded from both scalp and inside the skull. If a seizure focus is found, it is often possible to remove the offending brain tissue surgically. This operation is called *resection*; the skull is opened and a portion of the brain is sucked out with a vacuum device. The procedure can prevent the occurrence of both focal and generalized seizures. Unfortunately, some seizures have no identifiable focus; all parts of the brain seem to erupt simultaneously. Since Bob's seizures fell in this latter category and all other clinical interventions had failed, he elected to have the radical surgical procedure called *midline cerebral commissurotomy*, cutting the fiber system (*corpus callosum*) connecting the two brain hemispheres. In other words, much of the brain was cut down the middle, separating the hemispheres but leaving the brainstem intact as shown in Figure 2–1. This operation eliminates most cross-communication between the brain hemispheres but leaves both hemi-spheres otherwise functioning normally. The operation often succeeds in redu-cing seizures, perhaps by preventing the spread of electrical discharges between hemispheres or maybe by just reducing the overall level of synaptic excitation.

After the operation, Bob experienced a remarkable recovery. He was finally free of all seizures and appeared normal to his friends and family. Because his radical operation was very rare, a group of neuroscientists friendly with his surgeon asked Bob to participate in some scientific experiments to access the effects of the surgery on Bob's brain function. Bob (now labeled a *split-brain patient*) readily agreed and came to the scientist's lab for tests.

The tests designed for Bob were based on the known asymmetry of the brain hemispheres as indicated in Figure 2–1. Contrary to popular belief, specific functions such as language are not confined to one hemisphere. Rather, the neural tissue of one hemisphere may be critical for anything approaching normal function. For example, an isolated left hemisphere can carry out com-plex mental calculations, but the isolated right hemisphere is typically limited to simple additions of sums less than 20. Functional asymmetry apparently results from specialized methods of information processing in each hemisphere, or perhaps from only certain parts of each hemisphere. This picture is consistent with the existence of widespread regional networks associated with specific kinds of cognitive processing.

Any such network may extend into both hemispheres, but perhaps the *critical nodes* (*hubs*) are confined to only one hemisphere, as indicated in Figure 2–2. In this oversimplified model, an imagined network associated with, let's say, a specific language function is indicated. The small circles are nodes indicating brain tissue masses where substantial network connections occur; each node may consist of thousands of *neurons* (nerve cells). The critical node shown with many connections in the left hemisphere may be called a

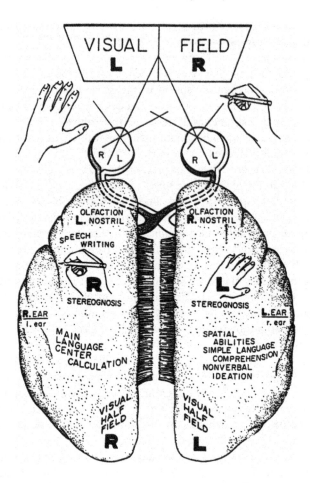

Figure 2–1   Brain functions separated by split-brain surgery.[2]

"hub" in the same sense that the Atlanta airport is the hub for Delta Airlines. One may guess that the hubs are fixed, but perhaps nodes change location over time. The brain-imaging technique fMRI (functional magnetic resonance imaging) may be able to locate major hubs (if these cause local increases in blood oxygen) but perhaps not the lesser nodes of extended networks.

Figure 2–1 shows that visual information from both eyes, but only the right visual field (appearing on the right side of the face), enters the left brain hemisphere. Conversely, objects in the left visual field (left side of the face) project only to the right hemisphere. In a similar manner, the right hand is connected to the left hemisphere, and the left hand is connected to the right hemisphere. In normally connected persons, objects in both visual fields (or in either hand) are available to both hemispheres because of signal transmission through the commissural fibers in the center connecting the two hemispheres. In split-brain

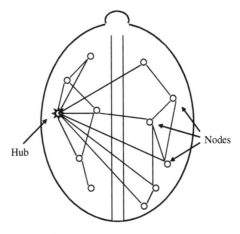

Figure 2–2   Imagined cortical network with several nodes and one hub.

patients, however, each hemisphere functions independently in most conscious activities. That is, each disconnected hemisphere appears to have "a mind of its own." The split-brain studies were pioneered by neuroscientist Roger Sperry who was awarded a Nobel Prize in 1981.[2] While "Bob" is a fictitious character in our little story, the following is an actual experiment carried out by Sperry and his colleagues; I have just substituted the name "Bob" for several patients in the study.

In one test, the word KEY was flashed to Bob's left visual field and the word RING flashed to his right visual field as indicated in Figure 2–3. We refer to Bob's right and left hemispheres as Bob(right) and Bob(left), respectively, noting that only Bob(left) can speak because of language dominance in the left hemisphere. When asked what he saw, Bob(left) reported having seen the word RING (presented in the right visual field), but he denied having seen the word KEY (presented to the left visual field).

In addition to the screens with flashing words, the experimental set-up in Figure 2–3 contains a number of objects on a table hidden from visual input to both hemispheres. When Bob(right plus left) is asked to retrieve the object flashed on the screen with his left hand, Bob(right) responds by feeling the objects and choosing the key even though Bob(left) denies having seen it.

Bob's unusual behavior was not confined to the laboratory. When asked how well he was recovering, Bob's wife indicated that he seemed fine except for the "sinister left hand" of Bob(right) that sometimes tried to push her away aggressively at the same time that Bob(left) asked her to come help him with something. This report may remind us of a famous scene from the movie *Dr. Strangelove* in which actor Peter Sellers plays a German scientist working for the U.S. government. He is not quite able to control one arm that insists, independent of the other parts of his self, on giving the Nazi salute at the most inappropriate times.

Our story of Billy Bob raises the deep problem of human identity, closely related to the consciousness question. Billy Bob began his existence as a single cell,

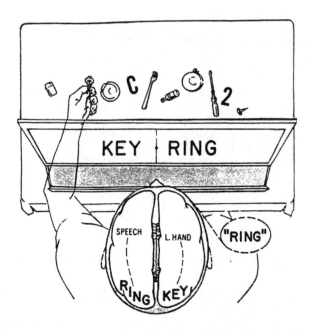

Figure 2–3   Example of split-brain responses.[2]

but that cell divided and later the identical twins Billy and Bob were born. This first division only poses an identity challenge for those who equate a fertilized egg to a person. However, as Billy and Bob age, all their cells change; some memories are erased and others are added. Just what is the essence of Billy or Bob? Suppose Billy contracts a fatal disease but is informed that an advanced technology can come to his "rescue" by downloading all his memories into a supercomputer. Does this offer make him feel any better about his plight? Religious persons may insist that Billy's essence is his soul, an immaterial entity that retains independent identity presumably in the face of all physical changes. Fair enough, but was the soul infused into Billy Bob right after conception? If so, did the soul split when the egg split? And what happened to Bob's soul when the split-brain operation was performed? Regardless of whether a religious or non religious perspective is followed, our normal intuition about the unity of consciousness within each individual is called into question. Are many of our ideas about consciousness just persistent cognitive illusions? Is there some deep connection between consciousness and the physical universe that might shed light on these questions? We will reconsider these issues in Chapters 9–12.

6. THE ABORTIONIST GOD?

Sue, Billy, and Bob are actors in my play chosen to illustrate issues of consciousness and the (usual) identity of self; however, their medical conditions and experiences are all real, and with the exception of the split-brain patient, quite commonplace. Our story demonstrates that the religious fundamentalist view that "life begins at conception" runs into multiple dilemmas. A zygote is certainly living tissue, but so are the unfertilized egg and the millions of sperm cells from a single male ejaculation that are destined to die in some lonely toilet. The zygote contains the genetic information (DNA) from both parents necessary to produce a child in the usual way, but cells in the appendix, stomach, and most other tissue also contain complete DNA, albeit from only one parent. It is then theoretically possible to have yourself cloned using only genetic information from, for example, a cell in your rectum. But contrary to what one might think based on all the provocative name-calling, no such rectal-clone currently exists.

In the first few days after the unfertilized egg (*oocyte*) absorbs the one lucky sperm, the egg divides into a group of cells with an inner and outer layer called a *blastocyst*. The inner group of cells will develop into the embryo, while the outer group will become membranes that nourish and protect it. The blastocyst implants into the wall of the uterus on about the sixth day following conception. The "life begins at conception" dogma runs up against the following wall of issues:

- Billy and Bob originated with a single conception. The division of the zygote Billy Bob occurred naturally in our story, but it could have been induced by fertility drugs. Drug-related zygote splitting often produces even more individuals, say Brett and Brad, in addition to Billy and Bob. The zygote might have been removed from the mother, divided mechanically in a Petri dish, and reimplanted, thereby allowing the lab scientist to "play God" by choosing the number of individuals to be developed from the original zygote. One conception can result in multiple humans.

- A clone may be created by *somatic cell* nuclear transfer. A somatic cell is any cell in the body other than the reproductive cells, egg and sperm. In mammals, somatic cells have two sets of chromosomes (complete DNA), whereas the egg and sperm have only one set. To produce the first artificial clone (Dolly, created from a somatic cell), the nucleus of a somatic cell from a white-faced sheep was transferred to the egg cell of a black-faced sheep in which the nucleus had been removed. The new nucleus contained the complete DNA of the white-faced sheep and behaved like a newly fertilized zygote when implanted in a black-faced sheep. The nucleus donor (the white-faced sheep) is then, in a sense, both father and mother to Dolly, whereas the other sheep served only as a safe container (surrogate mother) holding the embryo-fetus while Dolly developed from embryo to baby sheep. This same process is theoretically possible with humans; no conception would be required for the birth of a human clone in this case. I am not arguing that such creation should actually be produced, only that it could be done. Since human clones would not originate with conception, would religious fundamentalists claim they lacked "life?"

- We use the legal term "act of God" for events outside of human control such as hurricanes or other natural disasters. If we accept the idea that *human life begins at conception* and imply that embryos should be awarded a status equal or close to that given full-term babies, millions of spontaneous abortions every year certainly qualify as natural disaster. Thus, it would appear logical for religious "pro-life" persons to conclude that God is an abortionist, responsible for the murder of millions of "children" every year. According to the *Catholic Encyclopedia*, God does not store souls in his garage waiting for available bodies. Rather, God is supposed to create the soul at the time it is infused into the embryo. Perhaps religious leaders claiming communication with God should pass along the following suggestion: *Please delay soul infusion, at least until the target embryo proves to be viable, let's say after 8 weeks.*

- If embryos are given a status similar to that of full-term babies, it follows ethically that vigorous measures should be employed to prevent high-risk pregnancies, whether the risk is from spontaneous or induced abortions. The most effective means of preventing abortions seems to involve well-funded, comprehensive programs based on improved medical care, education, and most of all, birth control. Astonishingly, many conservative "pro-lifers" oppose the very birth control programs that would almost certainly lead to a substantial reduction in abortions, both spontaneous and induced. To my mind, the higher the value one places on embryos and fetuses, the more compelling is the ethical argument to support birth control programs.

- Modern science has accumulated a large body of evidence that correlates our conscious experiences to the structure and function of our brains. While there is much to learn, this evidence suggests that "human beings" develop gradually, and there is no magic time when human tissue suddenly turns into human being. My arguments are not meant to trivialize the wrenching decisions often forced on women with unwanted pregnancies. However, the choice whether or not to have an induced abortion should at least be based on the best available scientific and ethical considerations.

These arguments point to the critical need for expanded birth control. According to a report by the World Health Organization in 1992, sexual intercourse occurs about 100 million times daily, resulting in about 910,000 conceptions (0.9%) and 350,000 cases of sexually transmitted disease (0.35%). When used properly, condoms are very effective in preventing the spread of disease, and various forms of birth control are typically 99% effective in preventing unwanted pregnancy, again when used properly. Oral contraceptives ("The Pill") block the release of eggs from the ovaries. IUD's work by normally preventing sperm from reaching the egg in the fallopian tubes or, if conception does take place due to an unusually persistent sperm, by preventing the zygote from implanting in the uterus.

In his book, *The Language of God*,[3] medical doctor and geneticist Francis Collins, a devoted Christian and former head of the Human Genome Project, argues forcefully for the overwhelming evidence for evolution, and that belief in evolution is fully consistent with mainstream religious beliefs, labeling this position *theistic evolution*. Collins addresses the problem of when "human life" begins, conceding that no clear mechanism has yet been provided by today's science. He also provides a short overview of the ethical issues associated with stem cells derived from human embryos used in research, cloning, genetic disorders diagnosed by early removal of cells from embryos, and so forth. I think most scientists applaud his effort to bridge the scientific and religious communities, whether or not they share Collins's religious convictions. I keep Collins's book right next to Dawkins' book *The God Delusion* on my bookshelf; thus far, no spontaneous combustion has occurred!

7. WHEN TO PULL THE PLUG?

Our fictitious story of Billy Bob has profound ethical implications unrelated to the abortion issue. When Billy was comatose, ethical questions concerned his treatment and prospects for recovery. A common ethical argument suggests that comatose patients be kept on life support systems as long as there is some chance of eventual recovery, but just how low should we set the *recovery probability threshold* before "some chance" is interpreted as "essentially no chance?" In the United States, murder defendants may be sentenced to die if found guilty "beyond a reasonable doubt." Should a similar test be applied to comatose patients?

The American Medical Association decided in 1986 that it is ethical to withhold life-prolonging medical treatment, including food and water, from patients in irreversible coma, even if death is not imminent, provided that adequate safeguards confirm the accuracy of the hopeless prognosis. This ruling does not force physicians to remove IV's; rather, it suggests that family members should be allowed to make this decision.

Living wills and *do not resuscitate* orders are legal instruments that make a patient's treatment decisions known ahead of time; allowing patients to die based on such decisions is not considered to be *euthanasia*. Patients often make explicit their desire to receive care only to reduce pain and suffering. The legal instrument that seems best for protecting the patient's interests is *The Medical Durable Power of Attorney*, which designates an agent to make decisions in case of incapacity, and can give written guidance for end-of-life decisions. This feature differs from legal instruments that may require interpretation by physicians or even court-appointed guardians. The Medical Durable Power of Attorney takes the job of interpretation out of the hands of strangers and gives it to a person trusted by the patient.

A more troubling ethical dilemma occurs with *locked-in patients*. The locked-in state is a state of severe and permanent paralysis. Patients in the fully locked-in state suffer from a complete and irreversible loss of motor functions, making it impossible for them to acknowledge or communicate with others even though they may maintain near-normal levels of consciousness. They often understand what others are saying and doing, but they cannot respond.

The locked-in state can occur as a result of stroke or head injury. A stroke in the brainstem may cause complete paralysis by blocking all signals from brain to muscles but leave the cerebral cortex (and consciousness) fully intact. End-stage *amyotrophic lateral sclerosis (ALS)* is also a common cause of the locked-in state. This condition is also known as Lou Gehrig's Disease, after the famous baseball player of the 1920s and 30s. ALS attacks roughly one in a thousand people with no known cause. Today's most famous ALS patient is renowned theoretical physicist Stephen Hawking; unable to move or speak, he still communicates by using a little finger to choose words for his speech synthesizer. He has managed to produce numerous scientific papers and books on cosmology over more than 40 years after diagnosis. While applauding Hawking's astonishing scientific and personal accomplishments under such severe conditions, we should not fool ourselves that other ALS patients are likely to come close to duplicating his success. Hawking has survived his disease much longer than most other ALS patients who typically die within 2 to 5 years of diagnosis.

We can only speculate on the appalling experiences of patients in the locked-in state. Some patients appear to have normal consciousness. Others may be in a state of stupor, appearing halfway between coma and consciousness, only roused occasionally by appropriate stimulation. They are unable to tell their stories, which possibly contain rich mental experiences. Often the patient's wishes for life support are unknown. Patients are totally paralyzed; they can think, feel, and know but cannot express themselves in any manner. Only diagnostic tests like EEG and fMRI reliably distinguish between the fully locked-in state and the vegetative state. The locked-in patients are essentially strong *anti zombies*. Whereas strong zombies simulate human consciousness that they lack, locked-in patients simulate a lack of the consciousness that they actually possess. The phrases "living hell" or "buried alive" come immediately to my mind when I consider their plight. Current research in creating brain–computer interfaces attempts to use the patient's EEG as a means of direct communication to the outside world. The plight of the locked-in patients provides the strong motivation for such research to be outlined in Chapter 6.

Perhaps the 2nd most remarkable story of a semi-locked-in patient is that of Jean Bauby, once editor-in-chief of a French magazine. At age 42, Bauby suffered a massive brainstem stroke that left him paralyzed and speechless, able to move only one muscle, his left eyelid. Yet his mind remained active and alert. By signaling with his eyelid, he dictated an entire book titled *The Diving Bell and the Butterfly*,[4] blinking to indicate individual letters, a total of about two hundred thousand blinks. The book led to a movie with the same title. Bauby's book tells about life in the hospital, flights of fancy, and meals he can only eat in his imagination. His story is also concerned with his ability to invent a new inner life for himself while trapped in the proverbial diving bell, providing us with valuable insight into a unique kind of consciousness. Bauby died 5 days after the book's publication.

Thousands of patients now exist in irreversible conditions of deep coma, vegetative state, minimally conscious state, or locked-in state. Most are unable to communicate to family and caregivers whether, if they only had a choice, they would choose to continue living in such dire circumstances or assert their right to die. Since all of us are potential candidates for these conditions because of auto accidents, stroke, or diseases like ALS, recording our wishes in advance is essential. Such instructions to our designated agents or family members must consider several issues, including religion, worldview, age, financial capacity, and the law's limitations. In the case of locked-in patients, the potential anguish of being trapped in the proverbial diving bell or buried alive must be considered. Ideally everyone "at risk" (meaning *everyone*) will have created a personal *Medical Durable Power of Attorney* while still able. A few example instructions that I personally favor are provided in the Endnotes.[5]

8. SUMMARY

When science and religion are concerned with separate realms of reality, no conflict need occur. Often, however, the realms overlap as in the case of our challenge to understand more about consciousness. Conflicts between science and religion may be viewed as just one aspect of arguments about the structure of reality. What accounts for human existence? Evolution and natural selection have successfully addressed important parts of this question, but the origin of critical initial and boundary conditions remains a mystery. We must continuously remind the faithful of how much we know, and the scientists of how little we know.

Closely associated with the consciousness problem is the problem of identity. How do we define an individual who may experience substantial changes during his life or may exhibit multiple "selves," as in the case of split-brain patients? Serious ethical issues are raised in the context of consciousness study. At what point in human development does a person come into existence? When does life cease to be worth living in coma and locked-in patients? Who and what decides when to pull the plug?

Chapter 3

States of Mind

1. FOLK PSYCHOLOGY, SCIENCE, AND ENGINEERING

In my expanded version of Plato's cave allegory, science is represented by tiny flashlights allowing exploration into the proverbial tunnels of consciousness. But many tunnels are inaccessible, forcing us to fill knowledge gaps as best we can with intuition, hunches, and common sense. The common sense assumptions we make regarding the behavior and mental states of others are known by cognitive scientists and philosophers as *folk psychology* or *common sense psychology*. Folk psychology provides a conceptual framework for our social actions and judgments about the psychology of others, including relations between their behavior, mental states, and environment. If I see someone eating rapidly, I assume that person is hungry. When I observe a man introduce himself to an attractive woman in a bar, I don't assume he is interested in her cooking skills; I have an alternate theory of his mind.[1]

This chapter integrates scientific data with common sense; one field famous for this healthy combination is engineering. Engineers can be divided into two overlapping groups: those with strong common sense laboratory and "real-world" practical skills and those with a good command of mathematical theory. Competence in common sense engineering originates with a combination of hands-on experience and academic training. On the other hand, good engineering theory requires direct connections to both mathematical physics and the world's laboratories. Engineers obtain useful results with systems that are poorly known or controlled. Errors (*glitches*) are expected, so engineering systems are designed to work despite accidents and disorder. To avoid glitches and keep costs low, competent engineers follow the KISS principle, *Keep it Simple, Stupid!* Failures to "kiss" properly tend to be eliminated by *marketplace natural selection*. The capacity to combine common sense and intuition with rigorous science is also the hallmark of good medicine. It's no accident that many of my engineering students have attended medical school.

While my own inclinations and skills have tended toward the more mathematical end of the engineering spectrum, I have great respect for the abilities of my more hands-on and intuitive colleagues. Time spent in the laboratory facing the practical limitations of experimental science made me a better theoretician. In the philosopher's language, common sense engineering with minimal theoretical foundation might be labeled *folk engineering*. In order to illustrate the interrelated roles of intuition, hunches, common sense, and the unconscious, I have chosen several examples here from both science and folk psychology, some consisting of my personal social experiences and their implied lessons. These experiences also provide metaphors demonstrating challenges to common assumptions, including the perceived unity of consciousness and the widely assumed confinement of consciousness to brain boundaries.

2. THE CONSCIOUS, UNCONSCIOUS, AND PROVISIONALLY CONSCIOUS

Various categories of consciousness are summarized in Figure 3–1 where two-way communication with normal humans occurs only for brains to the right of the dashed center line.[2] This picture ranks brain states crudely in terms of their ability to produce physical action (motor functions) and internal awareness (cognitive functions). The labels represent both recognized clinical conditions and several speculations. This picture embodies a number of gray areas and controversies, including proper interpretation of the split-brain patients, but provides a good introduction to multiple conscious states.

- The *healthy alert* person (upper right corner) operates at high awareness and motor function, fully able to plan and carry out physical action. When *drowsy* his motor and cognitive skills are impaired. By contrast, under *hypnosis* he can concentrate intensely on a specific thought, memory, or feeling while blocking distractions. The *right brain* label refers to the apparent separate consciousness of an epilepsy patient having undergone the split-brain operation discussed in Chapter 2.

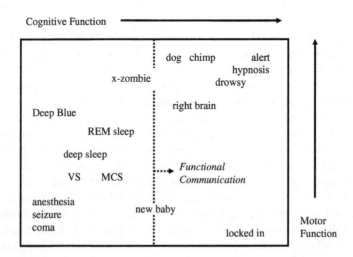

Figure 3–1   Various states of consciousness.[2]

- The *locked-in syndrome* is perhaps the most disturbing of all medical conditions as discussed in Chapter 2. The locked-in patient may be fully conscious but cannot move or communicate due to paralysis of all or nearly all voluntary muscles. The majority of locked-in patients never regain voluntary movement.
- Enthusiastic new mothers may object that I have located the *new baby* partly to the left of the dashed line, indicating lack of functional communication. But, this controversy is avoided by identifying some of the gestation period with the "baby" category for purposes of this plot.
- In *coma*, *anesthesia*, and *deep sleep*, we are mostly unaware and lack voluntary movement. The caveat "mostly" is based on evidence that the unconscious mind can store some information during these states.
- Most dreaming occurs in *REM sleep*, so labeled because of the *rapid eye movements* typically visible under the subject's closed eyelids. Dreaming is a kind of limited consciousness, one with minimal connections to waking reality. No one knows why we dream.
- VS is the clinical category called the *vegetative state* associated with severe brain injury, often caused by accident or stroke as discussed in Chapter 2. Some patients "awake" from coma, open their eyes, but remain unconscious. Wakefulness in this case means only that vegetative patients exhibit sleep and waking cycles revealed by EEG.
- Patients who recover from the vegetative state may gradually start making deliberate movements but remain unable to express thoughts and feelings. This level of functional recovery is categorized as MCS, the *minimally conscious state*. Like the vegetative state, the minimally consciousness state may be a transient condition on the way to full or partial recovery, or it may be permanent.
- *Deep Blue* is the name given by IBM to its chess-playing computer, which defeated human world champion Garry Kasparov in 1997. Cognitive scientist and philosopher Noam Chomsky has suggested that this achievement is no more interesting intellectually than the fact that a bulldozer can move more dirt than a man.
- The imagined *x-zombie* is like the philosophical zombie (p-zombie), except I use this term to indicate creatures on a continuum from weak zombies, more to the right in Figure 3–1 and having minimal consciousness, to strong zombies at the left, lacking all consciousness. The terms "weak" and "strong" in this instance refer to the strength of the central zombie concept, consistent with my use of these labels as modifiers for the terms *reductionism* and *anthropic principle*, the latter referring to cosmological issues of Chapter 9. These x-zombies are hypothetical creatures who lack full consciousness but behave otherwise just like normal persons.

The critical role of the observer in thought experiments is cited in Chapters 1 and 9–11. To follow up this idea in the context of consciousness, consider a stage production of a Shakespeare play. Actors say that a truly successful performance requires that they "become" the character whose part they are playing, as in the example of an actor playing Falstaff. The actor suspends awareness of his real self and lets the fictitious Falstaff character take over much of his mind. The actor also forms partnerships with audience members who agree to "forget" that the actor is just playing a role, a willing suspension of disbelief. Stronger partnerships lead to more enjoyment for both parts of this, dare we say, "extended consciousness?" As members of the audience, one part of our consciousness essentially "tells" another part to temporarily and selectively suspend some of our rational thought processes and just enjoy the play. The relationship of actor to audience member appears similar to the partnership between hypnotist and subject.

During the play's performance, Falstaff is similar to a zombie. To audience members willing and able to temporarily surrender rational parts of their own consciousness, Falstaff appears and acts just like a normal human, but in reality, no conscious Falstaff exists. The actor is conscious of course, but to the extent that he actually "becomes" Falstaff, one may argue that his normal conscious-ness is temporarily suspended. I enjoy the Star Trek TV series, but I might hesitate to visit the set or meet the actors for fear of spoiling my illusions at later viewings. Yes, I want to "boldly go" to a lot of places, but not where my favored illusions are shattered, at least not the harmless ones.

In Chapter 1, it was questioned whether strong zombies are possible based on thought experiments involving various tests of candidate zombies. Falstaff's story perhaps hints that such questions must carefully account for the observer's role in any such experiment. That is, the Turing and other tests that attempt to distinguish zombies from conscious creatures involve interactions between an observer and the creature under study. Can the observer's consciousness be fully separated from the creature's? In Chapters 9–12, we will address the persistent assumption that each consciousness is strictly confined to a single brain.

I credit my dog, a golden retriever named Savannah, with excellent motor function and at least rudimentary consciousness. Two-way communication between us is commonplace; she obeys commands and lets me know when she wants to chase a golf ball by "impatiently" nudging my hand holding the ball. At various times, she exhibits external behavior that we humans associate with excitement, sadness, fear, and even guilt. I include the *dog* with the *chimpanzee* in this putative example of non human consciousness (Figure 3–1) because of the domestic dog's evolutionary history with humans. Natural selection has favored dogs that communicated efficiently with their human companions, apparently over more than 10,000 years. A plausible conjecture is that this association has made the dog's internal experience more human-like than that of a wolf or perhaps even a chimp in the wild. Maybe Savannah is really just a zombie, but I doubt it.

Chimps share even more of their DNA and brain structure with humans than do dogs. They use tools, solve problems, and exhibit many other human-like behaviors. In the 1950s, I spent many Saturday afternoons at the local movie theater where admission was 9 cents and popcorn was 5 cents. The typical fare was two cowboy movies, five cartoons, and a serial. But sometimes one of the features was a movie starring Johnny Weissmuller as Tarzan and a chimp named Cheeta as himself. A new Cheeta, once identified as the original but recently exposed as an (apparently innocent) imposter, lives in a house in Palm Springs with his human companion, drinks Diet Coke, eats junk food, and watches TV. Despite these credentials seemingly at par with some of our politicians, Cheeta is ineligible to run for public office or even vote.

3. UNCONSCIOUS BRAIN PROCESSES

Many things happen in our brains that we are unaware of. The autonomic nervous system is controlled by a small group of cells deep in the brain that targets most body functions, including heart rate, blood pressure, digestion, and genital sexual response. Other unconscious events are more directly associated with mental activity. Negative comments in the operating room about a patient under general anesthesia can influence subsequent patient feelings, even though the patient expresses no awareness of the comments. Research subjects viewing rapid screen displays of pictures lasting only 10 milliseconds report no image awareness. But in later tests, these same subjects score well above chance when asked to pick target pictures from a larger collection, showing that the pictures impacted memory without the subject's awareness. Essentially the same process is repeated in our daily lives. Much of our knowledge, skills, experiences, and prejudices are acquired with no awareness of causal input to our brains.

Hitting baseballs or playing musical instruments requires intricate control of muscles carrying out complex tasks in series of steps. Yet they occur automatically in experienced players, outside of awareness. These tasks require a part of the mind that we cannot be fully aware of, but one that still exerts critical influences on thoughts and actions. Creativity also appears to originate with unconscious mental processes; solutions to difficult problems may appear to "pop out" of nowhere after an incubation period in the unconscious. *Intuitive feelings* or *hunches* are based on a perceived ability to sense something without reasoning. Acting without good reason might seem like a dubious life strategy; however, we encounter many fuzzy situations where choices must be made with very limited information. If our source of intuition is actually an experienced unconscious, following hunches would seem to constitute strategy far superior to random choices.

While the existence of unconscious brain processes is well established, there is much argument over the actual role of unconscious mind. In Freud's view, "the unconscious" does not include all that is not conscious; it consists only of knowledge that the conscious mind doesn't want to know. The conscious mind then actively represses this knowledge so that the two parts of consciousness are often in conflict. Many scientists disagree with Freud's model and assign different roles or less importance to the unconscious. Nevertheless, many instances have been reported in which "people see what they want to see." An experimental subject shown an especially disturbing picture may report seeing something quite different. Different witnesses to a crime may provide widely disparate reports to police and so forth. These erroneous mental pictures are often attributed to the unconscious, with or without Freudian interpretations. For our purposes we may define "the unconscious" as *brain phenomena that are closely related to and may influence conscious mental processes but lack the feature of awareness.*

4. BRAIN INPUT AND OUTPUT

The simplified view of brain function indicted in Figure 3–2 consists of a "gray box" with certain inputs and outputs. Inputs to the *peripheral nervous system* (represented by rectangle *A*) vary widely in normal daily experiences, composed of combinations of the five senses: sight, hearing, smell, touch, and taste. Stimuli from the external world first activate receptor cells, for example, in the retina or skin. This sensory input is then processed in several stages in the peripheral nervous system before reaching the brain. Stimuli can also cause rapid motor (muscle) action to occur before any brain involvement at all. Place your hand on a hot stove, and the reflex arc carries signals through your spinal cord, causing your hand to withdraw but bypassing conscious awareness. Only later does awareness of pain reach consciousness. In severe sports or war environments, we may train our brains to override such reflexes and suffer the consequences. Brain and spinal cord together constitute the *central nervous system*, but the brain mostly rules the spinal cord. Within the brain itself, either the conscious or unconscious systems may apparently rule in different situations.

A scientific experiment may be designed with a single controlled input like a succession of light flashes or auditory tones. Substantial processing of the input event occurs even before its signal reaches the brain; brain input is distributed over a longer time interval than the external stimulus. Alternately, the input might consist of electrical stimulation of a peripheral nerve or even direct stimulation of the brain itself in an animal or patient with electrodes implanted

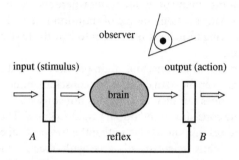

Figure 3–2   Sensory input and motor or cognitive output in the human brain.

for clinical purposes. Once inside the brain, the partly processed signal initiates a series of progressively more complex events: integration of different senses, inclusion of memory influences, emotional investment, and preparation for action. Brain output also passes through several peripheral stages (rectangle *B*) before external action takes place. Output may consist of a motor event like hitting a tennis ball or a cognitive event like answering a question. Scientists know quite a bit about input and output stages external to the brain, represented by rectangles *A* and *B* in Figure 3–2, but very little about the complex sequences of brain processing itself, reminding us again of *how much we know, but how little we know*. In Chapters 4, 7, and 12, we will explore the idea that much of internal brain processing of "information" involves fractal-like dynamic behavior, relying on interactions across spatial scales in the brain's nested hierarchy.

In scientific experiments, the observer typically controls external stimuli, leading to partial control of brain inputs; near full control is accomplished in the case of direct brain stimulation, that is, bypassing rectangle *A* in Figure 3–2. The observer may look inside the brain with various imaging techniques and correlate these data with observed actions and verbal responses. In this manner, relationships between specific brain actions or thought processes and various spatial-temporal patterns are studied. These brain patterns may consist of electric (EEG) or magnetic (MEG) fields, changes in blood oxygenation (fMRI), or tissue uptake of a metabolically active molecule (PET) to be discussed in Chapter 5. Each imaging method measures different brain events so we must be very cautious about commonly used terms like "activity" to describe brain patterns. Signal patterns obtained with one technique may or may not match patterns obtained with a different technique, not surprising since they measure different biological processes. It is best to avoid altogether the vague label "activity," an abstract concept that cannot ever be measured.

5. CONSCIOUSNESS TAKES TIME

Some of the most fascinating studies of consciousness were carried out by physiologist Benjamin Libet and colleagues.[3] His research focused on differences between a subject's *detection of a stimulus* and *conscious awareness of the stimulus*. Why are these two events not identical? The fact that they differ makes the research quite interesting because *unconscious mental functions operate over different time intervals than conscious mental functions*.

The first of Libet's experiments involved patients with brain surface electrodes implanted for clinical reasons. Electrical stimulation of brain regions reacting to sensory input (*somatosensory cortex*) in awake patients elicits conscious sensations like tingling feelings. These feelings are not perceived by the patient as originating in the brain; rather, they seem to come from specific body locations determined by neural pathways. Stimulation near the top of the brain near the midline (motor cortex) produces tingling in the leg; stimulation points on the side of the brain produce feelings from parts of the face, and so forth.

Libet's stimuli consisted of trains of electric pulses; the essential stimulus feature was found to be the duration of the stimulus. *Only when stimuli were turned on for about one-half second (500 milliseconds) or more did conscious sensations occur.* Experiments were also carried out by stimulating deep brain regions with similar results.

Why did these scientific studies require brain stimulation—why not just stimulate the skin? A short skin stimulus registers in our consciousness, as we experience when receiving a flu shot. How can Libet's results be consistent with this common experience? The answer is that skin stimulation passes through multiple processing stages in both the peripheral system and deep brain, resulting in input to the cerebral cortex that is spread out over time. Recording electrodes implanted in somatosensory cortex begin to show a response from a skin stimulus after 5 to 50 milliseconds, depending on stimulus location. Shorter latencies occur when the stimulus site is the head; stimulation of the foot takes much longer. These delays result mostly from signal propagation (*action potentials*) along peripheral nerves of differing lengths. The first electrical responses in the cortex, called *primary evoked potentials*, do not by themselves indicate conscious awareness; electrical responses must persist for much longer times for awareness to occur.

Libet's studies suggest that consciousness of an event is only associated with electric field patterns in neural tissue that persist for at least 500 milliseconds (ms). To check this idea, Libet and others carried out several versions of *backward masking* studies. The general experimental setup provides two distinct stimuli. If the second stimulus is applied between, let's say, 200 ms and 500 ms after the first stimulus, it can "mask" conscious awareness of the first stimulus, meaning the subject will report no knowledge of the first stimulus. Some have interpreted the effect of the second stimulus as blocking memory formation of the first stimulus. Libet showed that this interpretation is probably wrong with experiments involving two equal skin stimuli separated by 5 seconds (S_1 and S_2), and one cortical stimulus (C) applied between $T=50$ ms and 1000 ms after S_2 as indicated in Figure 3–3. *If the cortical stimulus was applied within 400 ms of S_2, its effect was to make the subjective feeling of stimulus S_2 stronger than S_1, and no loss of memory of S_1 occurred.* In other words, as consciousness of stimulus S_2 was forming in the subject's brain (in the interval after the S_2 stimulus), this incomplete conscious process was retroactively modified by stimulus C.

In still another set of Libet's experiments, subjects were advised to perform sudden wrist motions spontaneously. The subjects acted "whenever they felt like it" and recorded the time of their conscious intention to act. Electrodes on the wrist and scalp allowed the computer to record scalp potentials during the 2 to 3 second period prior to wrist movement, called the *readiness potential*. The following sequence of events occurred: *(1)* The readiness potential recorded from the scalp began about 550 ms before wrist movement. *(2)* The conscious wish to move occurred later, about 200 ms before movement. *(3)* Actual wrist movement occurred. Libet suggests that *the process leading to a voluntary act is initiated by the brain unconsciously, well before the conscious decision to act occurs.*

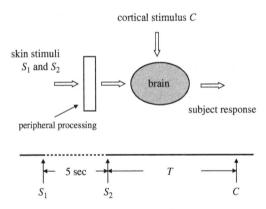

Figure 3–3 Consciousness of external events occurs only after about a half-second delay[3].

This raises the profound question of *free will*, a subject long debated by both philosophers and the faithful. In these limited experiments at least, the unconscious appears to act first, although alternate explanations are proposed below.

Time delay in our awareness of external events is an essential feature of many fields, for example, cosmology. The super giant star Betelgeuse is known to be unstable; it could explode as a supernova at any time and outshine the moon at night. In fact, the supernova may have already occurred. If the star exploded on the day of Isaac Newton's birth in 1643, humans cannot know of this event until the year 2073 since the star is (or was) located 430 light years from Earth. The internal delays of consciousness also have interesting consequences. Consider the typical tailgater driving on the highway at 68 mph (about 100 feet/second), closely following the car in front. During the time for a brake light signal to traverse the optic nerve and reach cerebral cortex, the car has traveled only about 1 foot. When the driver's foot first hits the brake pedal due to his unconscious reaction, the car has traveled at least 15 feet. Conscious awareness of the brake light does not occur until much later when the car has traveled about 50 feet, meaning that over a short interval of awareness, the driver could actually be unaware that he had already crashed into the car ahead.

Libet's experiments have interesting implications, especially in the context of EEG studies, cortical anatomy and physiology, and mathematical theory of cortical dynamics, to be discussed in Chapter 7. In particular, the questioning of free will opens a large can of worms with religious, ethical, and scientific implications. Based on a broader spectrum of evidence from several fields, my interpretation of Libet's data follows:

- Consciousness of an external event takes substantial time to develop. The early parts of a visual or auditory signal may reach neocortex in 10 ms, and it takes about 30 ms for signals to cross the entire brain on *corticocortical fibers*. These *white matter* fibers connect different parts of cerebral cortex to itself, the so-called *gray matter* forming the outer layer of the brain. The corticocortical fibers run just below the cerebral cortex and form most of the white matter layer in humans as shown in the upper half of Figure 3–4. The lower half of Figure 3–4 shows the *thalamus* as a black oval; the thalamus is the main sub cortical relay station for all sensory input except smell. It also supports two-way interactions (feedback) between itself and cortex, as indicated by several *thalamocortical fibers*. Humans have about 10^{10} corticocortical fibers and 10^8 thalamocortical fibers. The relative number of fibers in these two systems is more equal in lower mammals; an anatomical feature apparently related to the issue of *what makes the human brain human*, an issue to be considered in more depth in Chapter 4. Human brains appear to have stronger dynamic interactions between cortical regions than with midbrain regions, in contrast to lower mammals.

- If consciousness of external signals takes roughly 500 ms to develop, conscious awareness requires many passes of signals back and forth between multiple brain regions. In other words, the emergence of awareness requires the development of numerous feedback loops (in corticocortical, thalamocortical, and other fiber systems) involving widespread cortical and lower brain regions. *Consciousness of a sensory stimulus is apparently represented in the total activity of distributed cortical networks rather than any one network node.*

- Parts of the unconscious may be viewed as incompletely formed consciousness, that is, preconscious processes from which consciousness emerges after a few hundred milliseconds or so. Other parts of our unconscious remain forever hidden from awareness but exert important influences on our conscious mind; they affect our choices to act in certain

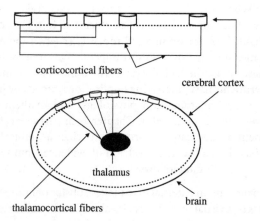

Figure 3–4   Corticocortical and thalamocortical fiber systems.

ways. Interactions occur in both directions; the conscious mind may influence the unconscious and vice versa.

- Initiation and guidance of voluntary acts by the unconscious is a common occurrence familiar to anyone who has ever played baseball or tennis. The complex responses required in sports are much more involved than simple reflexes. A basketball player attempting a jump shot makes split-second adjustments according to his location, velocity, and body angle as well as positions of his opponents. Conscious planning of quick action in sports or playing a musical instrument is typically detrimental to performance; it is best if our painfully slow consciousness relinquishes control to the faster unconscious. In Sections 8 and 9, I will suggest examples of the unconscious initiation of acts in several controlled social situations.

- My colleague Richard Silberstein, well-known for his cognitive experiments with EEG, has suggested the following interpretation of the experiment where subjects were asked to perform sudden wrist motions "whenever they felt like it." In Libet's interpretation, a subject's movements originate in the conscious system, but it appears more likely that the subject simply sets up an unconscious agent to respond to some random internal neural event. Richard conjectures that these neural events may originate in the basal ganglia (of the midbrain) as this system plays a role in timing, motor responses, and so forth. Figure 3–5 summarizes the suggested process. Unconscious processes (agents) may be activated by either an external stimulus or some internal neural event. In either case, the agent may act quickly to elicit a motor response, and conscious awareness occurs later. With Richard's interpretation, no violation of free will occurs.

- Several other mechanisms appear consistent with both free will and Libet's studies. First, the conscious will has about 100 to 150 ms to veto any unconscious impulse. This interval is the time between conscious awareness of an action and the act itself, at least in Libet's experiments.

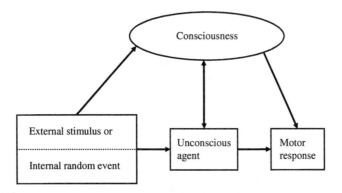

Figure 3–5   Postulated mechanisms involved with unconscious decisions in Libet's experiments.

Perhaps more importantly, it seems likely that our unconscious is placed under prior constraints by the conscious mind, depending on the expected external environment. In Figure 3–5, the unconscious agent(s) can be established by the conscious mind well in advance of possible events. If the conscious mind makes a decision to drive a car in traffic, it apparently places prior constraints on impulsive action by the unconscious. The impulse to suddenly rotate the steering wheel 90 degrees while traveling at 70 mph is unlikely to occur. On the other hand, the unconscious impulse to slam on brakes is allowed. In an emergency like a child running in front of the car, the foot can begin to move off the accelerator in about 150 ms, much too fast for the conscious mind to initiate the act. Actual awareness of the child does not occur for another 350 ms, even though there is no conscious awareness of any delay. I am suggesting that the conscious mind is in continuous communication with the unconscious (the double arrow in Fig. 3–5), providing updated information on the external environment and corresponding constraints on unconscious action. Sometimes we are aware of this communication as an internal dialog; most of the time it occurs below our level of awareness. Maybe our free will is not quite as free as we thought, but it still appears to be pretty "inexpensive."

6. A BLACK CLOUD OF CONSCIOUSNESS

We have argued that awareness of the present requires some time to emerge. Our subjective feeling of the present actually refers to times about 1/2 second in the past. Consciousness is distributed over time, and it is also distributed over space within the brain. In order to emphasize spatially distributed consciousness, a useful metaphor from one of my favorite science fiction stories comes to mind. In 1957, British astronomer Fred Hoyle published a novel called *The Black Cloud*,[4] stimulating the interests of two historical figures in a personal and professional relationship at the time: physicist Wolfgang Pauli and psychologist Carl Jung. Pauli later told Hoyle[5] that he discussed the philosophical implications of the novel with Jung and thought the novel was "better than your astronomical work." This was apparently a typical backhanded remark by Pauli, who as a lowly graduate student attending a visiting lecture by Einstein, began the question period with the quip, "What Professor Einstein has just said is not really as stupid as it may have sounded." Perhaps Pauli's conscious mind had neglected to provide his unconscious with normal prior constraints.

In Hoyle's novel, a black cloud of matter with diameter larger than the Earth–sun separation approaches our solar system. The heroic scientists make repeated attempts to study its physical properties by probing the cloud with electromagnetic signals of different frequencies, resulting in cloud behavior in violation of known physical laws. After eliminating all other possibilities, the scientists are forced to an astounding conclusion: the cloud is intelligent! The scientist's next question is whether the cloud contains a single consciousness or many little conscious entities. They decide that the cloud has developed highly effective means of internal communication by electromagnetic fields. Each small part of the cloud is able to send signals to other parts in select frequency bands. The imagined process is analogous to the Internet, but with a large fraction of the Earth's population online at all times and rapidly sending messages to an ever-changing subset of recipients.

The scientists decide that because the rate of information transfer between all parts of the cloud is so high, the sub clouds cannot be considered as having separate consciousnesses. Any thoughts or emotions experienced by a sub cloud are assumed to be quickly and fully transmitted to many other sub clouds. Thus, the black cloud is deemed to contain a single global consciousness. Individual sub clouds might be concerned with tasks like celestial navigation, memory storage, internal regulation of bodily functions, and so forth; however, for the cloud to behave as a single mind, the sub clouds must work in concert. Neuroscientists refer to the analogous brain processes as *functional segregation* and *functional integration*. Different brain regions do different things; they are segregated. At the same time, they cooperate to yield a unified behavior and (apparent) unified consciousness so they are integrated. The question of how this can be accomplished in human brains, known as the *binding problem* in neuroscience, will be considered in Chapters 6 and 7.

A fanciful representation of the black cloud's "nervous system," imagined to be composed of many sub clouds, is indicated in Figure 3–6. This picture also provides an idea of how human brains may operate by means of the interactions between many subsystems. Ovals of different size might represent tissue masses containing between, let's say, a hundred thousand and a hundred million neurons. The lines connecting ovals represent *functional connections* rather than fixed connections between tissue masses. While the human brain contains more than a hundred trillion (10^{14}) "hard-wired" fiber connections, the lines in Figure 3–6 represent only a snapshot of active connections at a fixed time; the functional connections turn on and off in fractions of a second. In the black cloud, this process of switching specific interactions between sub clouds is accomplished by tuning electromagnetic transmitter signals to match the *resonance* characteristic of the receivers, analogous to a gigantic system of broadcasting stations and TV tuners, which also operate on resonance principles. I conjecture that *resonant interactions* between brain masses may allow for an analogous selectivity of communication between brain subsystems, thereby addressing the so-called binding problem of brain science (see Chapter 7).

In Figure 3–6, I have extended the non controversial idea of multiple brain subsystems by picturing subsystems as nested hierarchies, small systems (black dots), within progressively larger systems (solid and dashed ovals) up to the scale of the entire brain. Interactions may occur between systems at the same level (*spatial scale*) or across scales, as indicated by lines between black dots and ovals, for example. Whenever several subsystems become functionally

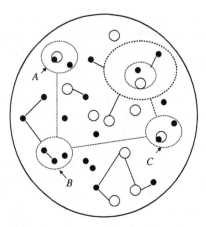

Figure 3–6   Symbolic representation of multiscale interactions in complex systems like our fanciful black cloud or the human brain.

connected, they temporarily form a single system. We may conjecture that none of the smaller subsystems are capable of individual consciousness; rather, a global consciousness may emerge gradually as more and more subsystems are recruited to become functionally connected across multiple scales. Time is also important in this process; consciousness requires that the subsystems remain functionally connected for at least a half second or so. Our proposed picture implies that some subsystems of moderate size may develop rudimentary consciousnesses that may or may not be subservient to the global consciousness. Perhaps we can identify the unconscious with one or more such subsystems. This general idea is, of course, not new, having been championed by such thinkers as William James, Sigmund Freud, Carl Jung, and Donald Hebb, although perhaps with much less emphasis on the *nested* feature of the hierarchy.

The imagined communication process used by the black cloud also nicely illustrates the general idea of *non-local interactions*, meaning generally that distant parts (say, A and B) of some system may selectively exchange information without affecting the parts located between A and B. For example, when I send a letter from New Orleans to London, the text is read only by the intended recipient and requires no serial information chain to relay the message. The letter's content has no direct influence on anyone but the recipient. My use of "non-local" here differs from the (non-hyphenated) label *nonlocal*, used in cosmology to indicate faster-than-light influences to be discussed in Chapters 11 and 12.

The corticocortical fibers of Figure 3–4 form a massive system of non-local connections. In Figure 3–6, the functional connections are mostly non-local. For example, the tissue represented by the dashed oval A has non-local interactions with tissue represented by oval B. On the other hand, interactions between A and

C are strictly local; they occur only by means of their common interaction through subsystem *B*. By contrast to these long-range interactions, the internal interactions inside the black dots occur only by means of *nearest neighbor connections*, in which each small tissue mass (smaller than the dots) interacts only with contiguous tissue. The black dots might conceivably represent cortical *minicolumns* or *macrocolumns*, brain structures containing about a hundred and a hundred thousand neurons, respectively, as will be described in Chapter 4. This distinction between non-local and nearest neighbor interactions is closely related to *small world phenomena* in general networks (Chapter 7) and has important implications for the dynamic behavior of complex systems, including brain dynamic behavior as measured with EEG.

7. EMERGENT PHENOMENA

In philosophy and science, *emergence* refers to novel holistic (or global) properties that arise in complex systems from relatively simple interactions between smaller-scale systems. In meteorology, *tornados* emerge from simpler interactions of small fluid masses. In some materials, *superconductivity* emerges from quantum field interactions between atoms and electrons. *Wars* between nations emerge from the interactions of social systems at multiple smaller scales forming nested hierarchies. Given these examples, we may naturally ask if consciousness emerges from interactions between so-called "neural networks," that is, cell assemblies perhaps organized in nested hierarchies at multiple spatial scales, something like the black cloud model of Figure 3–6. Let me stress that I am not claiming any comprehensive equivalence between consciousness and the emergent phenomena observed in physical systems. Rather, known complex systems may provide us with testable ideas about brain anatomy and physiology that may be necessary for consciousness to exist, to be argued in Chapter 4.

Several typical features of emergence are summarized using Figure 1–3: *(1)* The holistic properties *M* of the system *S* are observed at larger scales than the smaller scale entities *E* that make up the system *S*. *(2)* The holistic properties *M* of the system *S* cannot be accurately predicted even from excellent knowledge of the entities *E* and their interactions *I* "in practice." In strong emergence, *M* cannot even be predicted "in principle." *(3)* The properties of the elements *E* and interactions *I* may be simple or complex; however, the holistic system properties *M* differ substantially from properties of the elements *E*. *(4)* The system *S* exhibits *circular causality*; that is, both top-down and bottom-up interactions across hierarchical scales are critical to the observed holistic properties *M*.

Emergence may be nicely demonstrated by perhaps the most complex system that we know of, the human global system in which the elements *E* are the Earth's seven billion people interacting as individuals with rules represented by I_1, I_2, and so forth. Furthermore, the global system forms a huge nested hierarchy with humans organized in many ways and many levels, analogous to our fanciful black cloud picture in Figure 3–6. Interactions occur between individuals, ethnic groups, nations, and so forth. Very large-scale macroscopic properties $(M_1, M_2, \ldots)$ are associated with economic development, environmental effects, wars, and on and on. The system exhibits many examples of interrelated circular causality. Global economic conditions affect individuals from the top down, causing effects on person's actions that later work their way back up the hierarchy. Persons experiencing physical hardships, loss of pride, or attacks on their religion may choose extremist leaders, small-scale units, to be sure, but nevertheless critically important. Wars may then emerge from the bottom-up interactions initiated by such leaders; wars then provide strong top-down influences across spatial scales, causing even more hardship at the individual level and completing a vicious circle of causality. The bottom-up ascent of Adolf Hitler and the Nazi Party in 1933 was fueled by the devastating top-down effects of German hyperinflation (1921–23) in the Weimar Republic. World War II produced many adverse top-down effects on much of the global population, and so forth. In Chapter 4, I will propose the human global system as a metaphor in our attempts to understand human brain dynamic processes.

8. GAMES PEOPLE PLAY

I end this chapter with several personal stories demonstrating operations of the unconscious, intuition, emergence, and so forth. Also introduced is the speculative idea of intelligence on scales larger than the single brain. Unverified personal accounts are known among scientists as *anecdotes*, sometimes used as a derisive term suggesting questionable reliability. These stories of "personal experiments" depart from the repeatable type 1 experiments of Figure 1–2. But I make no attempt here to prove anything definitive about consciousness, only to introduce ideas to be examined in more depth in later chapters.

The academic field of *sociology* provides an excellent metaphor for brains composed of many interacting subsystems. Sociology focuses on how and why people are organized, either as individuals or as members of various groups in an extensive nested hierarchy. One important issue to be faced in all kinds of systems is the influence of boundary conditions. Scientific studies normally involve *controlled experiments*, in which most external influences on a system are fixed so that the effects of internal influences may be measured unambiguously. Due to the inherent complexity of social systems, such control is almost certain to be imperfect. One particular social system, the *poker game*, has the advantages of simplicity and (mostly) fixed boundary conditions, in which external influences are minimal and the players pursue a well-defined internal goal. For these reasons and because of my own experiences, I propose the poker game as a useful metaphor for the relative roles of mathematics, logic, and intuition in the big game of life. In Chapter 12 I will employ the poker deck metaphor to illustrate the idea of "dynamic memory patterns" in the context of human short-term memory.

Two years after a major career shift from engineering and theoretical physics to neuroscience, I found myself in a *soft money position* at the UCSD Medical School, meaning that I was paid only when successful in obtaining my own federal research grants. As a newcomer working on theoretical brain problems then considered well outside the mainstream, obtaining grant money was not easy. Five of my first ten years as a neuroscientist turned out to be self-supported rather than grant supported. My main source of income during these lean years was San Diego's small legal card rooms. By contrast to casinos, card room fees (called the "rake" or "rent") were kept modest by city regulation. This critical feature facilitated environments in which the top 0.1% to 1% of players might earn a reasonable living "wage" at the tables. In my case, 15 hours per week of play was sufficient to support an ascetic lifestyle, allowing time and mental energy to continue scientific research.

My friends often assumed that mathematical training allowed me to "beat the game" by calculating odds, but this had little to do with how money was actually made. The label "poker" refers to several different games; the importance of knowing odds differs substantially between games. San Diego's law allowed only one game, *five-card draw*, in which players are dealt five cards face down, followed by the first betting round. Players remaining after the first round then draw up to four new cards in exchange for an equal number of discards. After the draw, each player normally has a new hand of five cards, and the second and last round of betting takes place. Aside from modest fees, the essential features of this particular game are: *(1)* No cards are ever exposed, unlike games like stud poker or Texas hold'em currently popular in television coverage. *(2)* Many games are "no-limit," meaning that any player can bet any amount up to all his chips on the table. These features effectively eliminate most considerations of odds from game strategy since experienced players typically follow reasonable statistical strategies intuitively. Success depends almost exclusively on folk psychology, understanding the mental states and behavior of opponents, including an appreciation of how one's own self is perceived by his or her opponents. A good player must try to read the minds of opponents and see himself through their eyes. Each game is essentially a controlled experiment in folk psychology and unconscious action.

When I first started playing, I fundamentally misjudged the nature of the game by vastly underestimating its critical psychology component; one might characterize my play as "autistic" in this sub culture. Mathematical training was probably a handicap; I knew the rules and odds, but I was abysmally ignorant of the game's essence. Fortunately, I became aware of my error several years before poker became my night job. Later, as an experienced player, I often observed the same autistic play by scientists and mathematicians new to the game. It took me some time to finally understand how closely a player's chips represented his feelings of self-worth. Understanding the depth of this emotional involvement was essential. In some games, my chip stack represented 50% of my financial net worth, subject to loss in a single hand. Across the table from me might be a multimillionaire with very little of his net worth at risk, yet he typically seemed every bit as attached to his little pieces of plastic as I was to mine. The critical distinction between human financial and social goals in various "games" has only recently become fully appreciated in economics, especially in the relatively new field of *behavioral economics*. This distinction is nicely demonstrated when professional poker players appear on television, and the host suggests a demonstration game played for pennies or matchsticks. To appreciate the silliness of this idea, imagine challenging a tennis professional to a "match" played without balls. You swing your racquet, and I'll swing mine; we'll just pretend we're hitting the ball!

A full table consisted of eight players arranged in a circle; cards were dealt in turn by the players. My seven opponents might consist of five acquaintances and two strangers, but no friends. Although the players engaged in (mostly) civil conversation, these games differed greatly from the typical friendly home game. Regular players were labeled by colorful names that mysteriously emerged from the sub culture, names like Sailor Alan, Tomato John, Bicycle Bill, Dick the Contractor, and Blond Paul (me). Professionals were well known and mostly welcome, accepted members of a sub culture where status was partly defined by the ability to accumulate chips, a plausible minimodel of the "greed is good" American society.

The atmosphere of these games is perhaps illustrated by a story or two. There is an old joke about a player asked by a friend why he continues to play when he knows the game is crooked. The player answers, "Yes, I know, but it's the only game in town." One incident that sticks in my mind concerns Pigeon Pat, a player on a losing streak who kept borrowing more and more money from other players. When no one would extend additional credit, he abruptly left the game, shouting "save my seat!" Shortly after, he returned with substantial cash and resumed playing. About an hour later, the police came and arrested him. It turned out that he had walked around the block to the nearest bank, robbed it, and returned directly to the card room.

Good basic poker requires folding most hands, leaving plenty of time to observe other players closely. My decisions to play a hand, call a raise, or fold were based on both conscious and unconscious processes. The most important decisions depended on complicated information sets. Objective data included my opponents' positions relative to the dealer, sizes of their bets, number of cards drawn, and number of chips remaining in our stacks. Subjective data included (mostly) unconscious memories of past play, my best guess of how opponents expected me to act, their mannerisms, and perhaps other visual, auditory, and (possibly) even olfactory information available only to my unconscious. I typically made critical financial decisions in a second or two, based mostly on intuition apparently originating in my unconscious. Just as in sports play, it was often better to make choices without actually thinking about them. In my 5,000 hours or so of professional play, these choices were often wrong, but they were less wrong and wrong less often than most of my opponents' choices.

We are all faced with many analogous situations in our daily lives, in which choices must be based on very limited data. We rely on some combination of logic and intuition, but the world's complexity often overwhelms logic, and intuition must play a dominant role in decision making. In considering the issue of logic versus intuition, we can perhaps learn something from *game theory*, a subfield of mathematics and economics, in which players try to make optimal decisions in order to maximize returns. The RAND Corporation is known for developing game theory to help formulate national strategies, especially with regard to nuclear weapons policies. My tentative conclusions about the poker game described above are: *(1)* Game theory is unlikely to contribute directly to conscious decision making because the complexity of situations actually faced by the players goes far beyond the idealistic assumptions of game theory.[6] However, the unconscious might benefit substantially from leisurely study of game theory, leading to delayed influences on later intuitive decision making, in other words, creating unconscious agents like those of Figure 3–5. *(2)* No universal optimal poker strategy exists. A critical aspect of Tomato John's strategy depends upon each opponent's view of Tomato's "ripeness;" his folk theory of Tomato's mind. Optimal strategy varies for each pair of players. Perhaps these ideas provide some insight into the game of life, in which our choices stem from some combination of the conscious and unconscious. The famous mathematician and one of the original developers of game theory, John von Neumann, consistently lost playing poker with his friends[6]. A related issue is the question of how well an advanced computer program might play against human opponents. The answer depends critically on just which game is to be played.[7] There may be an optimal strategy for playing the game of life, but we are unlikely ever to find it. In a similar way, the label *high intelligence* may encompass a broad range of brain dynamic strategies to be considered in Chapter 6.

9. ENCOUNTER GROUPS AND SHARED CONSCIOUSNESS

As noted in the first three chapters, contemporary science suggests that consciousness consists of many interacting subsystems. Awareness may emerge only when a substantial number of subsystems become interconnected in some way; that is, some critical level of functional integration in the brain is attained. EEG experiments to be described in Chapters 5 and 6 provide additional support for this idea. Multiple non conscious or perhaps minimally conscious subsystems within a single brain somehow combine to form a single integrated consciousness. If we accept this framework, it seems reasonable to ask whether multiple brains can somehow combine to form consciousness on scales larger than a single brain. To introduce this idea for later chapters, I cite another personal experiment in folk psychology.

The *encounter group* is a social learning tool developed by psychologist Carl Rogers in the 1960s. It has been said that group therapy is for sick people wanting to get well, while encounter groups are for well people wanting to get even better. The encounter group phenomenon occurs within the larger field of *humanistic psychology*, considered by one of its founders Abraham Maslow as a third alternative to the two other main branches of psychology at that time, behaviorism and psychoanalysis[8]. I became interested in encounter groups in the late 1960s and attended several groups over the next 10 years, some meeting once weekly and others over weekends. As suggested in Figure 3–7, these social experiments occurred at the opposite end of the human spectrum of "internal transparency" from the poker game.

An encounter group is hard to define; it seems to be one of those events that one must experience to understand. Some common features in my experience were "staying in the here and now," meaning that participants agreed to talk only about what was going on among themselves in the present, not about past history or the external world. In other words, for the next few hours let's agree to the following: Pretend that this room is our universe. Let's say what we really think and feel, but try to do this in a way that doesn't attack others. Recognize that we have no direct experience of another person's consciousness, so expressions like "You *are* X (wrong, idiot, saint, coward, perfect...)" should be replaced by something like "Right now, *my impression* of you is X." The second choice tends to avoid defensive reactions and allows the respondent to focus more on your impression of him. Perhaps the impression is temporarily correct, but need not be a permanent condition that defines the person. One can perhaps admit to being "stupid" or a "coward" on special occasions, but we naturally resist these terms as permanent defining labels. Furthermore, it is far more honest to admit that you cannot know another's consciousness; you only know your own impressions of him.

This all may seem a bit flaky to those who have not experienced the encounter group process, but I observed it consistently breaking down the normal barriers between people, often leading participants to report profound experiences carried forward in their lives. One well-known encounter group

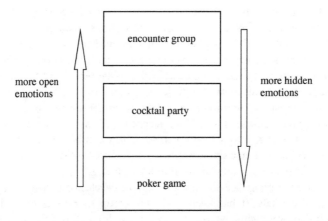

Figure 3–7 Three social environments with different "rules" about emotional transparency.

environment, based on Carl Roger's ideas, is the *La Jolla Program*, founded and run by Bruce Meador for the past 40 or so years. In 1981, I attended the 17-day program where I met my wife-to-be. The next year, we were asked to return as group facilitators, so I can make some modest claim to semiprofessional experience with both extremes of internal transparency shown in Figure 3–7.

The encounter group culture tends to frown on analysis of the group process, taking the holistic view that meaningful things "just happen" or emerge when the right environment is created. But as a scientist, I must at least attempt some analysis, so here is my personal view of the encounter group experience. Extending my metaphor of the black cloud, an important feature that allows us to remain individuals is our psychic boundary, the barrier to fully sharing our thoughts and emotions with others. Since maintaining this boundary seems essential if we are to survive as individuals, it should be expected that both our conscious and unconscious selves fight hard to keep most of this boundary in place. One aspect of the psychic boundary is illustrated by the word *mokita* from the Kiriwina language of New Guinea, meaning *that which we all know to be true, but agree not to discuss.*

In certain environments we allow little doors here and there in this boundary to open so that some integration with other consciousnesses occurs. Solders in combat, athletic teams, revival meetings, religious cults, mobs, and some marriages provide plausible examples. But opening barrier doors can lead to inner conflict; the marriage partner with cold feet just before his wedding date is perhaps an instance of conflict between the conscious and unconscious self. With friends the doors open a little; with strangers we normally keep the doors closed. However, the encounter group provides a novel environment where: *(1)* Members are strongly encouraged to open doors based on positive feedback from the facilitator and other group members. Some of the social rules of the outside world, especially those having to do with emotional transparency and honesty, are changed. Whatever we believe to be true can actually be discussed; *mokita* is *discouraged.* *(2)* All group members are aware that opening doors is only temporary. At the end of the group, members go back to the real world of mostly closed doors, but perhaps more comfortable in their interactions with others and less fearful of small-door openings. The limited time interval of the groups is critical. We definitely want to survive as individuals, but maybe we can give up part of our individual selves when we know it's only for a few hours or days.

10. GROUP CONSCIOUSNESS

Let me now pose a crazy-sounding question: Could a "room-scale" consciousness emerge from, let's say, 10 encounter group participants strongly interacting with enough of their barrier doors open? The idea may seem ridiculous, but suppose we imagine some progressive process where more and more barriers are purged so that the group becomes more and more functionally integrated. Is there any level of functional integration where the group might be considered a single consciousness? Does the fact that participants remain physically separated make a difference? Suppose we facilitate functional integration by progressively adding more physical connections between brains using an imagined advanced technology that selectively relays action potentials between brains. If a group consciousness were in fact created in this manner, what would happen to individual consciousnesses? Could group and individual consciousnesses coexist? If so, could each become aware of the other's existence? Would individual consciousnesses become subservient to the group, a sort of mob psychology? How similar are these questions to the issues raised in regard to conscious–unconscious interactions in single brains?

If this thought experiment seems a bit farfetched, I suggest an unequivocal example from real life. *Conjoined twins* (or Siamese twins) are identical twins formed in the uterus either by an incomplete splitting of the fertilized egg or a partial rejoining of an egg that had split earlier. This occurs roughly once in every 200,000 births; about 25% survive. My first example is the famed "Scottish brothers" of the 15th century, essentially two heads sharing the same body. They had separate brains, so we naturally grant them separate consciousnesses. But, they carried the same genes and were never physically separated, sharing the same environment all their lives. Can we perhaps infer some overlap in their consciousness? Were there ever periods when one could say they had a single consciousness?

My next example is twins joined at the head with partial brain sharing. Do they have one consciousness or two? It seems that the adjective "partial" is critical here. Lori and George (a she) Schappell, Americans born in 1961, are joined at their foreheads and share 30% of brain tissue. George has performed widely as a country singer and won music awards. During her sister's performances, Lori remains quiet and attempts to become "invisible." From these reports, Lori and George appear to have entirely separate consciousnesses. But, imagine several pairs of twins with progressively more brain in common; at what point do two consciousnesses become one? How similar are these questions about conjoined twins to issues concerning split-brain patients or conscious–unconscious interactions in single intact brains?

11. SUMMARY

Human brains exhibit multiple states of consciousness defined in terms of motor and cognitive functions: waking, sleep stages, coma, anesthesia, vegetative, and minimally conscious states. Unconscious processes are closely related to and may influence conscious mental processes but lack the feature of awareness. Conscious awareness of external events develops over about half a second, implying that consciousness resides in the global activity of distributed networks rather than isolated at any one location.

Intuitive feelings or hunches are based on a perceived ability to sense something without reasoning. In the real world, we encounter many ambiguous situations in which decisions must be based on minimal information. If intuition originates in an experienced unconscious, following hunches constitutes a life strategy superior to making random choices.

If progressively more connections are added, can such functional integration of multiple brains lead to a group consciousness? Can group and individual consciousnesses coexist in a nested hierarchy? Would individual consciousnesses become subservient to the whole, a sort of mob psychology? How similar are these questions to conscious–unconscious interactions in single brains?

Chapter 4

Why Hearts Don't Love and Brains Don't Pump

1. HUMAN BRAINS AS COMPLEX ADAPTIVE SYSTEMS

What makes human brains so special? How do they differ from hearts, livers, and other organs? The heart's central function is to pump blood, but it is not accurate to say that it is *just* a pump. Hearts and other organs are enormously complicated structures, able to continuously repair themselves and make detailed responses to external control by chemical or electrical input. Yet, only brains yield the amazing phenomenon of consciousness. In this chapter, I address one of the most fundamental issues of brain science: What distinguishes the brain from other organs, and what distinguishes the human brain from the brains of other mammals? Brains are complex and evidently human brains are, in some poorly understood sense, more complex than other animal brains. To help address this issue, I consider the scientific category known as *complex systems*, composed of smaller interacting parts and exhibiting emergent behavior not obviously predictable from knowledge of the individual parts. *Complex adaptive systems* have the added capacity to "learn" from experience and change their global behavior by means of feedback processes. Examples include stock markets, ecosystems, and living systems.

This brief overview of neurophysiology and neuroanatomy emphasizes several general features distinguishing human brains from other organs, including the hallmarks *hierarchical and non-local interactions*. I suggest here that *(1)* brains are highly complex adaptive systems, and *(2)* the features required for healthy brain function have some common ground with known complex adaptive physical and social systems. With these tentative ideas in mind, I propose the *human global social system* as one of several convenient brain analogs. Some may object to this choice of analog since its small-scale parts are creatures that appear to be fully conscious in the absence of external interactions; however, I propose this analog system in order to describe the kinds of dynamic behavior one might look for in any complex system, be it biologic, economic, or physical. The fact that the small-scale units are themselves conscious does not detract from its usefulness as a *dynamic* metaphor.

By contrast to alternate analogs like holograms or spin glasses, special magnets with complex internal interactions, our global society is familiar to all. More importantly, the global social system is more complex than any single brain if the social system's full fractal-like features down to the smallest (sub molecular) scales are included. Cooperation and conflicts between individuals, cities, and nations serve as convenient metaphors for dynamic neural interactions on multiple levels (*scales*), a process that might be labeled *neuron sociology*. Interactions in modern social systems often occur between distant points without directly altering the dynamics of structures in between; this is the definition of "non-local," a concept closely related to the *small world phenomena* discussed in Chapter 7. Mathematical models of non-local systems differ fundamentally from local systems, the former typically modeled by integral equations, the latter by differential equations; I will outline this distinction in Chapter 7. In Chapters 9–12, I will drop the hyphen and adopt the label *nonlocal* as used in quantum mechanics, meaning faster-than-light influences. In this book we are dealing with the intersections of many different areas of human knowledge, each with its own jargon; sometimes similar labels occur with entirely different meanings.

Brains also provide for non-local dynamic interactions in the time domain when information is retrieved from long-term memory. *Conditional probability* is the chance that some event A will occur given that event B has already occurred. A system in which the *conditional probability* of future states depends only on the current state (not on its earlier history) is known as a *Markovian process* in probability theory. For example, given the location and velocity of a baseball leaving a pitcher's hand, we could predict the probability that it will cross the strike zone; such prediction is independent of any earlier motion of the same baseball.

If long-term memory, stored chemically or in synaptic contact strengths, is separate from brain dynamics, brain dynamics is non-Markovian in this sense. That is, given an exact description of the dynamic state of a brain at some initial time, we could not predict, even in principle, future states, as these would depend partly on the content of memory retrieval (we are describing a thought experiment, not a real experiment). In an analogous manner, our global social system dynamics is non-Markovian since the long dead communicate to us through books, films, and so forth, arguably making the future even more unpredictable than it would be otherwise. The "temples of the dead" that we label *libraries* are the analogs of brain memory traces. Perhaps brain scientists have nearly as much to learn from historians, economists, and sociologists as they do from physicists.

2. THE HUMAN BRAIN AT LARGE SCALES

The *central nervous system* consists of brain and spinal chord. The *peripheral nervous system* has two parts: The *somatic system* consists of nerve fibers in the skin, joints, and muscles under voluntary control. The *autonomic system* includes nerve fibers that send and receive messages from internal organs, regulating things like heart rate and blood pressure. The autonomic system also relays emotional influences from brain to facial displays like laughing, blushing, or crying.[1]

The three main parts of the human brain are *brainstem, cerebellum,* and *cerebrum* as indicated in Figure 4–1a. The brainstem, which sits at the top of the spinal cord, relays signals (*action potentials*) along nerve fibers in both directions between spinal cord and higher brain centers. The *cerebellum,* located at the top and to the back of the brainstem, is associated with fine control of physical (*motor*) movements: threading a needle, hitting a baseball, and so forth. The cerebellum also contributes to cognitive functions.

The large remaining part of the brain is the cerebrum, divided into two halves or *cerebral hemispheres.* The outer layer of the cerebrum is the *cerebral cortex,* a folded, wrinkled structure with the average thickness of a five cent coin

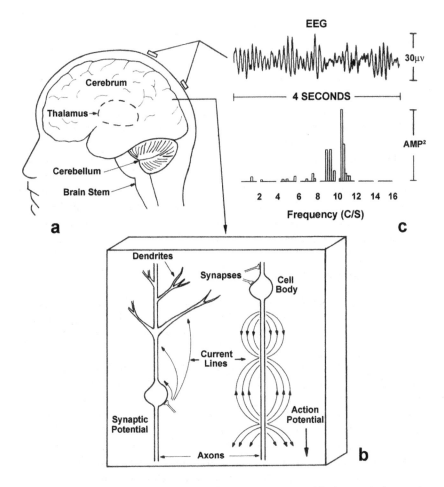

Figure 4–1   Human alpha rhythm and frequency spectrum (c) plus cortical synaptic action at small scales (b).[2]

(2 to 4 mm) and containing roughly ten billion (10^{10}) *neurons*. Neurons are nerve cells with many branches similar to a tree or bush. Long branches called *axons* carry electrical signals away from the cell to other neurons. The ends of axons consist of *synapses* that send chemical *neurotransmitters* to the tree-like branches (*dendrites*) or cell body (*soma*) of target neurons as indicated in Figure 4–1b. The surface of a large cortical neuron may be covered with ten thousand or more synapses transmitting electrical and chemical signals from other neurons. Much of our conscious experience involves the interaction of cortical neurons, but this dynamic process of neural network (*cell assembly*) behavior is poorly understood. The cerebral cortex also generates most of the electric (EEG) and magnetic (MEG) fields recorded at the scalp. Many drugs including caffeine, nicotine, and alcohol alter brain function; drugs work by interacting with specific chemical (*neurotransmitter*) systems.

Figure 4–1c depicts 4 seconds of an electroencephalographic (EEG) record, the electric potentials recorded from a person with electrodes held against his scalp by elastic caps or bands.[2] Also shown is the corresponding *frequency spectrum*, produced by a common signal transformation (called the *Fourier transform* or *spectral analysis*) that reveals the dominant frequencies in the signal; in this case the oscillations are near 10 cycles per second, units given the shorter label Hertz (Hz). EEG is a non invasive and painless procedure to be described in Chapter 5. Some of the current generated by neurons in the cerebral cortex crosses the skull into the scalp and produces scalp currents and electric potentials typically in the 50 microvolt range, signals about 100 times smaller than chest potentials generated by the heart (EKG). The subjects of clinical EEG studies are often epilepsy patients with recordings carried out by technicians under the direction of *neurologists* specially trained in EEG. By contrast, EEG studies in *psychology* and *cognitive science* rely on healthy volunteer subjects, often the scientists themselves and their students.

3. BRAIN INPUTS AND OUTPUTS

Figure 3–2 demonstrates a very simplified view of central nervous system function with (input) sensory information like the usual sights and sounds of our daily lives, leading to (output) motor activity like applying car brakes, waving to a friend, or answering a question. Signals move mainly from left to right in the diagram, but lateral neural connections and feedback signals from right to left also occur. Identical sensory information can take many possible paths between input and output. The number of synaptic relay stations between (input) sensory receptors in the retina, inner ear, nose, tongue, or skin and (output) muscles producing physical action can be very large or as few as two or three in the case of the *spinal cord reflex*. The time required for inputs to produce outputs can range from roughly 100 milliseconds to a lifetime, but outputs that take long times can no longer be identified with well-defined inputs.

This simplified view of the brain as a *black box* in engineering terminology or *stimulus-response system* in the behavioral psychologist's parlance is quite limited. It masks the point that inputs to parts of our consciousness and unconscious can be internally generated. Human outputs often occur with no discernible input, and many stimuli elicit no immediate motor response. You can call someone a "dirty SOB," and he may not hit you in the face immediately, but later, in your favorite sleazy bar, he could produce a very unpleasant response. Sensory input passes through multiple preprocessing stages that determine details of the stimulus features. The modified signals are then integrated with other sensory information so that the sights and sounds from the external world are combined in some way to form a unified pattern of information. Next, this new information is combined with old information from memory systems and assigned an emotional tone. Finally, preparation for motor output occurs in the context of both internal and external factors. The methods by which these signal integrations occur are largely unknown. This knowledge gap is known as the *binding problem* of brain science. We know quite a bit about the input and output ends in Figure 3–2, but much less about the workings of brain regions in between.

Some years ago I was body surfing off a remote Mexican beach where a friend and I were camping. I was alone in the water about 100 yards out and the day was overcast, contributing to some uneasiness. Suddenly, something big and black appeared in the water about 10 yards away, startling me, but my view was blocked by a passing wave. The unknown black object caused visual input that activated (in sequence) photoreceptor, bipolar, and ganglion cells in my retina, followed by activation of the million neurons that form my *optic nerve*. Generally, information from more than 100 million receptors converges on these one million axons, indicating that early retinal stages involve substantial visual processing well before signals reach the brain.

Optic nerves from both eyes meet and cross at the optic chiasm at the underside of the brain as indicated in Figure 2–1. Information coming from both eyes is combined and then splits and crosses over according to *visual field*. Right and left visual fields consist of everything I see to the right and left of my nose (with some overlap). If an object appears on my right side, information in the form of axon signals (action potentials) is sent to the left side of my brain. The right side of my brain deals with the left half of the *field of view from both eyes*, and similarly for the left side of my brain. Most of the axons in the optic nerve end in synapses in the thalamus (Fig. 4–1). Signals are then relayed up the visual pathway to *primary visual cortex*, located in the *occipital region* near the back of the brain.

In the next stages, signals from primary visual cortex are transmitted to other visual areas of cortex along two major corticocortical fiber pathways called the *dorsal* and *ventral streams*. The dorsal stream carries signals toward the front of the brain along the upper portion in each hemisphere. The ventral stream carries signals forward toward the lower part of the two temporal lobes. This picture of successive activation of neural structures up the visual pathway breaks down in less than 100 milliseconds from the visual stimulus when multiple cortical feedback systems evidently dominate cortical dynamic behavior. At later times, signals are transmitted back and forth between multiple brain regions. Corticocortical action potentials can traverse the entire brain on long fibers, say from occipital to frontal cortex, in about 30 milliseconds.

My unconscious mind evidently became aware that the stimulus was caused by a large black object after 200 to 300 milliseconds, apparently because of multiple feedback signals between cortical regions and between cortex and midbrain structures, including my limbic system associated with memory and emotion (in this case, terror!). My unconscious then alerted my *autonomic system* to increase heart rate and blood pressure in preparation for action. Lower animals have also evolved limbic systems responsible for this so-called *fight or flight response* to perceived danger, a feature of rats as well as humans. Widely distributed cell assemblies are believed to produce both unconscious processes and conscious awareness, although we have little information about their (possibly overlapping) brain locations. My conscious awareness of whether or not the object was a genuine threat and my decision to take action were delayed several seconds before the passing wave allowed me to get a good look at the object. Frontal cortical regions play a critical role in this decision-making process but evidently integrate their actions with a whole constellation of rapidly changing cell assemblies throughout the brain. As the wave passed, this global dynamic brain process allowed me to identify the object as a rather passive-looking sea lion, but by that time my fear and flight responses were in full operation. I was swimming toward shore as fast as I could; I was no better than a rat.

4. CHEMICAL CONTROL OF BRAIN AND BEHAVIOR

Neurons and cell assemblies communicate both electrically and chemically. Electrical signals (*action potentials*) travel along axons to their synaptic endings, and the synapses release chemical neurotransmitters that produce specific responses in each target cell (the *postsynaptic neuron*); the type of response is determined by the particular neurotransmitter. Each neurotransmitter exerts its postsynaptic influence by binding to specific *receptors*, chemical structures in cell membranes that bind only to matching chemicals, analogous to metal screws accepting only matching bolts.

Drugs, chemicals introduced into the body to alter its function, also work by binding to receptors. One important class is the *opiates*, associated with euphoria and pain relief and including *morphine* and *heroin*. Research funding on opiate receptors in the early 1970s occurred largely because of heroin addiction by American soldiers in Vietnam.[1] Subsequent scientific discovery of opiate receptors raised the question of why such human receptors exist in the first place; after all, we are not born with morphine in our bodies. Might opiate receptors match a new class of neurotransmitters that regulate pain and emotional states? This conjecture was indeed verified: neurotransmitters labeled *endorphins* were discovered; they are produced during strenuous exercise, excitement, and orgasm. Endorphins are produced by the *pituitary gland* and *hypothalamus*, small structures at the brain base just below the thalamus.

Endorphins resemble opiates in their abilities to produce a sense of well-being and pain reduction; they work as natural pain killers, with effects potentially enhanced by other medications. Endorphins might provide a scientific explanation for the *runner's high* reported by athletes.

Hormones are chemical messengers that carry signals from cells of the *endocrine system* to other cells in the body through the blood. Hormones regulate the function of target cells having receptors matching the particular hormone as indicated in Figure 4–2. The net effect of hormones is determined by several factors including their pattern of secretion and the response of the receiving tissue. Hormone levels are correlated with mood and behavior, including performance in cognitive tasks, sensory sensitivity, and sexual activity. Women's moods often change during menstrual periods as a result of *estrogen* increases. Men with high *testosterone* levels may be more competitive and aggressive. *Clinical depression* has been related to several hormones, including melatonin and thyroid hormones.

The *hypothalamus* connects the endocrine and nervous systems and is responsible for regulating sleep, hunger, thirst, sexual desire, and emotional and stress responses. The hypothalamus also controls the pituitary gland, which, in turn, controls the release of hormones from other glands in the endocrine system. The *neuromodulators* are a class of neurotransmitters that regulate widely dispersed populations of neurons. Like hormones, they are chemical messengers, but neuromodulators act only on the central nervous system. By contrast to synaptic transmission of neurotransmitters, in which a presynaptic neuron directly influences only its target neuron, neuromodulators are secreted by small groups of neurons and diffuse through large areas of the nervous system, producing global effects on multiple neurons. Neuromodulators are not reabsorbed by presynaptic neurons or broken down into different chemicals, unlike other neurotransmitters. They spend substantial time in the cerebrospinal fluid (CSF) influencing the overall activity of the brain. Several neurotransmitters, including *serotonin* and *acetylcholine*, can also act as neuromodulators.

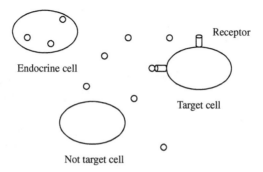

Figure 4–2 Chemical messengers (hormones) produced by an endocrine cell bind to specific cell receptors on target cells.

5. ELECTRICAL TRANSMISSION

While chemical control mechanisms are relatively slow and long lasting, electrical events turn on and off much more quickly. Electrical transmission over long distances is by means of action potentials that travel along axons at speeds of about 100 meters/second in the peripheral nervous system, 6 to 9 meters/second in the corticocortical axons (white matter), and much slower within cortical tissue (gray matter). The remarkable physiological process of action potential propagation is analogous to electromagnetic wave propagation along transmission lines or TV cables, although the underlying physical basis is quite different. Action potentials travel along axons to their synaptic endings, releasing chemical transmitters that produce membrane changes in the target (*postsynaptic*) neurons.

Synaptic inputs to a target neuron are of two types: those which produce *excitatory postsynaptic potentials* (EPSPs) across the membrane of the target neuron, thereby making it easier for the target neuron to fire its own action potential and the *inhibitory postsynaptic potentials* (IPSPs), which act in the opposite manner on the target neuron. EPSPs produce local membrane *current sinks* with corresponding distributed passive sources to preserve current conservation. IPSPs produce local membrane *current sources* with more distant distributed passive sinks as depicted by the current lines in Figure 4–1c. All tissue current forms closed loops. IPSPs cause (positively charged) potassium ions to pass from inside to outside the target cell just below the input synapse (active source current). The ions re-enter the cell at some distant location (passive sink current). EPSPs cause (negatively charged) chlorine ions to contribute to local active sinks and distant passive sources as indicated in Figure 4–3. Action potentials also produce source and sink regions along axons as shown in Figure 4–1b; several other interaction mechanisms between

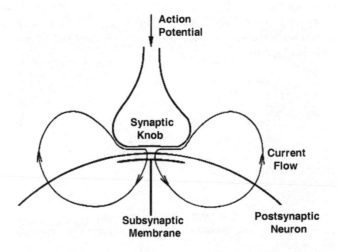

Figure 4–3 An excitatory action potential arriving at a synapse causes the release of a neurotransmitter that causes a local current sink in the target cell.

adjacent cells are also known. Much of our conscious experience must involve, in some largely unknown manner, the interaction of cortical neurons. The cerebral cortex is also believed to be the structure that generates most of the electric potentials measured on the scalp (EEG).

6. CEREBRAL CORTEX

The cerebral cortex consists of *neocortex*, the outer layer of mammalian brains plus smaller, deeper structures that form part of the *limbic system*. The prefix "neo" indicates "new" in the evolutionary sense; neocortex is relatively larger and more important in animals that evolved later. I will use *cerebral cortex*, *cortex*, and *neocortex* interchangeably in this book unless noted otherwise. Cortex is composed mostly of cells lacking myelin wrapping and is often referred to as "gray matter," indicating its color when treated by anatomists with a special stain, but cortex is actually pink when alive. Cortex consists mainly of about 80% excitatory *pyramidal cells* (neurons) and 20% inhibitory neurons. Pyramidal cells tend to occupy narrow cylindrical volumes like tall skinny trees, as opposed to the more spherical basket cells that are more like little bushes. Each pyramidal cell generally sends an axon to the underlying white matter layer; the axon connects to other parts of cortex or to deeper structures. Cortex surrounds the inner layer of white matter, consisting mostly of *myelinated axons*. Myelin consists of special cells that wrap around axons and increase the propagation speed of action potentials, typically by factors of 5 to 10. Cortex exhibits a layered structure labeled I through VI (outside to inside) defined by cell structure; for example, more of the larger pyramidal cell bodies are found in layer V. This layered structure holds for all mammals.

Figure 4–4 depicts a large pyramidal cell within a *macrocolumn* of cortical tissue, a scale defined by the spatial extent of axon branches (E) that remain within the cortex and send excitatory input to nearby neurons. Each pyramidal cell also sends an axon (G) into the white matter layer. In humans more than 95% of these axons are corticocortical fibers targeting the same (*ipsilateral*) cortical hemisphere. The remaining few percent are *thalamocortical fibers* connecting to the thalamus or callosal fibers targeting the opposite (*contralateral*) cortical hemisphere. A probe (A) used to record small-scale potentials through the cortical depth is also shown in Figure 4–4. The dendrites (C) provide the surfaces for synaptic input from other neurons, and J represents the diffuse current density across the cortex resulting from the membrane current sources and sinks as represented by the expanded picture (F). The macrocolumn of Figure 4–4 actually contains about a million tightly packed neurons and ten billion or so synapses; if all neurons were shown, this picture would be solid black. Anatomists are able to identify individual neurons only with a special stain that darkens only a small fraction of the total.

Neuroscience over the past century has been strongly influenced by the idea that the brain has developed in *phylogeny*, meaning its evolutionary history is characterized by the successive addition of more parts. In this view each new

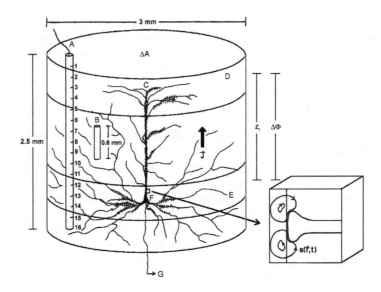

Figure 4–4   A cortical macrocolumn with depth electrode (A) and corticocortical axon (G).[2]

structural addition has added more complex behavior and at the same time imposed regulation on the more primitive (lower) parts of the brain. The brainstem, limbic system, and cerebral cortex form three distinct levels both in spatial organization and in evolutionary development as suggested in Figure 4–5. In this oversimplified picture, the brainstem, often called the reptilian brain, or limbic system might be prevented by the cortex from taking certain actions, say rape and murder, an idea with obvious connections to Freud's id and super ego. In the colorful language of writer Arthur Koestler, psychiatrists actually treat three patients in each session, an alligator, horse, and a man, representing progressively more advanced brain structures. A scientific view, expressed by famous neuroscientist Vernon Mountcastle,[3] retains much of this classical idea but emphasizes that the dynamic interplay between many subsystems in all three evolutionary structures is the very essence of brain function.

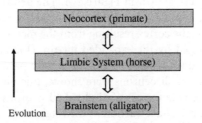

Figure 4–5   The evolutionary development of major structures roughly matches their spatial depth in the human brain.[2]

7. THE NESTED HIERARCHY OF NEOCORTEX: MULTIPLE SCALES OF BRAIN TISSUE

The 10 billion or so cortical neurons are arranged in columns at various scales defined by anatomical and physiological criteria, as indicated in Figure 4–6 and Table 4–1.[3] The *cortical minicolumn* is defined by the spatial extent of intracortical inhibitory connections, approximately 0.03 mm or roughly the diameter of a human hair. Minicolumns extend through the cortical depth, so their heights are about 100 times their diameters. Each minicolumn contains about 100 pyramidal cells. Inhibitory connections typically originate with the smaller and more spherical basket cells. Inhibitory action tends to \occur more in the middle (in depth) cortical layers, labeled III, IV, and V.

The *cortical module* (or *corticocortical column*) is defined by the spatial spread of (excitatory) subcortical input fibers (mostly *afferent* corticocortical axons) that enter the cortex from the white matter below. Modules contain about

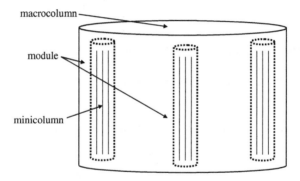

Figure 4–6   Three distinct structural scales of cortical columns defined both anatomically and physiologically.

Table 4–1   Spatial Scales of Cortical Tissue Structure and Function

Structure	Diameter mm	# Neurons	Description
Minicolumn	0.03	10^2	Spatial extent of inhibitory connections
CC column	0.3	10^4	Input scale for corticocortical fibers
Macrocolumn	3.0	10^6	Intracortical spread of pyramidal cell
Region	50	10^9	Brodmann area
Lobe	170	10^{10}	Areas bordered by major cortical folds
Hemisphere	400	10^{11}	Half-brain

10,000 neurons and 100 minicolums. This extracortical input from other, often remote, cortical regions, is excitatory and tends to spread more in the upper and lower cortical layers (I and VI). The selective actions of inhibitory and excitatory processes in different layers could account for global behavior in response to different neurotransmitters as will be discussed in Chapter 6.

The *cortical macrocolumn* is defined by the intracortical spread of individual pyramidal cells.[4] As indicated in Figure 4–7, pyramidal cells send axons from the cell body that spread out within the local cortex over a typical diameter of 3 mm. This picture was obtained by using a special preparation that stains only a few cells viewed in a transparent background of unstained tissue. The actual density of axon branches in this preparation is greater than 1 kilometer per cubic millimeter! If all neurons were stained, the picture would be solid black. In addition to the intracortical axons, each pyramidal cell sends one axon into the white matter; in humans, most of these re-enter the cortex at some distant location. Macrocolumns contain about a million neurons or about ten thousand minicolumns.

Inhibitory interactions occur mostly in the middle cortical layers, and excitatory interactions are more common in the upper and lower layers; this has important implications for cortical dynamics. Healthy brains seem to operate between the extremes of global coherence (all parts of cortex doing similar things) and functional isolation (each small part doing its own thing). Different neuromodulators tend to operate selectively on the different kinds of neurons at different cortical depths. *Neuromodulators can apparently act to*

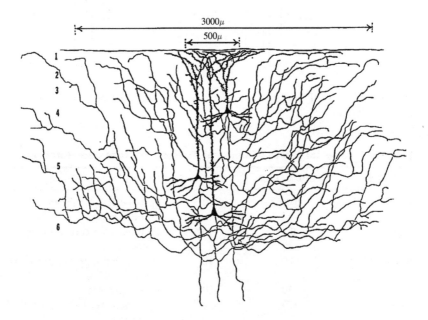

Figure 4–7 A macrocolumn showing three cortical pyramidal cells in cerebral cortex with layers 1–6 (or I–VI).[4]

control the large-scale dynamics of cortex by shifting it between the extremes of global coherence and full functional segregation. This idea has important implications for several brain diseases, and I will return to this topic in Chapter 6.

An overview of cortical structure (*morphology*) reveals neurons within minicolumns, within modules, within macrocolumns, within Brodmann regions, within lobes, within hemispheres—a nested hierarchy of tissue. A plausible conjecture is that each of these structures interacts with other structures at the same scale (level) as in neuron-to-neuron interactions or minicolumn-to-minicolumn interactions. If inhibitory processes within a column are swamped by excitation (too many EPSPs and not enough IPSPs), this overexcited column may spread its excitation to other columns in the runaway positive feedback process called *epilepsy.*

Cross-scale interactions also occur. Small cell groups produce chemical neuromodulators that act (bottom up) on neurons in the entire cortex. External sensory stimuli reach small groups of cells in primary sensory cortex that elicit (bottom up) global brain responses. When your alarm clock goes off, you hop out of bed, begin to plan your day, and so forth. Extended brain networks are activated involving memory and emotion; this global dynamics acts (top down) to produce action in specific muscle groups, causing you to open a door, call a friend, and so on. The information storage in memory must be enormous, not only for things purposely memorized, but for the many other things we take for granted like how to dress, walk, open doors, brush teeth, and distinguish a mouse from a spouse.

The morphology of cerebral cortex, in which complex structure occurs at multiple scales, reminds us of *fractals,* geometric shapes that exhibit fine structure at smaller and smaller scales. Natural objects that often approximate fractals include coastlines, clouds, and mountain ranges. We need not be concerned here with precise fractal definitions, which include a mathematical property called *self-similarity,* meaning statistically similar properties at multiple levels of magnification. Rather, we note that cerebral cortex has a *fractal-like structure* and exhibits *fractal-like dynamic patterns,* meaning dynamic patterns exhibit fine structure at multiple scales. Intracranial measurements of electric potential can be expected to depend strongly on the sizes and locations of recording electrodes, as in Figure 4–4.

The scientific practice of *electrophysiology,* which consists of recording electric potentials in tissue, spans about five orders of magnitude of spatial scale. Measured potentials at any so-called "point" necessarily represent space averages over the volume of the electrode tip. With electrodes of different sizes, potentials are recorded inside cells (0.0001 cm), within the cortical depths (0.01 cm), on the brain surface (0.1 cm), and on the scalp (2 to 10 cm). Scalp electrodes are about 1 centimeter (cm) in diameter, but recorded potentials are space averaged over much larger source regions because of volume conduction and physical separation from sources as will be discussed in Chapter 5. Scalp potentials (EEG) are exclusively large scale, generated by the space-averaged synaptic activity in tissue masses typically containing 100 million to 1 billion neurons.

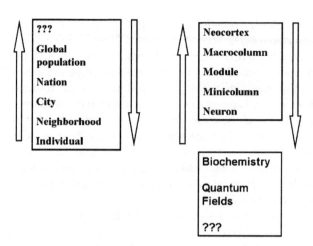

Figure 4–8   A nested hierarchy containing human and brain structures at distinct scales; the arrows emphasize the critical cross-scale interactions[2].

Top-down and bottom-up hierarchical interactions across spatial scales occur in many systems, such phenomena are a hallmark of complex systems. Complex dynamic phenomena have been studied in physical, biological, social, and financial systems under the rubric *synergetics*, the so-called *science of cooperation*, a field of science developed by physicist Hermann Haken. Hermann has labeled top down/bottom up interactions in dynamic systems, including our postulated cortical interactions, as *circular causality*. Small-scale events cause new events to occur at larger scales, which, in turn, influence smaller scales, and so forth. In the global social system, families, neighborhoods, cities, and nations interact with each other, at the same scales and across scales as indicated by Figure 4–8. National leaders like the U.S. president or chairman of the Federal Reserve exert strong (bottom-up) influences on humans worldwide. These influences are called "bottom-up" because they are initiated by small-scale entities (single humans); the fact that they are powerful persons increases their influence on the global system but is still in the "bottom-up" category. At the same time, actions of these leaders are constrained or perhaps even dictated (top down) by global events like wars and financial crises. One may guess that such cross-scale interactions are essential to brain function, including electrical and chemical dynamic behavior and even consciousness itself.

8. CORTICOCORTICAL CONNECTIONS ARE NON-LOCAL

The upper portion of Figure 3–4 depicts a few cortical macrocolumns and corticocortical fibers; note, however, that these columns actually overlap so column boundaries are only determined in relation to designated pyramidal cells. The axons that enter the white matter and form connections with other cortical areas in the same hemisphere are the corticocortical fibers, perhaps 97% of all white matter fibers in humans. The remaining white matter fibers are either thalamocortical (perhaps 2%) connecting cortex to the deeper thalamus in the "radial" direction, or callosal fibers (perhaps 1%) connecting one cortical hemisphere to the other. In addition to the long (1 to 15 cm) *non-local* corticocortical fibers, neurons are connected by short-range (less than a few mm) *local* intracortical fibers as indicated in Figures 4–4 and 4–7.

The actual corticocortical fibers shown in Figure 4–9 were dissected from a fresh human brain immediately after its unfortunate owner was executed for murder in the 1940s. While the donor (reportedly) gave his brain willingly, similar procedures are unlikely to be repeated in today's ethical environment. The average length of the corticocortical fibers is a few centimeters (*regional or Brodmann scale*), and the longest fibers are roughly 15 to 20 cm (*lobe scale*). Cerebral cortex is divided into 50 Brodmann areas based on relatively minor differences in cell layers and structures, which in some cases are known to correspond to distinct physiological functions, for example, in *visual, auditory, somatosensory,* and *motor cortex.* Touch some part of the body and the matching area of somatosensory cortex responds; motor cortex initiates signals sent to muscles. The 10 billion corticocortical fibers are sufficiently numerous to allow every macrocolumn (3 mm diameter) to be connected to every other macro-column in an idealized homogeneous system. Because of connection specificity (some columns more densely interconnected than others), actual full inter-connectivity occurs at a somewhat larger scale, but probably less than 1 cm.

While specificity of fiber tracts prevents full connectivity at the macro-column scale, a pair of cortical neurons is typically separated by a *path length*

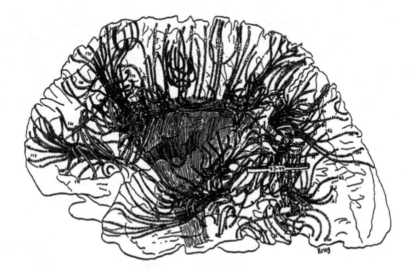

Figure 4–9   A few of the 10 billion human corticocortical axons obtained by tedious brain dissection.[6]

of no more than two or three synapses. That is, an action potential from a neuron targets a secondary neuron, which, in turn, targets a third neuron, and so forth. Only two or three such steps are required for influences from one region to spread to the entire cortex. The corticocortical network's path length is analogous to the global human social network with its so-called *six degrees of separation* between any two humans, meaning a path length of no more than six social contacts worldwide. Pick someone at random, say a Mr. Dong from China. You probably know someone, who knows someone, and so forth, who knows Mr. Dong, with perhaps only six acquaintance steps needed to complete the path. We humans live in a *small world* social network. Small world phenomena are studied in a branch of mathematics called *graph theory* and also appear widely in physical systems. I will revisit small worlds in the context of cortical connectivity in Chapter 7.

8. WHAT MAKES THE HUMAN BRAIN "HUMAN?"

What distinguishes the human brain from the brains of other mammals? This question presents an apparent paradox: Cognitive processing, indeed, most of our conscious experience, depends critically on the dynamic operations of cerebral cortex. But there is very little difference between the cortical structures (*morphology*) of different mammals; all contain similar cell types and distinct cortical layers I through VI. This striking similarity even includes a constant number of cells within the minicolumn. Larger brains will, of course, have more neurons and columns to interact with one another. While brain size surely counts for something, it fails to explain why humans seem more intelligent than elephants, dolphins, and whales, at least based on our biased human measures. Dolphins don't get PhDs, but maybe they just have better things to do. These species all have larger brains covered by folded cortices that look much like human brains. While humans do enjoy the largest ratios of brain weight to body weight, such measure contributes little to the fundamental question of why human brains produce more complex behavior. I have gained weight since high school, but I don't think this has made me dumber; rather it's probably the other way around.

To address the problem of "brain humanness," we first note the words of Vernon Mountcastle, "the dynamic interaction between brain subsystems lies at the very essence of brain function," suggesting emphasis on interconnections between subsystems rather than just the anatomy of the subsystems themselves. Neuroscientist Valentino Braitenberg[5] has emphasized an important quantitative difference in the brains of different species of mammals. Suppose we count the number of axons entering and leaving a patch of the underside of neocortex. Some fibers connect cortex to cortex (corticocortical fibers); others connect cortex to deep (midbrain) structures, especially the thalamus. Some years ago my colleague Ron Katznelson[2] consulted the anatomical literature to estimate the following ratio

$$Ratio = \frac{number\ of\ corticocortical\ fibers}{number\ of\ corticomidbrain\ fibers}$$

In the human brain, this ratio is large, perhaps in the range of roughly 20 to 50, meaning that only about 2% to 5% of human fibers entering or leaving cortex connect to midbrain structures. As indicated in Figure 4–10, a cortical column of one square millimeter sends about 100,000 axons to other parts of cortex and receives cortical input from about the same number, but only about 2,000 fibers connect to the thalamus and other midbrain structures. In contrast to this human anatomy, the relative density of thalamocortical compared to corticocortical fibers is substantially higher in other mammals. Data from several mammals are summarized in Figure 4–11, indicating that the fraction of corticocortical fibers becomes progressively larger as mammals become capable of more complex behavior. Unfortunately, we do not have corresponding estimates of this ratio for elephants, dolphins, and whales, data which may or may not support these ideas.

The estimates of Figure 4–11 provide an intriguing, but tentative and incomplete, explanation for human brain *humanness* that makes intuitive sense in several ways. I think I am smarter than my dog Savannah, but in what sense am I smarter? My olfactory cortex is a *moron* compared to Savannah's. She experiences a whole world of distinct smells that I can barely imagine; I go sightseeing, she goes smell-sniffing. She finds golf balls in tall grass and under water by *smellor* technology, the doggy version of infrared sensing. In some way that we don't understand, our humanness seems to originate from global interactions of multiple cortical neurons and columns at different scales within the nested hierarchy of cortical tissue. Dynamic feedback between cortex and midbrain may be relatively less important in humans than in lower mammals, but this does not negate the critical influence of midbrain chemical control acting on longer time scales. We are more human-like than horse-like or alligator-like (at least most of us).

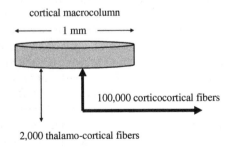

Figure 4–10 The approximate numbers of corticocortical and thalamocortical axons entering or leaving the underside of a macrocolumn patch of cerebral cortex.

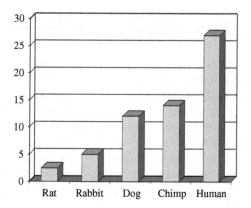

Figure 4–11   An estimate of the ratios of corticocortical to thalamocortical axons (Fig. 4–10) in several mammals.

Imagine that we know nothing of the dynamic behavior of electric potentials in cortex, the spatial and temporal patterns measured on the scalp with EEG or within the brain using small electrodes. Given the basic anatomy and physiology of cortex discussed in this chapter, can we make any tentative predictions about expected dynamic behavior? In the following sections, I list several qualitative predictions of cortical dynamic behavior based only on the basic cortical physiology and anatomy outlined in this chapter.

9. INFLUENCE OF HIERARCHICAL STRUCTURE ON CORTICAL BEHAVIOR

The nested hierarchical cortical structure consists of neurons within minicolumns within modules within macrocolumns inside cerebral cortex lobes. We then expect to observe fractal-like electric potential patterns; the closer we look with smaller and smaller electrodes, the more detail we expect to see. Recording potentials inside the cortex yields space averages of potential over the volume of the electrode tip and time averages over the sample time. Instead of recording the quantity $V(\mathbf{r}, t)$, the potential at a so-called "point" $\mathbf{r}$ and time t, we actually measure $V(\mathbf{r}, t; R, \tau)$, where R is radius of a spherical volume of tissue surrounding point $\mathbf{r}$, and τ is the time over which the time average potential is recorded. We expect potential maps obtained with our experiments to be scale dependent. The recorded potential oscillations of $V(\mathbf{r}, t; R, \tau)$ must depend on the spatial scale R, which determines the numbers of excitatory and inhibitory processes contributing to the measurement. Preferred frequency ranges of (scalp-recorded) EEG are associated with certain behaviors and tasks, but there is no guarantee that these same preferred frequencies will exhibit the same relationships when recorded with small electrodes inside the skull. The critical dependence of measurements on the spatial and temporal scales of observation is a familiar issue. In Chapter 1, I contrasted dynamic behaviors of small and large corporations in our economy. Human activity can be measured for individuals, families, cities, nations, or the entire world, multiple spatial scales of observation. In addition, one can follow human activity on daily, yearly, or century time scales.

Both top-down and bottom-up interactions across spatial scales, the process known as *circular causality*, are expected in neocortex. Think of the dynamic behavior of a familiar physical system, global weather. *Meteorology*, the study of the dynamic patterns of atmospheric pressure, temperature, and water vapor, has several sub classifications depending on the spatial and temporal scales of description, ranging from local to global and days to weeks. Global-scale weather dynamics over long time scales (years) is the province of *climatology*. Large-scale weather systems act top-down to influence local dynamics, helping to create local events like *tornados*. Large-scale systems always rotate counter-clockwise in the northern hemisphere due to the *Coriolis effect*, a mechanical influence of the earth's rotation on objects moving tangentially to its surface. Most, but not all, tornados rotate in the same direction even though Coriolis forces on tornados are negligible because of their small size. Rotation and other tornado properties are strongly influenced top-down by global effects. A common myth is that Coriolis forces cause water entering bathtub drains to rotate counterclockwise and clockwise in the northern and southern hemi-spheres, respectively. I informally tested this idea in my oversized tub and spa, circulating the water by hand, and then waiting several minutes until all visible circulation disappeared; dirty water and my favorite tiny rubber ducks facili-tated this observation. When I pulled the plug, no circulation was apparent until the tub was nearly empty, at which time water rotation matched my (top-down) rotation by hand, either clockwise or counterclockwise.

Perhaps neuroscience's most prominent advocate of the brain as a complex adaptive system is UC Berkeley Professor Walter Freeman,[7] the experimental and theoretical neuroscientist who has championed theoretical modeling of the nervous system since the early 1960s. Walter's early contributions include identification and strong emphasis on the nested hierarchy of neuron popula-tions (labeled *K sets*) and treatment of larger-scale neural structures as neural masses. In many disparate systems with multiple interacting parts, the later step is often necessary to develop tractable models, analogous to treating, for example, a large number of gas molecules as a continuous fluid. When I first entered neuroscience from physics and engineering in 1971, treatment of cortical tissue as a continuous medium seemed like the natural approach to modeling large-scale phenomena like EEG. I was initially discouraged, however, as many neuroscientists seemed to view the neural mass concept with skepti-cism if not outright hostility. After reading Walter's papers, I was strongly encouraged to go forward with the EEG modeling. Over the years, Walter has offered many apparent connections between complex systems and genuine neural systems, including considerations of general network behavior to be discussed in Chapter 7.

My colleague, the physicist and neuroscientist Lester Ingber,[8] emphasizes that theories of complex systems (spin glasses, lasers, chemical mixes, weather, ecology, and so forth) typically employ *mesoscopic-scale* mathematics to bridge gaps between microscopic and macroscopic descriptions. This occurs even in the absence of fixed mesoscopic structures in these (mostly) physical systems. Neocortex is especially interesting in this context because of the distinct meso- scopic tissue scales, both anatomically (fixed columnar structure) and physio- logically (scale-dependent inhibitory and excitatory interactions). Lester has developed an ambitious theory of *statistical mechanics of neocortical interactions* based on modern methods of mathematical physics applied to genuine cortical tissue. Lester has held several conventional professorial and government posi- tions, but for 15 of the early years he supported his esoteric neuroscience work by running a karate school in California (Lester holds a black belt). Later he acted for several years as a director of research in the financial services industry, applying his mathematical methods to futures and options markets.

As similar mathematical tools appear appropriate for disparate complex systems, we can reasonably search for analogous dynamic behavior in brains. Cortical analogs provide intriguing hints of possible behavior to be searched for experimentally: multiscale interactions, standing waves, neural networks, holo- graphic phenomena, chaos, and so forth. The S&P 500 stock index provides one brain analog; the index is composed of markets and associated corporations, made up of separate parts composed of individuals, a multiscale complex system. Same-scale interactions occur between individuals and markets; cross-scale inter- actions are both top-down and bottom-up. Non-local interactions are common- place. Variables like prices, profits, index level, and so forth are analogous to multiscale measures of electric potential. Global economic conditions provide an environment in which the corporations are embedded. The economy acts top- down on corporations, which act bottom-up on the economy; circular causality is omnipresent. Lester has emphasized mathematical similarities between brains and human systems—financial markets, military hierarchies, and so forth. Such efforts in neuroscience to identify plausible analogs with genuine mathematical theory are likely to persist into future generations.

10. INFLUENCE OF SYNAPTIC DELAYS ON CORTICAL BEHAVIOR

Another prediction of cortical dynamic behavior follows from the extreme interconnectedness of cortex. Each large pyramidal cell receives ten thousand or so synaptic inputs, from contiguous cortical neurons, distant cortical neu- rons, and neurons in the midbrain. We might then expect to see similar dynamic behavior in widespread cortical regions due to the general global nature of the system. We might, in fact, wonder how any part of the brain can ever become functionally segregated. Perhaps we might guess that inhibitory synapses can effectively "wall-off" minicolumns from their neighbors, while at the same time allowing excitatory input from distant minicolumns via cortico- cortical axons.

Still other anticipated behavior follows from local delays of cortical and white matter tissue. When a synapse sends its neurotransmitter to the dendrite of the target (postsynaptic) neuron, the maximum influence of this input on the cell body occurs only after a delay called the *postsynaptic potential rise time*, typically a few milliseconds. Furthermore, such influence diminishes over a longer delay called the *postsynaptic potential decay time*. We might expect multiple neural networks to form on different scales, involving interactions between cortex and thalamus as well as interactions between cortical regions. If several inhibitory and excitatory neurons form a temporary local network in cortex or in cortex and thalamus, we might predict oscillations of electric potential with dominant frequencies based on serial postsynaptic potential delays at several stages. The occurrence of such *local network oscillations* evidently require substantial functional isolation from other tissue, otherwise they could no longer be classified as "local."

11. INFLUENCE OF NON-LOCAL INTERACTIONS WITH AXONAL DELAYS ON CORTICAL BEHAVIOR

I use the label *non-local interaction* here to indicate that synaptic and action potentials at one cortical location influence cortical tissue in other locations without altering the intervening cortical tissue. Intuitively, this seems to allow for much more complex dynamic patterns than could occur with strictly local (intracortical) interactions, as will be argued in the context of *graph theory* and *small world phenomena* in Chapter 7.

Global axonal delays are distinct from local synaptic delays and occur because the speed of action potentials carrying signals through the white matter is not infinite. *Occipital cortex* (near the back of the brain) can directly influence frontal cortex by means of action potentials carried by corticocortical axons, after delays in the 30 millisecond range. Mathematical theories based on either local (postsynaptic) delays or global (axonal) delays are able to predict oscillations with frequencies in the general range of dominant EEG rhythms. When I first proposed a theory of *standing brain waves* based only on axonal delays in 1972, the few existing EEG theories were all based on postsynaptic potential delays.[9] Some controversy over these (partly) competing views remains to this day, although there are good reasons to believe that both local and axonal (global) delay mechanisms contribute substantially to EEG dynamics. One may guess that in particular brain states, frequency bands, or scales of observation, either local or global delay phenomena may be more evident in the collected data.

Postsynaptic and axonal delays, which I label here as local and global delays, respectively, are analogous to several familiar physical phenomena. A simple oscillatory electric network with some preferred (resonant) frequency typically has a characteristic delay time depending only on network elements like resistors and capacitors. Delays are fully determined by local elements, thus, if the physical size of the network is increased by increasing the length of its connecting wires, the characteristic delay and corresponding resonant frequency are essentially unchanged. If, however, the network is made very large by connecting elements with, let's say, coast-to-coast transmission lines, multiple resonant frequencies can be expected, and these will depend on both the local network elements and the physical size of the system; characteristic delays then have both local and global origins. Such global delays are well understood in transmission line systems. In Chapter 7, I will show that global delays are also important in genuine (as opposed to toy) spatially extended chaotic systems.

The earth-ionosphere system (a *resonant cavity*) shown in Figure 4–12 is a physical system with global delays causing the so-called *Schumann resonances*. Lightning bolts provide electric field sources producing ongoing electromagnetic *traveling waves* in the spherical shell between the earth's surface and the inner layer of ionosphere. Lightning consists of *noise*, that is, electric field oscillations with broad frequency mixtures. But, as a result of the spherical shell geometry, the induced electromagnetic waves combine (*interfere*) such that only standing waves with preferred wavelengths persist. The fundamentals of wave phenomena involve close relations between wave frequencies and spatial wavelengths, thus the selection of preferred wavelengths by the system geometry implies preferred (resonant) frequencies, called the *normal modes of oscillation*. The lowest predicted frequency (*fundamental mode*) of the Schumann resonances is determined only by the speed of light c and the earth's radius a

$$f_1 = \frac{c\sqrt{2}}{2\pi a} \tag{4.1}$$

The higher resonant frequencies are *overtones*, which in this and in most oscillatory systems are not *harmonics* (multiples) of the fundamental. The Schumann standing wave mechanism is very similar to that of a vibrating guitar or piano string. The main difference is that in vibrating strings, reflection of traveling waves from boundaries causes wave interference and

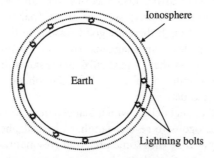

Figure 4–12 The Schumann resonances are standing electromagnetic waves in the earth-ionosphere shell caused by ongoing lightning strikes.

the preferred standing waves. By contrast, Schumann wave interference occurs due to waves traveling around the closed shell; standing waves occur due to the *periodic boundary conditions* of the closed shell geometry (see also Figs. 7–4 and 7–5). These standing waves are, by the way, mathematically very similar to the standing wave functions of quantum mechanics that yield electron energy levels in atoms, except that in the atmosphere tangential but not radial standing waves occur. Quantum waves will be discussed in Chapter 10.

Do the Schumann resonances have anything to do with *brain waves*? Consider any closed shell of arbitrary shape containing some material medium in which wave interference can occur. The existence of standing waves and corresponding resonant frequencies requires only that the material medium supports traveling waves that do not fade away too quickly (*weakly damped waves*) so that interference can do its job. Canceling of excitatory and inhibitory synaptic action in cortical columns may produce such interference in cerebral cortex.

Each cortical hemisphere is topologically equivalent to a spherical shell, implying that the wrinkled surface of each hemisphere can be reshaped or mentally inflated (as with a balloon) to create an equivalent spherical shell with effective radius *a* related to its surface area by the relation

$$a \sim \sqrt{\frac{A}{4\pi}} \tag{4.2}$$

Thus, cerebral cortex and its white matter system of (mostly) corticocortical fibers is a system somewhat analogous the earth-ionosphere shell as indicated in Figure 4–13 (see also Fig. 7–4). Cortical signals are carried (non-locally) just below the cortex, leading to some differences as will be discussed in Chapter 7. With a brain hemispheric surface area $A \sim 1000 - 1500\,\text{cm}^2$ and

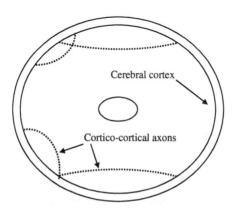

Figure 4–13 Standing brain waves, analogous to Schumann resonances, are postulated based on axon speeds and (topologically equivalent) spherical shell geometry.

characteristic corticocortical axon propagation speed $v \sim 600 - 900$ cm/sec, the
fundamental cortical frequency predicted by the *naïve application* of (4.1) is

$$f_1 \sim 12 - 23\,\text{Hz} \qquad (4.3)$$

I call this estimate "naïve" because the fundamental mode frequency depends
on both the physical shape and material properties of the wave medium. Thus,
Equation 4.1 cannot be expected to represent genuine brain waves, even if the
cortex were actually a spherical shell; postulated brain waves have little to do with
electromagnetic waves. The ideas of this section do not, by any wild stretch of the
imagination, constitute a brain theory; rather, they simply suggest a hypothesis
and related experiments to test for traveling and standing *brain waves*. If the
estimate (Eq. 4.3) had been obtained before the discovery of the 10 Hz human
alpha rhythm in the 1920s, it would have provided a plausible, testable prediction.
The appropriate experimental question would have been, *Can brain states be
found in which neural network activity is sufficiently suppressed to allow observation
of simple standing waves?* Such putative experiments would have found the
predicted EEG oscillations in the 8–13 Hz band in relaxed subjects (minimal
mental load) with closed eyes to minimize the processing of visual information.

Generic waves originating at 8 epicenters (one on the back side in the first
plot), each traveling outward from its own central origin in a spherical shell, are
illustrated in Figure 4–14. Each epicenter might represent a simultaneous
lighting strike or a cortical location where strong excitatory synaptic activity

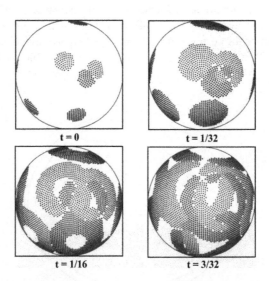

t = 0	t = 1/32
t = 1/16	t = 3/32

Figure 4–14   Generic traveling waves in a spherical shell spread from eight epicenters
and later interfere to form standing waves; the light and dark points represent negative
and positive perturbations of the field variable, respectively. The time $t = 1/2$ is required
by a wave packet to move from its epicenter to the opposite pole.[2]

originates. Darker and lighter regions might represent positive and negative fluctuations about some constant background field, say, pressure perturbations (sound waves), electromagnetic field perturbations, or positive and negative fluctuations of mass synaptic action (brain waves). After an initial transient period ($t < 1/2$), the traveling waves combine to form standing waves with preferred (resonant) frequencies determined by medium properties and the spherical shell geometry.

I avoid technical detail here but will provide the genuine theory outline and experimental evidence for standing brain waves of *synaptic action* in the context of *field theories* of cortical dynamics in the Endnotes section (under Chapter 7) at the end of the book. Neural network (cell assembly) and global field descriptions (including standing waves) constitute complementary models of cortical reality. Neural networks may be pictured as embedded in cortical fields in a manner analogous to social networks embedded in cultures. I will suggest in several parts of Chapters 6 through 8 that standing brain waves can facilitate more regular (less chaotic) dynamic behavior and coordinate the simultaneous operation of multiple networks. This idea addresses the so-called *binding problem* of brain science: how the unity of conscious perception is created by distinct neural systems processing vision, sound, memory, and so forth. Field theories suggest how distinct neural networks can be *bound by resonance* is some frequency bands while, at the same time, operating independently at other frequencies, to be discussed in Chapter 7.

12. SUMMARY

Sensory input to a brain may or may not elicit an output, typically a perceptual or motor response. We know quite a bit about the input and output ends of this gray box, but much less about the workings of regions in between. Human brains are made up of hundreds of substructures, including the gray matter of cerebral cortex, and the deeper white matter layer, consisting mostly of corticocortical fibers connecting different parts of cortex to itself. The high density of these long axons in humans compared to lower mammals may be an important aspect of our humanness.

Neurons and cell assemblies communicate both electrically and chemically. The *neuromodulators* are a class of neurotransmitters regulating widely dispersed neural populations. Like hormones, neuromodulators are chemical messengers but act only on the central nervous system. By contrast to the local synaptic transmission of neurotransmitters in which a presynaptic neuron directly influences only its target neuron, neuromodulators are secreted by small groups of neurons and diffuse through large areas of the nervous system, producing global effects on multiple neurons.

While chemical control mechanisms are relatively slow and long lasting, electrical events turn on and off much more quickly. Electrical transmission over long distances is by means of action potentials that travel along axons at speeds as high as 100 meters/sec in the peripheral nervous system, 6 to 9 meters/

sec in the corticocortical axons (white matter), and much slower on non-myelinated axons within cortical tissue.

Based only on basic anatomy and physiology of cortex, tentative predictions of dynamic behaviors in cerebral cortex are advanced here. Experience with other complex systems suggests that the nested hierarchical structure of cortical columns may have profound influence on cross-scale interactions, both top-down and bottom-up. Cortical dynamics is expected to be fractal-like. Inhibitory processes may allow functional segregation of selected cortical tissue, effectively walling off portions of tissue that participate in discrete networks. Neural networks (cell assemblies) are expected to form at multiple spatial scales and operate over multiple time scales. Synaptic delays in local networks may produce some of the characteristic oscillation frequencies recorded with electrodes of various size and location. Non-local interactions by means of the corticocortical fibers apparently allow for much more complex dynamics than would be possible with only local interactions.

The cortical–white matter system of each brain hemisphere is topologically equivalent to a spherical shell. The white matter medium carries signals with finite speeds, suggesting the possible occurrence of *standing waves* with frequencies in roughly the EEG range. Standing brain waves (with embedded networks) address the so-called *binding problem* of brain science, how the unity of conscious perception is created by distinct neural systems. Brain waves are predicted by a *field theory* of cortical dynamics. Neural network and global field descriptions constitute complementary models of cortical reality. I suggest that these are *not* simply optional ways of looking at the same thing, but rather that both models are required for a deeper understanding of dynamic behavior. In the philosophical version of *complementarity*, two views are complementary only if they provide non overlapping insights. If the two neural models are combined, *neural networks may be pictured as embedded in cortical fields, analogous to social networks embedded in human cultures.*

Inhibitory and excitatory processes occur in selective cortical layers. Similarly, different neuromodulators tend to operate selectively on the different kinds of neurons at different depths. Healthy brains seem to operate between the extremes of global coherence and functional isolation (segregation). Thus, neuromodulators can apparently act to control the large-scale dynamics of cortex by providing for shifts between more global coherence and more functional isolation, an idea with implications for several brain diseases as will be described in Chapter 6.

Chapter 5

EEG: A Window on the Mind

1. IMAGING BRAIN AND MIND

Brain imaging may reveal either structure or function. Structural or static imaging is accomplished with *computed tomography* (*CT*) or *magnetic resonance imaging* (MRI); the latter provides better contrast than CT in pictures of soft tissue. My label "static imaging" indicates changes on yearly time scales in healthy brains or perhaps weeks or months in the case of growing tumors. By contrast, intermediate timescale methods like *functional magnetic resonance imaging* (*fMRI*) and *positron emission tomography* (*PET*) track brain changes over seconds or minutes. Still more rapid dynamic measures are *electroence-phalography* (*EEG*) and *magnetoencephalography* (*MEG*), which operate on millisecond time scales, providing dynamic images *faster than the speed of thought*.

fMRI is a technique for measuring blood oxygen level in small tissue volumes (*voxels*), little tissue cubes a few millimeters on a side. In cortex, such *voxels* contain ten million or so neurons and perhaps a hundred billion synapses. The relationship between blood oxygen level and action or synaptic potentials is not well understood; however, this *BOLD* (blood oxygen level–dependent) signal provides an important local measure of one kind of brain activity. Typical fMRI studies look for differences in BOLD signal between some mental task and a control condition using statistical tests applied on a voxel-by-voxel basis. Recognition of human faces, for example, may be represented as small red spots on 3D brain images. fMRI is a *tip of the iceberg measure* in the sense of finding locations with BOLD signals elevated by a few percent during the task, rather than exclusive locations of brain activity as sometimes erroneously interpreted by the general public. One plausible interpretation of such "hot spots" is that they may identify major hubs of extended neural networks as depicted in Figure 2–2.

PET is another important imaging technique that can measure several kinds of local metabolic (biochemical) activity in tissue. PET and fMRI provide excellent spatial resolution but poor temporal resolution. These measures are complementary to EEG, which provides poor spatial resolution and excellent (millisecond) temporal resolution. MEG is still another technique for observing thinking brains, recording tiny magnetic fields 2–3 centimeters above the scalp, produced by synaptic current sources in cortex. MEG is similar to EEG in this regard but is mostly sensitive to sources in cortical folds (*fissures* and *sulci*), whereas EEG is more sensitive to sources in the outer smooth part of the cortical surface (*gyri*). In this limited sense of differential sensitivity to source location, EEG and MEG are complementary measures, but the similarity of spatial and temporal resolutions implies considerable overlap.[1]

2. EEG RECORDING

The first EEG recordings from the human scalp were obtained in the early 1920s by the German psychiatrist Hans Berger. Berger's subjects were often his teenage children; his studies revealed near sinusoidal voltage oscillations (*alpha rhythms*) in awake, relaxed states with eyes closed. Opening the eyes or performing mental calculations often caused substantial amplitude reduction, findings verified in modern studies. Unfortunately, it took more than 10 years for the scientific community to accept Berger's scalp potentials as genuine brain signals rather than system noise or biological *artifact* like eye or muscle potentials. By 1950, EEG was widely viewed as a genuine *window on the mind*, with important applications in neurosurgery, neurology, and psychology.[2]

My focus on the quick dynamics of consciousness motivates emphasis on EEG with its excellent temporal resolution, while acknowledging the importance of complementary measures applied at different time and space scales. Figure 5–1 indicates several similarities and contrasts between today's EEG and earlier systems. The upper photograph shows me (standing) in 1976 pasting electrodes on the scalp of my assistant using a glue-like substance dried with an air gun. The scalp was abraded by a blunt needle causing minor discomfort, and conductive gel injected through a hole in the electrode. EEG channels sampling 16 scalp sites were displayed on a paper chart and stored on a primitive computer. My goal in this particular study was to see if dominant alpha frequencies were negatively correlated with brain size as would be expected if alpha rhythms were (at least partly) standing brain waves. The picture was taken by a reporter from a local newspaper that helped us with subject recruitment by writing an article on our research.

After recording sessions in the medical school of the University of California at San Diego, I would often drive across town to a remote Navy laboratory where a sympathetic friend converted our primitive computer tape to IBM tape. The new tape was then submitted to UCSD's IBM mainframe to carry out several kinds of mathematical analysis. Computer time in those days was expensive. I once made a critical programming error, accidentally erasing much of my meager salary for the year. I timidly approached the computer center director with my impoverished tale; thankfully the charges were reversed and I was able to keep up my rent payments and regular cans of tuna for supper. The lower photograph shows me at UC Irvine in 2005 sitting before a cheap, modern computer while my colleague Ramesh Srinivasan fits an elastic net containing 128 electrodes to the subject's head. The combination of dense electrode array and sophisticated computer algorithms allows for substantial improvement in modern spatial resolution, a process known as *high-resolution EEG*.

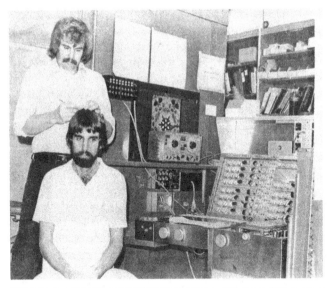

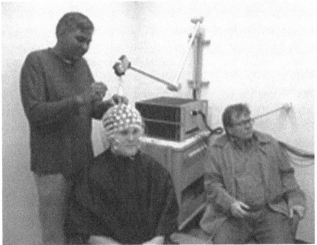

Figure 5-1 (Upper) Paul Nunez is shown placing electrodes on assistant Larry Reid in 1976.[2] (Lower) Ramesh Srinivasan is fitting an electrode array on Sam Thorp in 2005 while Nunez checks the computer monitor.[2]

One of my projects in the 1970s was to test experimentally the general concept of standing brain waves. As suggested by Equation 4.1, if alpha rhythms are (at least partly) composed of standing waves, brain size should be negatively correlated with the dominant alpha frequency. I had no way to measure brain sizes directly in living subjects. Even had MRI been available, no funding agency would have supported such a "crazy" idea. Fortunately, head size is strongly correlated with brain size, so I was able to estimate brain size with three simple tape measurements. Another obstacle was the fact that human head sizes do not vary over a sufficiently wide range to test my hypothesis easily. Resonant frequencies of all kinds of standing waves increase with propagation speed; thus, children were excluded because their corticocortical axon propagation speeds increase substantially with progressive axon myelination as they age. To get good statistics on the postulated relationship between head size and alpha frequency, I needed a lot of subjects with exceptionally small or large heads. Our EEG technician enthusiastically dubbed this the "pin head, fat head project."

My initial recruiting strategy was to attend a lot of parties in San Diego armed with my tape measure. Whenever a promising subject appeared, I would ask permission to measure his or her head; I can't remember anyone ever refusing the measurement. Surprisingly, some even failed to ask *why* I wanted to measure their heads; it just seemed a cool thing to do (California in the 1970s was atypical). Subjects were later brought to the lab where EEG was recorded. Eventually, local newspapers became aware of the project and efficiently recruited many more subjects for us. One paper produced a headline in bold black letters, "Scientist Seeks More Heads (Can Remain Attached!)" Eventually, I published an article in the respected EEG journal showing a small but statistically significant ($p = 0.01$ to 0.02) negative correlation between peak alpha frequency and head size, providing some preliminary support for the standing wave hypothesis.[3] This so-called "p value" means essentially that there is a 1% or 2% chance that our estimated negative correlation was just an accident. The negative correlation between head size and alpha frequency has been independently replicated in a more recent study[3]. I will discuss other contributions to EEG frequencies in Chapter 7 that explain why size provides only a small influence.

3. SIGNAL OSCILLATIONS: AMPLITUDE, FREQUENCY, AND PHASE

A short overview of elementary signal analysis is relevant here. Each of the two sine waves in Figure 5–2 (upper) shows three oscillations in 0.3 seconds, or 10 oscillations per second (10 Hz). The two upper waveforms differ only by a small *phase difference*; that is, peaks of the dashed curve occur a little earlier than peaks of the solid curve. Two waveforms 180° out of phase are shown in Figure 5–2 (lower). If each of the lower traces were to represent a distinct source strength at nearly the same cortical location, the corresponding scalp potential would be essentially zero due to cancellation of positive and negative contributions. If, on the other hand, these traces were to represent variations of some quantity with spatial location (say excitatory and inhibitory synaptic action along the cortical surface), the two waveforms would also cancel due to *wave interference*.

Every "sine wave" (*sinusoidal oscillation*) is fully determined by just three features—its amplitude, frequency, and phase. Physical and biological signals,

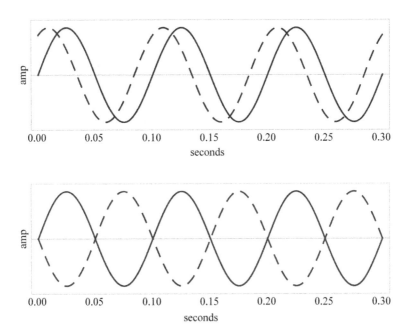

Figure 5–2 The two sine waves are nearly synchronous in the upper plot with only a small phase offset, but fully asynchronous in the lower plot.

including EEG, are generally composed of mixtures of multiple frequencies, each possessing its own amplitude and phase. Often we wish to know the contributions of different frequencies to our signals, a measure especially important in EEG because different frequency bands provide selective information about different brain states. A computer algorithm (*fast Fourier transform*) may be used to decompose any waveform, no matter how complicated, into its composite frequency components. This procedure, called *spectral analysis*, is analogous to atmospheric decomposition of white light (containing many frequencies) into distinct rainbow colors, each belonging to a specific frequency band of electromagnetic field oscillations. Figure 5–3 (upper) shows a waveform consisting of a little noise plus a mixture of three frequencies (5, 9, and 11 Hz), each with a different amplitude and phase. These three frequencies are revealed by peaks in the frequency spectrum in Figure 5–3 (lower). The broadening of spectral peaks is partly due to added noise but is mainly caused by application of the Fourier transform to a relatively short time period. Longer periods of analysis result in sharper spectral peaks (*better frequency resolution*).

The EEG community uses labels to characterize waveforms according to frequency band: *delta* (1–4 Hz), *theta* (4–8 Hz), *alpha* (8–13 Hz), *beta* (13–20 Hz), and *gamma* (roughly greater than 20 Hz, with emphasis often near 40 Hz). These categories should be taken with a pound of salt as EEG is typically composed of mixtures of frequencies. In particular, so-called "beta activity"

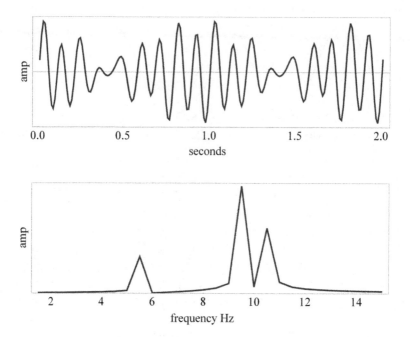

Figure 5–3   The upper plot shows an artificial signal composed of three frequencies, 5, 9, and 11 Hz, as revealed in the lower spectral plot.

may actually be composed of small amplitude beta oscillations superimposed on larger amplitude alpha. This confusion originates mainly from times before the 1970s when spectral analysis came to more common use in EEG. Before that, frequencies were defined only by the primitive method of simply counting the number of zero crossings of the waveform.

The phase of a single signal is of no interest if, as is often the case, the definition of zero time is arbitrary. By contrast, when multiple signals are analyzed, the *relative phases* between signals can be of great importance, as in multichannel EEG. When two signals are lined up with zero phase offset (or nearly so), the signals are said to be *synchronous*. If two signals maintain a (mostly) fixed phase relationship over a long time, the signals are said to be *coherent*. Based only on these short periods, the waveforms in Figure 5–2 are apparently coherent and nearly synchronous (upper) and coherent and asynchronous (lower), but these labels are usually applied to much longer records when dealing with genuine brain signals.

To demonstrate the distinction between synchrony and coherence, suppose the identical twins Jean (living in New Orleans) and Jacques (living in Paris) have identical eating and drinking habits. Each starts dinner with a glass of red wine at 6 p.m. local time, a second glass at 8 p.m., a beer for breakfast at 8 a.m., and so on. Their blood alcohol signals will not be synchronous because of the time difference between their homes; however, we expect their blood signals to be coherent at a frequency equal to 1/24th of an hour or approximately 10^{-5} Hz. The importance of local influences may be estimated with *coherence*, a statistical measure of the phase consistency between signal pairs. Coherence is a correlation coefficient (squared) expressed as a function of frequency. Generally, any signal may be synchronous or coherent in one frequency band while, at the same time, asynchronous or incoherent in other bands. All perfectly synchronous signals are coherent (coherence equal to one), but the reverse need not be true as in the blood of Jean and Jacques. In Chapters 6 and 7, I conjecture that such multiband coherence patterns may allow for cooperative behavior of distinct neural networks and more unified consciousness. That is, any pair of networks may be coupled in one sense (one frequency band) and, at the same time, operate as isolated networks in another band, an idea addressing the so-called *binding problem* of brain science.

4. EEG PATTERNS IN TIME

Suppose you and a friend recruit me to serve as your experimental subject. Your friend attaches a pair of electrodes to my scalp, a simple and painless procedure. My EEG is recorded overnight while I lie in a comfortable bed. EEG is transmitted to an isolated location with a computer screen showing both my ongoing brain oscillations and a record of my conscious state. Even though you may be unfamiliar with EEG, its general relationship to my mental state will become quite apparent. During *deep sleep* my EEG has larger amplitudes and contains much more low-frequency content. During REM sleep, when my eyelids reveal rapid eye movements associated with dreaming, my EEG contains more fast-frequency content. When I am awake and relaxed with closed eyes, oscillations repeating about 10 times per second (10 Hz) are evident. More sophisticated monitoring allows for identification of distinct *sleep stages, depth of anesthesia, seizures,* and other *neurological disorders.* Other methods reveal EEG correlations with cognitive tasks like *mental calculations, working memory,* and *selective attention.* Of course, EEG will not tell you what I am thinking or if my dream is erotic or simply exotic.

Scientists are now so accustomed to these EEG correlations with brain state that they sometimes forget just how remarkable they are. EEG provides very large-scale and robust measures of cortical dynamic function. A single electrode provides estimates of synaptic action averaged over tissue masses containing between roughly ten million and one billion neurons. The space averaging of brain potentials resulting from scalp recordings is unavoidable, forced by current spreading through the head (*volume conduction*). Much more detailed local information may be obtained from intracranial recordings in animals and epileptic patients, potentials recorded from the brain surface or within its depths. But, intracranial electrodes implanted in living brains provide only very sparse spatial coverage, thereby failing to record the "big picture" of brain function. Furthermore, the dynamic behavior of intracranial recordings is fractal-like, depending on the measurement scale determined mostly by electrode size. Different electrode sizes and locations result in substantial differences in recorded dynamic behavior, including frequency content and coherence. By contrast, EEG is essentially independent of electrode size because space averaging has already occurred when brain currents reach the scalp. Depending on scale, intracranial recordings can see the proverbial trees and bushes, and maybe even some of the ants on branches. By contrast, EEG sees the whole forest, but misses most of the detail. As in all of science, measurement scale is a critical issue. Studying this book with a microscope may cause you to miss the large-scale information content of its words. *Intracranial data provide different information, not more information, than is obtained from the scalp.*

5. EEG ANIMALS IN THE RHYTHMIC ZOO

Two famous early EEG pioneers are neuroscientist Herbert Jasper and his colleague neurosurgeon Wilder Penfield, well known for his electrical stimulation of cortical tissue, a procedure that sometimes evoked past memories in his epileptic patients. Cortical stimulation of conscious patients is needed even today to identify critical *network hubs* like speech centers to be spared from the surgeon's knife. The brain has no pain receptors, so this procedure is carried out in awake patients under a local anesthetic. Numerous EEG (scalp) and ECoG (cortical surface) recordings of epilepsy surgery patients were obtained by Jasper and Penfield in the 1940s and 50s. This work is summarized in their classic work *Epilepsy and the Functional Anatomy of the Human Brain*[4]. Several scalp-recorded normal rhythms from this text are shown in Figure 5–4. Note the changes of vertical scale; bars at the right of each waveform indicate 50 μV (microvolt) amplitudes. The resting alpha rhythm (labeled "relaxed") occurs mainly with closed eyes and has typical amplitudes of about 40 μV, whereas deep sleep and coma may exceed 200 μV.

The labels "drowsy," asleep, and deep sleep are now called stages 1, 2, and 3 or 4 sleep, respectively. Not shown is REM (rapid eye movement) sleep indicating dreaming, a state containing substantial high-frequency content similar to the "excited" trace. Erections of the penis and clitoris typically occur in normal REM sleep (even with non erotic dreams) along with greatly reduced muscle tone over the entire body, the latter usually preventing sleepwalking and other activities. We can dream away, but not much physical action is likely to come of it. Each of us has perhaps four or five periods of REM sleep per night, 1 or 2 hours in total, but most dreams are not remembered in the morning. What good are dreams? Nobody is really sure.

The example labeled "excited" could have occurred in any of several behavioral conditions, including performance of complicated mental tasks. The transition down the page from the more alert and aware states to progressively deeper states of unconsciousness occurs with generally lower frequency content and larger amplitudes. This general rule has held up quite well in modern studies, although partial exceptions occur. Two such cases are *alpha coma* and *halothane anesthesia*, in both cases very large amplitude, perhaps 100 to 200

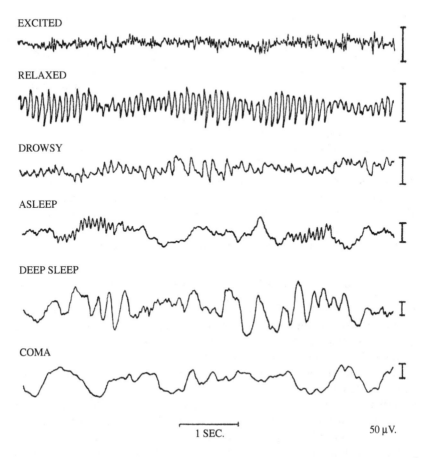

EXCITED

RELAXED

DROWSY

ASLEEP

DEEP SLEEP

COMA

1 SEC.   50 μV.

Figure 5–4   Several examples of normal scalp-recorded EEG in different brain states.[4]

microvolts (μV), alpha rhythms occur over the entire scalp. With halothane, the brain may be "tuned" to any dominant frequency between about 4 and 16 Hz by increasing blood concentration of halothane (depth of anesthesia). Deeper halothane anesthesia again results in larger amplitudes and lower frequencies. Halothane rhythms may be the best candidates for nearly pure standing waves, with minimal distortion from local networks. Other anesthetics have their own characteristic EEG signatures, typically similar to the deep sleep or coma traces.

Penfield and Jasper's extensive cortical recordings indicate that ECoG dynamic behavior between cortical areas largely disappears during anesthesia. That is, transitions from normal waking to anesthesia states appear to correspond to transitions from more local to more global dynamic states. A large variety of EEG behavior may be observed depending on depth and type of anesthesia as well as type of coma. These include sinusoidal oscillations and complex waveforms (combinations of frequencies) in the delta, theta, alpha, and beta bands. As a *general rule of head*, lower frequency oscillations tend to occur with larger amplitudes in a wide range of brain states. *Local differences in waveforms tend to disappear with deeper anesthesia, indicating transitions from more local (functionally segregated) to more global dynamic behavior.* This observation fits nicely within our conceptual framework of cognitive networks embedded in global fields, which tend to be more evident when mental processing is minimal.

The EEG traces shown in Figure 5–4 indicate only part of a much larger "zoo" of EEG rhythms, some having no known clinical correlates. Many abnormal rhythms have been recorded from the cortex and scalps of epileptic patients. These include unusually large rhythms in the delta, theta, alpha, beta, and gamma bands. A 14 Hz rhythm normally occurs during REM sleep; a regular 3 Hz rhythm might occur in epilepsy or in certain comas. A classical epilepsy signature is the 3 Hz *spike and wave*, which often occurs globally over the entire scalp, a (nonlinear) standing wave candidate. Global spike and wave traces typically occur during non convulsive absence seizures in which awareness is lost for seconds or minutes.

6. CLINICAL AND COGNITIVE APPLICATIONS OF EEG

EEG in patients is typically recorded by technicians directed by neurologists with advanced training in electroencephalography, thereby providing neurologists and neurosurgeons with an important clinical tool to follow and treat illnesses. Brain tumors, strokes, epilepsies, infectious diseases, mental retardation, severe head injury, drug overdose, sleep problems, metabolic disorders, and ultimately brain death are some of the conditions that may show up as abnormal EEG. EEG also provides measures of depth of anesthesia and severity of coma. Evoked and event-related potentials, which occur in response to an auditory or visual stimulus like a light flash or flicker, are used in the diagnosis and treatment of central nervous system diseases as well as illuminating cognitive processes. But EEG abnormalities are often nonspecific, perhaps only confirming diagnoses obtained with independent clinical tests.

A summary of clinical and research EEG is provided by Figure 5–5. Arrows indicate common relations between subfields. Numbered superscripts in the boxes indicate the following: (1) Physiologists record electric potentials (*local field potentials*) from inside animal skulls using electrodes with diameters typically ranging from about 0.01 to 1 millimeter. Dynamic behavior recorded in these studies generally depends on location and measurement scale, determined mostly by electrode size for intracranial recordings. Scalp-recorded EEG dynamics is exclusively large scale and independent of electrode size. (2) Human spontaneous EEG occurs in the absence of specific sensory stimuli but may be easily altered by such stimuli. (3) Averaged (transient) *evoked potentials* (EPs) are associated with sensory stimuli like repeated light flashes, auditory tones, finger pressure, or mild electric shocks. EPs are typically recorded by time averaging of single-stimulus waveforms to remove the spontaneous EEG. Cortical evoked potentials occur roughly 10 to 300 milliseconds after the stimulus. (4) *Event-related potentials* (ERPs) are recorded in the same

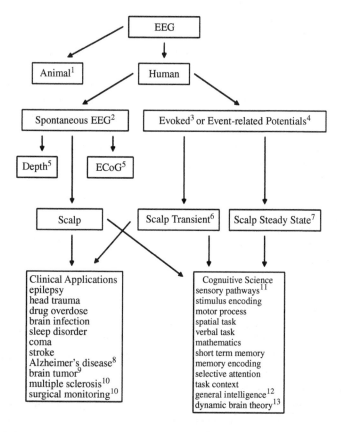

Figure 5–5   An overview of EEG applications; numbers refer to application discussed in the text.[2]

way as EPs, but normally occur after longer delays from stimuli (perhaps 200 to 500 milliseconds) and are more associated with the subject's mental condition (*endogenous brain state*). *(5)* Because of ethical considerations, EEG recorded in brain depth or on the brain surface (ECoG) of humans is limited to patients, often candidates for epilepsy surgery. *(6)* With transient EPs or ERPs, the stimuli consist of repeated short stimuli, usually light flashes or auditory tones. The number of stimuli may be anything between about ten and several thousand; the response to each stimulus is averaged over the individual pulses. The EP or ERP in any experiment consists of a waveform containing a series of characteristic peaks (local maxima or minima), occurring less than 0.5 seconds after presentation of each stimulus. The amplitude, latency from the stimulus, or covariance (a time delayed correlation measure obtained with multiple electrode sites) of each component may be studied in connection with a cognitive task (ERP) or with no task (EP). *(7)* Steady-state visually evoked potentials (SSVEP) use a continuous flickering light superimposed in front of a computer monitor providing a cognitive task like mental rotation of a three-dimensional figure or recognizing special patterns on the screen. The brain response in a narrow-frequency band containing the stimulus frequency is measured, and its magnitude, phase, and coherence (in the case of multiple electrode sites) related to different parts of the cognitive task. *(8)* Alzheimer's disease and other dementia typically cause substantial slowing of normal alpha rhythms. Thus far, however, traditional EEG has been of little use in the dementias because EEG changes are often evident only late in the illness when other clinical signs are obvious. *(9)* Cortical tumors that involve the white matter layer (just below cortex) cause substantial low-frequency (delta) activity over the hemisphere with the tumor. Use of EEG in tumor diagnosis has been mostly replaced by MRI, which reveals structural abnormalities in tissue. *(10)* Multiple sclerosis and surgical monitoring may employ evoked potentials. *(11)* Studies of sensory pathways involve very early components of evoked potentials (latency from stimuli less than roughly 10 milliseconds). *(12)* The study of *general intelligence* associated with IQ tests is controversial; however, many studies have reported significant correlations between scores on written tests and various EEG measures. *(13)* Both competing and complementary mathematical models of large-scale brain function are used to explain or predict observed properties of EEG in terms of basic physiology and anatomy. Any such models must represent a vast oversimplification of genuine brain function; however, they contribute to our conceptual framework and guide the design of new experiments to test this framework.

EEG has not yet proven to be clinically useful in the following diseases or trauma: mild or moderate closed head injury, learning disabilities, attention disorders, schizophrenia, depression, and Alzheimer's disease. Given the crude methods of data analysis of most clinical settings, we simply do not now know if these brain abnormalities produce EEGs containing clinically useful information. There is some reason to be optimistic about future clinical developments because quantitative methods to recognize spatial-temporal EEG patterns have been studied only sporadically. For example, coherence and other measures related to phase synchronization, which estimate the amount of functional isolation (segregation) versus integration between brain regions, are rarely applied in clinical settings. Perhaps this will change before too long.

7. EEG SOURCES AND SYNAPTIC ACTION FIELDS

The cortical sources of EEG are conveniently pictured in terms of *synaptic action fields*, the numbers of active excitatory and inhibitory synapses per unit volume of tissue (or unit surface area of cortex), independent of their possible participation in neural networks. A minicolumn of cortex contains about a hundred pyramidal cells and a million synapses, with perhaps six excitatory synapses for each inhibitory synapse. If we assume that 10% of all synapses are active at some given time, the excitatory and inhibitory synaptic action densities are about 80,000 and 14,000 per area of minicolumn, respectively. The number densities of active excitatory and inhibitory synapses, expressed as functions of time and cortical location, are assigned the symbols $\Psi_e(\mathbf{r}, t)$ and $\Psi_i(\mathbf{r}, t)$, respectively; these are *field variables*. I caution readers about my use of the word "field," sometimes confusing to biological scientists. A field is just a mathematical function (usually continuous or "smooth") representing some real quantity: pressure (sound wave), human population density (perhaps shown on a world map), and so forth. *The synaptic action fields are distinct from the electric and magnetic fields that they generate.* The synaptic field description is simply an efficient way of picturing established phenomena, for example, in the case of coherent synaptic activity in a tissue mass acting "top-down" on a neural network.

Each active inhibitory synapse produces a local current *source* at a membrane surface plus additional membrane *sinks* (negative sources) required by current conservation. Each active excitatory synapse produces a local negative source (sink) plus distributed membrane sources in a similar manner. The magnitude of electric potential at the local scalp generated by a cortical column depends mainly on the distribution of synaptic and return sources over its depth and the *synchrony* of synaptic activation. As a general "rule of head," about 6 cm^2 of cortical gyri tissue, containing about six hundred thousand minicolumns or sixty million neurons forming an extended sheet of cortical sources (*dipole layer*), must be synchronously active to produce recordable scalp potentials without averaging.

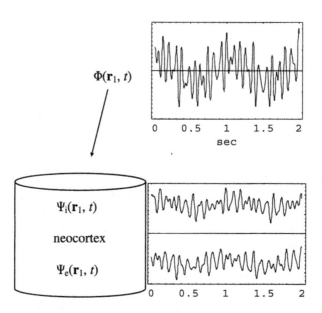

Figure 5–6   Simulated oscillations of excitatory and inhibitory synaptic action potential fields $\Psi_e(\mathbf{r}_1, t)$ and $\Psi_i(\mathbf{r}_1, t)$ at different cortical depths yielding cortical surface potential $\Phi(\mathbf{r}_1, t)^2$.

EEG is believed to be due to the modulation of synaptic action fields about background levels. To use a simple example, consider a simplified cortical model in which superficial and deep cortical layers are dominated by inhibitory $\Psi_i(\mathbf{r}, t)$ and excitatory $\Psi_e(\mathbf{r}, t)$ synaptic action, respectively, consistent with superficial current sources and deep current sinks. A short-time modulation of the synaptic action fields around background levels at horizontal cortical location $\mathbf{r}_1$ is simulated in Figure 5–6. The symbol $\Phi(\mathbf{r}_1, t)$ refers to an intermediate scale (*mesoscopic*) potential generated by the synaptic action fields in the local column. The parallel alignment of cortical pyramidal cells is an important feature, both for formation of columnar structure and for facilitating relatively large potentials from coordinated synaptic action within the columns. Observed scalp potentials are due to contributions from many such cortical columns.

8. SPATIAL PATTERNS AND HIGH-RESOLUTION EEG

The critical importance of measurement scale in electrophysiology can be emphasized by reference to a sociological metaphor. Data representing averages over large metropolitan areas will generally differ from data collected at the city, neighborhood, family, and person scales. Similarly, we expect brain electrical dynamics to vary substantially across spatial scales. Unprocessed EEG signals provide estimates of cortical signals space averaged over something like 30 to 100 square centimeters of (smooth) cortical surface because of two effects—current spreading due to the physical separation between cortical sources and scalp electrodes and the high electrical resistance of the skull. Each scalp electrode records the activity in a tissue mass containing perhaps 50 million to 1 billion neurons with an average of more than 10,000 local synaptic sources located on each neuron. The (millisecond) temporal resolution of EEG is excellent, but its spatial resolution is quite coarse.

Any spatial pattern may be decomposed into its spatial-frequency components, transformations analogous to spectral analysis of time-domain patterns of a single EEG data channel. The main difference is that spatial maps are composed of two sets of spatial frequencies, one for each direction on a two-dimensional surface. Decomposition of the scalp map into its spatial frequencies (essentially by Fourier transform in two surface dimensions) reveals that the major contributors to the scalp map have low spatial frequencies. In other words, the higher spatial frequencies present in the cortical map have been filtered out between cortex and scalp by the natural, passive tissue smearing-out process (*volume conduction*) of cortical currents and potentials.

In the practice of EEG, we would like to estimate the cortical map using our only available data, the scalp map, but we cannot put back information that has been removed by volume conduction. What we can do, however, is to selectively filter out low spatial frequencies in our scalp map in a manner that approximates the relative contributions of different spatial frequency components in the cortical map, provided our head model is sufficiently accurate. High-resolution

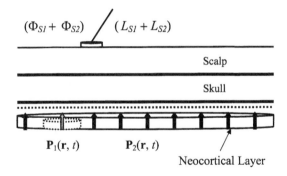

Figure 5–7   Two overlapping cortical source regions (dipole layers) are represented by the source vectors $\mathbf{P}_1$ and $\mathbf{P}_2$ that generate both low- (Φ) and high- (L) resolution scalp signals.[2]

EEG is based on this idea. Dense electrode arrays and computer algorithms are used to "project" scalp potentials to the cortical surface, allowing estimation of source activity in roughly 4 to 10 square centimeter patches of cortex. A major shortcoming of this procedure is that it necessarily underestimates the possible presence of genuine low spatial frequencies in the cortical map. In summary, we filter out low spatial frequencies in the scalp map, but we cannot distinguish low spatial frequency dominance (at the scalp) due only to volume conduction from genuine low spatial frequency cortical source activity.

Scalp data may be studied at two (mostly) distinct spatial scales, but both scales are much larger than the scales of intracranial recordings. Figure 5–7 represents two overlapping cortical source regions (*dipole layers*), labeled $\mathbf{P}_1(\mathbf{r}, t)$ and $\mathbf{P}_2(\mathbf{r}, t)$, the millimeter-scale (*mesoscopic*) source functions (*dipole moments per unit volume*). This idealized picture of cortical sources treats only sources in the cortical gyri (smooth cortex); sources in cortical folds generally make much smaller contributions to scalp potentials and don't change our general picture. Cortical source regions are assumed here to be internally synchronous in some frequency band of interest throughout each region (layer), but asynchronous between different regions (otherwise the small layer would simply be part of the large layer). Scalp potentials generated by both source regions are simply the sum of the separate contributions from each region, $\Phi_S = \Phi_{S1} + \Phi_{S2}$. Similarly, high-resolution estimates at the same scalp location yield $L_S = L_{S1} + L_{S2}$, where L stands for *Laplacian*, one of several approaches to high-resolution EEG. All other effects being equal, the larger source region contributes more to the unprocessed potential Φ_S, whereas the smaller region contributes more to L_S.

The selective sensitivity of conventional (unprocessed) and high-resolution measures is demonstrated in Figure 5–8 where the whole head has been approximated by a model consisting of concentric spherical shells. The horizontal axis indicates the radii of "circular" dipole layers, forming spherical

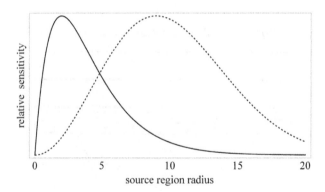

Figure 5–8   The selective sensitivity of scalp potential (dashed line) and high-resolution (solid line) measures as a function of the radii (cm) of circular source regions.[2]

caps analogous to the region between the North Pole (90° N) and, let's say, latitude 60° N. The vertical axis represents relative sensitivity as a function of dipole layer size; absolute sensitivity depends on other properties of the volume conductor. These plots show why high-resolution methods are more sensitive to the small source region in Figure 5–7, which might represent a local cortical network or part of a thalamocortical network. Such network (cell assembly) is said to be *embedded* in the large region. By contrast, unprocessed EEG is more sensitive to the large source region. Since these source regions are, by definition, internally synchronous at some frequency f_1, they can be considered distinct at f_1, but at the same time, just separate parts of the same source region at a different frequency f_2.

9. HUMAN ALPHA RHYTHMS

The so-called "alpha rhythm" is an important human EEG category that actually embodies several distinct kinds of alpha rhythms, usually identified as near-sinusoidal oscillations at frequencies near 10 Hz. Alpha rhythm in an awake and relaxed human subject is illustrated by the temporal plots and corresponding frequency spectrum in Figure 4–1. Alpha rhythm amplitudes are typically somewhat larger near the back of the brain (*occipital cortex*) and smaller over frontal regions, depending partly on the subject's state of relaxation.

Other alpha rhythms occur in other brain states, for example in *alpha coma* or in patients under halothane anesthesia; in these cases, large amplitude frontal alpha rhythms occur. In addition to alpha rhythms, a wide variety of human EEG activity has been recorded, a proverbial zoo of dynamic signatures, each waveform dependent in its own way on time and scalp location. Normal resting alpha rhythms may be substantially reduced in amplitude by eye opening, drowsiness, and by mental tasks. Alpha rhythms, like most EEG phenomena, typically exhibit an inverse relationship between amplitude and frequency. Hyperventilation and some drugs (alcohol) may cause lowering of alpha frequencies and increased amplitudes. Other drugs (barbiturates) are associated with increased amplitude of low-amplitude beta activity typically superimposed on alpha rhythms. The physiological bases for the inverse relation between amplitude and frequency and most other properties of EEG are unknown, although physiologically based dynamic theories have provided several tentative explanations, as outlined in the Endnotes and Chapter 7.

Alpha rhythms provide an appropriate starting point for clinical EEG exams. Some clinical questions are: Does the patient show an alpha rhythm with eyes closed, especially over posterior scalp? Are its spatial-temporal characteristics appropriate for the patient's age? How does it react to eyes opening, hyperventilation, drowsiness, and so forth? Pathology is often associated with pronounced differences recorded over opposite (*contralateral*) hemispheres or with very low alpha frequencies. A resting alpha frequency lower than about 8 Hz in adults is considered abnormal in all but the very old. Human alpha rhythms are part of a complex process apparently involving both local networks and global fields.

My studies of alpha rhythm span more than 37 years and continue in collaboration with my former student Ramesh Srinivasan at his lab at UC Irvine; he now does all the hard work and I claim part of the credit. In a typical study, Kim, a psychology student, has agreed to come to the lab and serve as a research subject. She takes a seat in a comfortable chair. We place a net containing 128 sensor pads on Kim's head and ask her to close her eyes and relax. The surface dots in Figure 5–9 show sensor locations on her scalp, and the black dots indicate nine locations along the midline of her scalp where we display 2 seconds of her alpha rhythm. We note several classic features of Kim's

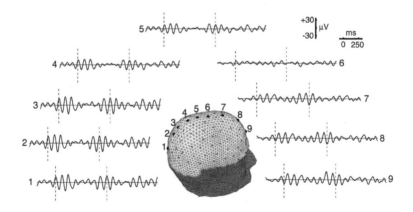

Figure 5–9   Nine electrode sites (out of 111) of alpha EEG recorded in a resting subject with closed eyes.[2] The front and back signals are 180° out of phase as indicated by the time slice (dashed lines), suggesting a standing wave.

rhythms. They exhibit amplitude variations over the 2-second period (waxing and waning) but are essentially oscillation with frequencies near 10 Hz. This alpha rhythm is evident at all midline sensor locations and nearly all other sensor locations (not shown), suggesting that the alpha sources originate from widespread locations in the cerebral cortex. That is, this alpha rhythm appears from this view to be much more of a global than local phenomenon. The dashed vertical lines indicate fixed time slices in Figure 5–9, showing that waveforms in the front (7–9) and back (1–3) of the head tend to be 180° out of phase. Amplitudes are largest at these same locations and smaller in middle sites (4–6). The spatial distribution of alpha rhythm is approximately that of a standing wave with a node (point of zero amplitude) near the center of the array, with one-half of the wave appearing on the scalp and one-half postulated to occupy the underside (*mesial surface*) of cortex.[5]

This general picture of global cortical sources is, however, partly clouded by amplitude differences between waveforms recorded at different scalp locations. In order to shed more light on the origins of this alpha rhythm, we construct high-resolution estimates of this same EEG data. To accomplish this, we pass the recorded waveforms from all 111 chosen sensors (lower edge sites are excluded for technical reasons) to a computer algorithm that "knows" the physics of current spread through brain, skull, and scalp tissue. The computer algorithm filters out the very large-scale (low spatial frequency) scalp potentials, which consist of some (generally) unknown combination of passive current spread and genuine large-scale cortical source activity.

The high-resolution estimate obtained from the same (Figure 5–9) data set is shown in Figure 5–10. Notably, the largest high-resolution signals occur at middle sites 5 and 6 where the unprocessed potentials are smallest. The

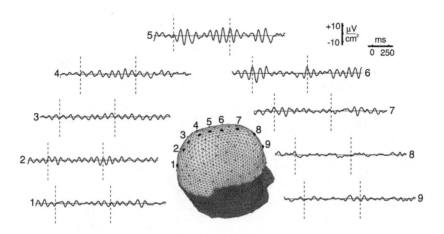

Figure 5–10   The same data shown in Figure 5–9 transformed to high-resolution EEG using all 111 data channels.[2] A local (non wave) patch of cortical source region near electrode site 5 is implied.

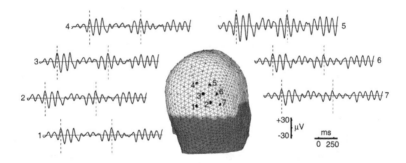

Figure 5–11   The same data shown in Figure 5–9 for electrode sites over occipital cortex.[2]

apparent explanation follows from Figures 5–7 and 5–8; high-resolution estimates are more sensitive to sources in smaller patches (dipole layers) of cortex. Kim's alpha rhythms apparently have multiple contributions, including a global standing wave and a local source region near the middle of the electrode array. This local oscillation, sometimes called the *mu rhythm*, may be blocked by movement because of its proximity to motor cortex. Other studies have shown that sources in local regions may oscillate at frequencies that differ slightly from global alpha oscillations, even though the local oscillations still occur within the alpha band (8–13 Hz).

Unprocessed EEG from the same 2-second period is shown at a group of seven occipital scalp sites in Figure 5–11, indicating in-phase potential oscillations over the entire occipital region, consistent with the standing wave interpretation. By contrast, the corresponding high-resolution estimate in Figure 5–12 suggests an additional (local) contribution from a source region near scalp site 5. Note that sites 4 and 5 are 180° (out of phase in the high-resolution estimate, further

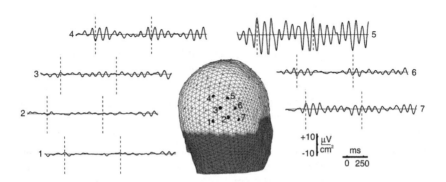

Figure 5–12   The same data transformed to high-resolution EEG using all 111 data channels[2]. Electrode site 5 makes a local contribution that adds to the global (apparent standing wave) contributions shown in Figure 5–11.

supporting the interpretation of site 5 as a local event. In Chapter 6, we will see that many such patches of local sources occur, oscillating both within and outside the alpha band. Our tentative interpretation is that these patches are parts of local networks (possibly including the thalamus) *embedded* in the global field, with the field contribution perhaps composed of standing waves.

10. SUMMARY

Brain imaging can be classified broadly in terms of spatial and temporal resolution. *Computed tomography (CT)* and *magnetic resonance imaging (MRI)* provide static high-resolution images of brain structure. *Functional magnetic resonance imaging (fMRI)* and *positron emission tomography (PET)* track brain changes with good spatial resolution over seconds or minutes. *Electroencephalography (EEG)* and *magnetoencephalography (MEG)* have coarse spatial resolution but operate on millisecond time scales, allowing observation of brain dynamics at the speed of thought. Tumors, strokes, epilepsies, infectious diseases, mental retardation, head injury, drug overdose, sleep problems, metabolic disorders, coma, and ultimately brain death may show up as abnormal EEG. Some EEG abnormalities are nonspecific, perhaps only confirming diagnoses obtained with independent clinical tests.

The frequency content of EEG has traditionally provided signatures of brain illnesses. EEG waveforms are labeled according to frequency band: *delta* (1–4 Hz), *theta* (4–8 Hz), *alpha* (8–13 Hz), *beta* (13–20 Hz), and *gamma* (greater than 20 Hz), but EEG is typically composed of mixed frequencies. The *fast Fourier transform* decomposes EEG records into composite frequency components. In multichannel EEG, the relative phases of signals provide important information in addition to frequency content. When two signals are lined up with zero phase offset, the signals are said to be *synchronous*. If two signals maintain a fixed phase relationship over a long time, the signals are said to be *coherent*. Functional relationships between source (or network) activity in different cortical locations are estimated with *coherence*, a statistical measure of the phase consistency between signals.

A wide range of human EEG activity may be recorded, a proverbial zoo of dynamic signatures, each waveform dependent in its own way on time and scalp location. Alpha rhythms provide a starting point for clinical exams. Like most EEG phenomena, they typically exhibit an inverse relationship between amplitude and frequency. Alpha rhythms are part of a complex process involving both local cortical source regions and global source fields, the latter may appear as standing waves. Raw (unprocessed) EEG and *high-resolution EEG* are selectively sensitive to different spatial scales of source regions, providing complementary measures of dynamic processes in the cortex. Oscillations in very large cortical regions (~100 cm^2) contribute more to raw EEG; smaller regions (~10 cm^2) are more likely to be picked up by high-resolution EEG. Local alpha sources are pictured as embedded in a global alpha field. In addition to their selective sensitivities to high- and low-resolution EEG, the two processes may be distinguished by small frequency differences, spatial distribution, phase relationship, or selective response to mental or physical actions[2].

Recordings from widespread cortical surface areas in many patients (most suffering from epilepsy) were carried out by EEG pioneers Herbert Jasper, Wilder Penfield, and Grey Walter in the 1945–1965 period. These early studies may enjoy important advantages over some modern studies, partly because the patient's natural rhythms may have been much less altered by anticonvulsant drugs. The early studies showed conclusively that human alpha rhythms occur over nearly the entire surface of accessible cortex. Furthermore, the alpha band was found to encompass multiple complex phenomena: Some rhythms were blocked by eye opening and some were not. Some responded in some fashion to mental activity and some did not.

The alpha rhythms recorded at the scalp with conventional (low-resolution) EEG represent only the subset of alpha phenomena that are synchronous over wide cortical areas. For example, an imagined scalp recording of the simulated source distribution in Figure 6–1 would show only a very smooth potential change from positive (bottom or occipital cortex) to negative (top or frontal cortex); the small-scale pattern details would be lost entirely between cortex and scalp. Embedded small-scale (< 1 or 2 cm diameter) alpha source regions cannot be observed directly in EEG scalp recordings. But with high-resolution EEG, we can now pick out distinct synchronous rhythms in cortical patches as small as 2–3 cm from the global rhythms. The combined high- and low-resolution methods described here, as well as many other modern studies,[2] essentially reconfirm much of the early pioneering work.

After about 1975 or 1980, for some reason that I cannot fully explain, parts of the EEG community developed a collective amnesia to the early cortical studies. Even today the EEG and MEG literature contains at lot of misinformation about the nature of alpha rhythm sources. One apparent origin of this misleading material is a persistent obsession with source localization: the idea that brain science should focus on finding a few isolated "equivalent sources" that are supposedly responsible for widely distributed complex phenomena. But Einstein's famous scientific advice suggests adoption of a more physiologically realistic conceptual framework, one that is *as simple as possible, but not simpler.*

Chapter 6

Dynamic Patterns as Shadows of Thought

1. DYNAMIC PATTERNS IN TIME AND SPACE

The EEG patterns discussed in Chapter 5 are characterized mainly by temporal frequency content—labeled delta, theta, alpha, beta, or gamma rhythms. More detailed descriptions employ picturesque descriptions like *spike and wave, sharp wave*, and so forth, or more nuanced frequency content using spectral analysis. The first 50 years or so of EEG focused mainly on temporal patterns. Some early success was achieved in finding approximate locations of cortical tumors and epileptic foci, but typically spatial analysis was limited to categorizing sources as either isolated (local or *focal*, as in focal seizures) or widely distributed. Early analysis of source locations or source distributions were severely impeded by practical limitations including sparse (electrode) sampling of scalp sites and primitive computational options.

EEG spatial properties are evidently just as important as its temporal properties. Modern systems typically record potentials at 64 to 130 or more electrode sites, with (center-to-center) electrode spacing in the 2 to 3 cm range. Computer algorithms estimate brain source locations in the few special applications where the sources of interest are actually confined to relatively "small" tissue volumes (say 5 to 10 cm^3). In the much more common occurrence of widely distributed sources, high-resolution EEG algorithms project scalp potentials to the cortical surface based on mathematical models of current spreading in tissue (*volume conduction*) as discussed in Chapter 5. These computer methods yield dynamic maps of cortical potential distributions analogous to the ever changing weather patterns over the earth.

We are not so concerned here with *spatial AND temporal patterns*, but rather with *spatial-temporal patterns*, emphasizing that spatial and temporal properties of cerebral cortex are interrelated. Generally in complex systems, changes in temporal patterns are expected to force changes in spatial patterns and vice versa. The spatial-temporal connection of dynamic properties occurs with simple wave phenomena and is also a hallmark of complex systems, including chaotic systems as will be demonstrated in Chapter 7 and the related Endnotes. Typically, we expect interplay between temporal patterns and spatial structures. Global dynamic patterns providing local influences (top-down) are routinely evidenced by the changing temperature and pressure maps as viewed on your TV weather channel; tornadoes provide a dramatic example of local events

111

produced largely by global dynamics. Since the brain is a complex system, we should anticipate analogous top-down global influences on local dynamics.

2. STATIC SPATIAL PATTERNS

We humans easily recognize simple spatial patterns like Zebra stripes, mountain ranges, and cloud formations, but our facility with complex patterns is mixed. Natural selection has endowed humans with exceptional skill in distinguishing human faces, but complex spatial patterns typically contain a wealth of information that is far too subtle for our limited brains. The raw data from an MRI or radar system constitute patterns that must be transformed by computer before we can make sense of them. The general area of *pattern recognition* aims to classify patterns based on prior knowledge of the system or, in the case of poorly understood systems, statistical information extracted from the patterns. Pattern recognition is used in computer science, psychology, and medicine, including computer-aided diagnosis.

A spatial pattern of cortical source activity is simulated in Figure 6–1, where the image symbolizes the area over a single cortical hemisphere (nose at the top). Real people are not blockheads, so the cortical surface is not really rectangular; the plot is idealized for simplicity. Each black and gray dot represents a snapshot (time slice) of positive and negative *source* activity, respectively, at the macrocolumn scale (~1 to 3 mm). Current passes from positive source regions into negative regions (*sinks*). Most current generated by these sources remains inside the skull, but just a little current enters the scalp where it is recorded as EEG. Each current source at the macrocolumn scale represents the net activity of between a hundred thousand and a million neurons, with an average of ten thousand or so synapses per neuron. In order to keep our discussion simple, only sources in smooth cortex (*gyri*) are considered here; if I were to include sources in cortical folds (*fissures* and *sulci*), the general argument would be largely unchanged.

Figure 6–1 represents a standing wave with embedded local source activity. The mostly positive and mostly negative source regions occur near the vertical coordinates 0 and 30, respectively. The long circumference of each hemisphere (including the underside of the brain) is about twice as long as shown in the image. This image represents one-half of a standing wave with a 60 cm wavelength, corresponding to oscillations of the fundamental mode in an idealized one-dimensional closed loop (see also Figure 7–5). In actual brains, such large patches of synchronous sources could be relatively pure standing waves or quasi-local activity influenced (top down) by global boundary conditions, that is, "quasi-standing" waves. Or, they could be something else altogether, maybe occurring with cortical source synchrony caused mainly by synchronous thalamic input (from the midbrain).

In practice, we never achieve information about cortical source distribution with detail that is anything close to the simulation shown in Figure 6–1. We have, however, many reasons to believe that this general picture is qualitatively

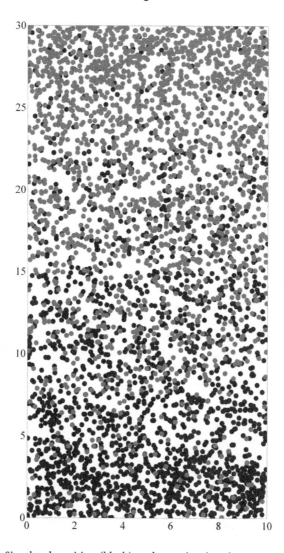

Figure 6–1   Simulated positive (black) and negative (gray) sources at the macro-column (3 mm) scale in a rectangular region (10 × 30 cm) representing the upper surface of one cortical hemisphere (nose at top). The pattern corresponds to a 60 cm long standing wave with embedded local random sources.[11]

correct. For example, ECoG (cortical) amplitudes are typically two to six times larger than the corresponding EEG (scalp). If cortex produced only small synchronous source patches, this ratio of cortical to scalp potentials magnitudes would be closer to 100. Recordable scalp potential require clumps or patches of (partly) synchronous sources with cortical areas of about 6 to 100 cm^2 or more, depending on the actual amount of synchrony within the patches.

3. ALPHA WAVE TOPOGRAPHY

A typical snapshot of alpha rhythm topography at the scalp, obtained with 2 cm electrode spacing, is shown in Figure 6–2, indicating maximum positive potential near the back of the head and maximum negative potential near the front. While this potential distribution (over both hemispheres) is similar to the standing wave source distribution of Figure 6–1, we must be cautious about such interpretation. *Scalp potential maps* are necessarily blurred representations of cortical potential due to volume conduction. In other words, the passage of cortical currents through skull and scalp tissue and the spatial separation of electrodes from brain sources act to filter out high spatial frequencies. Consider this analogy: Get too far away from a rough surface, and it will appear smooth because you don't see the high spatial frequencies. This lost spatial information cannot be restored; however, we can employ computers to remove low spatial frequencies from scalp maps to obtain high-resolution estimates of cortical potential. That is, we remove both the erroneous low spatial frequencies due only to volume conduction and the genuine low spatial frequencies in the original cortical map. Unfortunately, we cannot distinguish between these two contributors to the scalp map.

The high-resolution estimate of the same snapshot of alpha rhythm is shown in Figure 6–3, indicating a complex pattern of alternating positive and negative source regions. High-resolution EEG represents high-pass (spatially) filtered

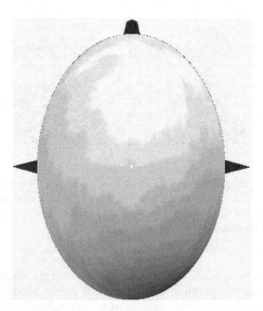

Figure 6–2   Typical instantaneous potential map of alpha rhythm generated by interpolation of data from 128 electrode sites.[1] The front and back of the head are roughly 180° out of phase.

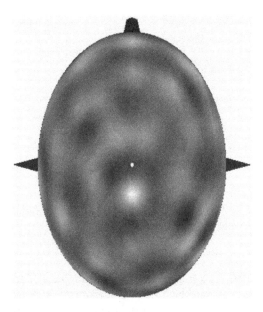

Figure 6–3   The same data shown in Figure 6–2 transformed to high-resolution EEG by high-pass spatial filtering.[1] The long wavelength part of the signal, due to both volume conduction and genuine cortical source distribution, is removed leaving only smaller scale features.

versions of scalp maps, but band pass estimates of the cortical maps. That is, the high spatial frequencies in cortical maps (ECoG) are irretrievably lost between cortex and scalp; the high-resolution computer algorithm then removes the very low spatial frequencies from scalp potential maps. The remaining high-resolution map consists only of the intermediate spatial frequencies in the original cortical map. The two filtering stages, first by natural tissue volume conduction and second by a high-resolution computer algorithm, are depicted in Figure 6–4.

Since high spatial frequencies in the cortical map are forever lost and cannot be restored, Figure 6–3 can only show details of the alpha rhythm map at the scale of several centimeters; this lower scale is limited by the physical separation (~1 cm) between cortex and scalp and the high electrical resistance of the skull. Were we actually able to view progressively smaller scales, fractal-like cortical potential maps like Figure 6–1 would be expected, with finer and finer detail discovered down to sub millimeter scales. The closer we look, the more detail we would expect to see.

Figures 6–2 and 6–3 provide two distinct estimates of the actual cortical source distribution of the alpha rhythm that are complementary, but far from complete because they omit smaller scale details. The high-resolution map of Figure 6–3 might indicate standing waves with spatial frequencies higher than

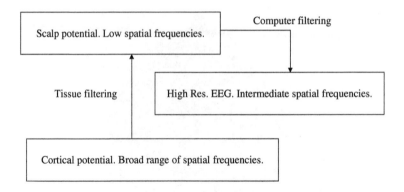

Figure 6–4   Summary of two-step spatial filtering: (natural) tissue filtering followed by the computer filtering of high-resolution EEG.

the fundamental (the wave overtones), or it may be evidence of underlying networks. My guess is that these maps show some combination of these two processes, raising the conjecture that the *spatial patterns formed by neural networks are influenced (top down) by the global boundary conditions*. Some of the general reasons leading to this conjecture will be discussed in Chapter 7 and a related discussion in the Endnotes on the influence of boundary conditions on chaos in complex systems.

EEG scientists have often focused on the amplitude distribution of potential, the so-called scalp potential map. This straightforward strategy makes good sense when brain sources are actually located in small areas; the obvious goal is then simply to find source locations. Some even seem to believe that brain source localization *is* brain science, a frequent source of frustration for me over the past 30 years or so. The overwhelming body of evidence suggests that cognitive processing involves widely distributed source constellations, forming cell assemblies (neural networks) that form and dissolve on 100 millisecond or so time scales. Thinking brains have associated sources that can be anywhere and everywhere; source localization is largely irrelevant in these cases. We should be most interested in finding relationships between the dynamic patterns revealed with EEG (and other measures) and behavioral or cognitive brain states, thereby decoding some of the brain's challenging language. Neuroscientist Sir Charles Sherrington made the case early in the 20th century with these famous poetic lines:

> It is as if the Milky Way entered upon some cosmic dance. Swiftly the brain becomes an enchanted loom where millions of flashing shuttles weave a dissolving pattern, always a meaningful pattern though never an abiding one, a shifting harmony of sub patterns.

A central question to be posed about any dynamic system is this: Is it composed of multiple subsystems with minimal communication, dominated by *functional isolation*? Or, is it more *globally coherent*, with all parts of the system acting in a similar manner? In some studies, the local (isolated) end of this range of dynamic behavior seems to occur with more substantial mental processing, the global end occurring more in states of anesthesia and global seizures. In other studies, mental processing seems to occur with enhanced global coherence, but only in selective, narrow frequency bands. This apparent paradox may be at least partly resolved by noting that dynamic processes can be coherent in one frequency band, and at the same time, incoherent in another band. Furthermore, I have greatly oversimplified this description of very complex processes in which large (regional) networks and genuine global dynamic behavior (including standing waves) are, in actual practice, not easily distinguished with EEG. One hallmark of complex systems is their ability to perform their dynamic dances near either end of the extremes of functional isolation (localization) or global coherence and most everything in between. It is suggested in this chapter that mental illness may owe at least part of its origins to lack of an appropriate local/global balance. For these reasons, a number of neuroscientists (including me) now focus on *dynamic correlations* between cortical sites, estimated with the measures *coherence* and *covariance*, as discussed in the following sections.

4. MOSES DELIVERS HIS MAGIC TABLET

In order to add to our sophistication with complex dynamic patterns, I adopt a little fable of a magic tablet, serving as a metaphor in our quest to read the *language of the brain* from potential maps. A mysterious fellow calling himself Moses and claiming to be from the distant planet Sinai appears suddenly on CNN. He provides Earth with a magic tablet that can provide information to cure human diseases, if only we can learn to read the tablet's responses to our questions. Moses then vanishes in a puff of smoke. The tablet's surface contains a 5×5 matrix of flickering lights, as shown in Figure 6–5. Moses' celebrated appearance leads to an eruption of talk show babble, readings by astrologers, predictions of the apocalypse, and mountaintop sermons. Universities rush to offer new PhD programs in *tablet science*; worldwide scientific efforts are focused on the tablet's dynamic patterns.

When the magic tablet is presented with unequivocal yes/no questions, it is soon discovered that higher flicker frequencies at matrix sites seem to code mostly as yes answers, but deciphering more subtle aspects of the tablet's language proves far more challenging. Spectral analysis reveals that flickering light patterns typically oscillate with multiple mixed frequencies, which may or may not be constant across the tablet's matrix. Most questions result in responses in the guise of complex patterns. The filled circles in Figure 6–5 might indicate different local flicker amplitudes, frequencies, phases, or any combination of these features. Any pair of matrix sites may produce oscillations that are synchronous at, let's say, 9 Hz, but at the same time, asynchronous at 5 Hz. Much early emphasis is placed on simple amplitude patterns, but this focus

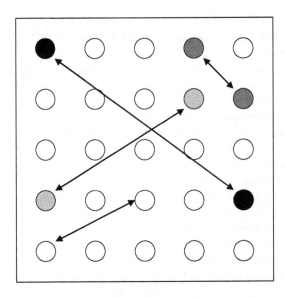

Figure 6–5   The magic tablet serves as a crude cortical analog with its flashing lights
producing many kinds of spatial-temporal patterns, including correlations (coherence or
covariance) between sites indicated by the arrows.

yields very limited success in decoding tablet language. The tablet is much more
complex than first assumed; scientists become painfully aware of *the fallacy of
the easy first step.*

The complexity of the magic tablet opens the door for many plausible
sounding, but ultimately false, claims. Some imagine coded patterns where
none exist, guided by good intentions but *fooled by randomness.* Others
obtain valid information, but vastly oversimplify these data, following unpro-
ductive scientific trails based on preconceived theories of how the tablet *should*
work according to the esteemed holders of PhDs in tablet science. Funding
agencies and private investors have trouble sorting the good science from the
bad; the reputation of tablet science is compromised and funding sources dry
up. False prophets spread rumors of new tablets operating with simpler languages and the promise of easy decoding.

Despite these obstacles to progress, some promising tablet information is
obtained from measures of *correlation* between matrix sites. These dynamic
correlation measures (*covariance* and *coherence*) reveal functional connections.
Covariance or coherence express correlations in terms of time lag or frequency
band, respectively. The 25 matrix sites have (25 × 24/2) or 300 paired coherence values for each frequency in the flickering lights. In Figure 6–5, dynamically correlated sites in one frequency band are indicated by arrows, a pattern
that is generally different for other frequency bands. Some coherence values
increase while others decrease in response to questions, but what do these

coherence patterns really mean? Many years after Moses' visit, the tablet's language remains largely undeciphered.

What does my little fable have to do with genuine EEG science? The magic tablet's matrix sites correspond to scalp electrode locations, but because of the poor spatial resolution of unprocessed EEG signals, the number of effective sites can be no more than about 20, similar to the spatial resolution of the tablet. By contrast, high-resolution EEG allows for sampling of 100 or more sites, yielding ($100 \times 99/2$) or 4,950 or more paired coherence values for each frequency band.

In 1998-2000, I enjoyed a fantastic sabbatical experience at the Brain Sciences Institute in Melbourne, Australia, participating in an experimental program with my graduate student Brett Wingeier and the institute director, Richard Silberstein. One of our goals was to see how coherence patterns change when subjects perform mental tasks like mental rotation of 3D objects, matching spatial patterns, or performing calculations. In one simple study, the subjects started with a small number and progressively added the numbers 1, 2, 3, and so on to the running total, for example, 7,8,10,13,17,22, ... up to sums of several hundred in each of a sequence of 1-minute periods, alternating with resting periods.[1] We then compared coherence patterns based on 10 periods alternating between resting and calculating states. Typically, coherence consistently increased between many scalp sites in the theta (4–7 Hz) and upper alpha (10–13 Hz) bands during calculation periods, while decreasing in the lower alpha band (8–9 Hz). These data are consistent with the recruitment of overlapping cortical "calculation" networks operating in select frequency bands, together with a reduction in standing wave activity near 8–9 Hz.

How can a pair of cortical locations be strongly correlated at one frequency (high coherence) and, at the same time, uncorrelated at another frequency (low coherence)? To provide some idea of why this kind of dynamic behavior might occur in an arbitrary complex system, I again recruit the famous twins Jean and Jacques from Chapter 5. Every drink consumed by Jacques is matched by Jean in his daily routine; their blood alcohol signals are highly coherent at the frequency of once per day or about 0.000011 Hz. In Paris, Jacques limits his intake to this daily routine. But, Jean lives in New Orleans and makes weekly visits to his favorite bar on Bourbon Street, consuming prodigious quantities of alcohol in addition to his normal daily intake. Jean's blood alcohol signal peaks at a frequency of once per week or about 0.0000017 Hz, but Jean and Jacques's signals are incoherent at this lower frequency. In other words, we infer from blood signals that Jean and Jacques' dynamic behavior is correlated at one frequency (once per day), but uncorrelated at a lower frequency (once per week). The coherence measure tells us of the existence of functional connections in dynamic systems but does not reveal their causes. Nevertheless, we can guess that high blood alcohol coherence at once per day is caused by similar daily routines.

5. SHADOWS OF THOUGHT

The strong experimental emphasis on EEG correlations between scalp sites originated with Mikhail Livanov, who in 1933, became head of the electrophysiology laboratory at The Institute of the Human Brain in Moscow.[2] While Livanov's pioneering work was limited by the technology available in his day, he reported many interesting spatial correlation patterns between scalp locations that could be attributed to cortical network formation during task performance. Depending on the specific experiment, his correlations were estimated in the time domain (covariance) or frequency domain (coherence).

The next actor in our story is Alan Gevins, a second generation pioneer investigating scalp correlations.[3] Alan became head of the EEG laboratory at the Langley Porter Neuropsychiatric Institute, a department of the University of California at San Francisco in 1974, and formed the *EEG Systems Lab* (now *The San Francisco Brain Research Institute*) as a nonprofit institute in 1980, independent of UCSF. He started *SAM Technology* in 1986 (named after Uncle Sam, his benefactor) in order to obtain small business federal grants to develop the EEG technology supporting his research. Alan and his colleagues focused on high-resolution estimates of *event related potentials*. One such experiment is depicted in Figure 6–6; the subject is given a cue (the first *event*) to prepare for an instruction coming one second later. The instruction is a number that informs the subject how hard to push a button. The accuracy of response is revealed to the subject by a computer monitor (the feedback *event*). Evoked scalp potentials are recorded over many sub second intervals, including: *(1)* the interval before the presentation of the number; and *(2)* the interval after the subject's accuracy is revealed.

Using high-resolution methods to minimize volume conduction effects, these experiments reveal characteristic patterns of *covariance*, essentially correlations between evoked potential waveforms as a function of time lag. To take an example from economics, increases in U.S. money supply may be uncorrelated with the official inflation rate in the same year, but correlated with inflation perhaps 3 years later; the economic variables then exhibit strong covariance after a 3-year delay. Alan's event-related covariances between posterior and frontal regions typically peak at 30 to 80 millisecond delays, reflecting processing times, including axonal delays, between cortical systems. Like the

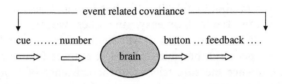

Figure 6–6   Summary of experimental set-up used by Alan Gevins to find event-related covariances in cerebral cortex.

coherence measure, covariance provides a measure of functional relations between cortical locations. Alan's covariance patterns in the preparation and feedback intervals suggest neural network (cell assembly) formations on sub second time scales.

Interestingly, covariance patterns in both recording periods depend on button push accuracy. Thus, the subject's performance accuracy can be predicted in a short period just before the button is pushed when brain *preparatory networks* evidently form. Figure 6–7 shows a covariance pattern formed in preparation for an accurate response with the right hand; lines between pairs of electrode sites indicate statistically significant covariances. Widely separated regions of both hemispheres are typically involved in the preparatory patterns. Alan tags his covariance patterns *shadows of thought*, with Plato's allegory of the cave in mind.

Alan has applied his sophisticated EEG systems to pharmacology by measuring the effects of drugs on mental task performance including functions like short-term memory. Drugs under study include caffeine, diphenhydramine (Benadryl—which produces drowsiness), alcohol, marijuana, and prescription medications used to treat a variety of neurological diseases such as epilepsy, sleep disorders, dementia, and ADHD (*attention deficit hyperactivity disorder*). Critical questions with drug treatments include: *How does a particular patient react to a particular drug, and what are the appropriate dosages?* The appropriate

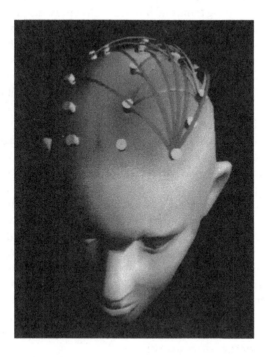

Figure 6–7   An Alan Gevins-recorded covariance pattern set up in preparation for an accurate response with the right hand.[3]

EEG tests can apparently provide immediate quantitative measures of drug effectiveness on individual patients; I have more to say about EEG applications in pharmacology in the following sections.

6. COHERENCE PATTERNS AND MENTAL TASKS

The next several sections are concerned with a branch of EEG called *steady-state visually evoked potentials* (SSVEP). The general goal remains one of finding correlations between potentials recorded at different scalp sites, but now the stimulus consists of a flickering light superimposed on a computer monitor displaying some visual task. The motivations behind this approach are both technical (increase of signal-to-noise ratio) and physiological (brains do special things in specific frequency bands). This technology was pioneered in the 1970s by Canadian scientist, David Regan.[4]

The next actor in our narrative is my colleague, Richard Silberstein, founder of the *Brain Sciences Institute* of Swinburne University in Melbourne, Australia. Richard was born in Poland during the Second World War, two years after his father and mother escaped from a cattle train headed to the Majdanek concentration camp, where the Nazis murdered tens of thousands of Polish Jews and captured Soviet soldiers. His father had miraculously discovered a hacksaw blade hidden in the train carriage. The prisoners sawed their way through the bars, jumped from the moving train, and hid with Polish peasants in the forest. One of the prisoners later became Richard's mother. Richard has advanced SSVEP methods substantially over the past 20 years by applying high-resolution and coherence measures in a number of clinical and cognitive studies including aging, ADHD, mood disorders, and drug addiction.[5]

Figure 6–8 shows one experimental set up in Richard's lab. Subjects were given a standard IQ test (*Wechler Adult Intelligence Scale-III*) and then fitted with goggles producing a flickering light. They were presented with a series of problems on a computer monitor; images were clearly visible through the flickering light. Each of the problems consisted of a matrix of shapes with one matrix location blank, another IQ-related test called *Raven's Progressive Matrices*. With each problem presentation, subjects were presented with six possible choices ("probes") for the empty matrix space; subjects responded with a "yes" or "no" using right- or left-hand button pushes. Processing speed (inverse of reaction time) was positively correlated with IQ score. A group of electrode sites in frontal and central regions exhibited large intersite coherences during the processing periods, peaking about 2 seconds after probe presentation. Subjects who responded more quickly to the probes were those who exhibited highest intersite coherences at the flicker frequency of 13 Hz. These findings again suggest formation of cortical networks associated with solving pattern recognition problems; the stronger the apparent binding of these networks (higher intersite coherences), the faster the correct answers were obtained.

The purpose of the flickering light in this and other SSVEP experiments is to eliminate scalp potentials not originating in the brain, that is, to increase

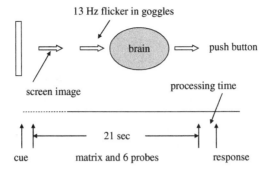

Figure 6–8 Summary of experimental set-up used by Richard Silberstein to find coherence patterns in cerebral cortex while the subject performs a mental task.

signal-to-noise ratio. EEG studies in cognitive science have long been plagued by *artifact,* scalp potentials due to muscles, eye movements, EKG, and so forth. Many EEG experiments, especially those involving high-frequency (gamma) rhythms recorded from the scalp, should be placed in the "adolescent" type 2 experimental category described in Chapter 1. As one colleague expresses it, *in our lab we don't call it "gamma," we call is "muscle."* By contrast to the artifact-plagued studies, SSVEP allows brain responses to be recorded in very narrow frequency bands, typically less than 0.1 Hz bracketing the light flicker frequency. Because artifact is broadband, it contributes very little to this narrow band signal.

7. OVERCORRELATED AND UNDERCORRELATED BRAINS: A TENTATIVE DISEASE MODEL

Throughout this book, I have emphasized the distinction between the extreme dynamic states of full functional isolation (localization) versus states of complete global coherence. This picture is, of course, a huge oversimplification, but a useful one that helps us choose the best methods to decipher the brain's difficult language. Complex systems are generally able to exhibit both extreme kinds of behavior and everything in between. Some complex systems are more complex than others, and complex systems sometimes enter states in which they act very simply for limited periods. Within this general conceptual framework, Gerald Edelman, head of the Neurosciences Institute in La Jolla, California, and Giulio Tononi of the University of Wisconsin have proposed a *quantitative measure of dynamic complexity* having some common ground with graph theory and small world networks to be outlined in Chapter 7. The most complex brain states then occur between the extremes of fully localized and fully global behavior. As these scientists express it:[6]

> ... high values of complexity correspond to an optimal synthesis of functional specialization and functional integration within a system. This is clearly the case for systems like the brain—different areas and different neurons do different

things (they are differentiated) at the same time they interact to give rise to a unified conscious scene and to unified behaviors (they are integrated).

Richard Silberstein has taken this general dynamic picture a step further in the physiological and clinical directions by showing how brainstem *neurotransmitter systems* may act generally to move the brain to different places along the local—global gamut of dynamic behavior. Different neurotransmitters may alter coupling between distinct cortical areas by selective actions at different cortical depths. For example, the neurotransmitter *dopamine* appears to be well positioned in the appropriate cortical layers to reduce corticocortical coupling and at the same time increase local network (cortical or thalamocortical) coupling. This may produce a shift from more global to more locally dominated dynamics, a shift from more over correlated (*hypercoupled*) to more under correlated (*hypocoupled*) brain states. In contrast, the neurotransmitter *serotonin* (5-HT) could move the cortex to a more hypercoupled state. Richard further conjectures that several diseases may be manifestations of hypercoupled or hypocoupled dynamic states brought on by faulty neurotransmitter action. For example, the association of (positive) schizophrenia symptoms with hypocoupled states is consistent with observations of a therapeutic response to dopamine receptor blockers and prominent beta activity likely due to enhanced local networks. Again, *a healthy consciousness is associated with a proper balance between local, regional, and global mechanisms.*

8. BINOCULAR RIVALRY, CONSCIOUS PERCEPTION, AND BRAIN INTEGRATION

Ramesh Srinivasan completed his PhD in Biomedical Engineering with me at Tulane University in the early 1990s. He then expanded his horizons, turning himself into a first-class cognitive scientist by first training at the University of Oregon and then working for the Neurosciences Institute in La Jolla. For the past 10 years or so, he has been a member of the prestigious Cognitive Science faculty at UC Irvine, where he operates the EEG lab (see Figure 5–1). Here I outline some of Ramesh's studies of consciousness using *binocular rivalry.*[7]

When two different images are presented, one to each eye, conscious perception alternates between the images (*conscious percepts*). Special goggles are used to present flickering blue (8 Hz) and red (10 Hz) lights simultaneously to the subject's left and right eyes (Fig. 6–9), a procedure also known as *frequency tagging*. The images are also distinguished by spatial patterns like horizontal and vertical lines. The subject indicates periods when he perceives only a blue or red image with response switches; typically either purely red or purely blue images are perceived 80% of the time. Evoked brain responses (SSVEP) are analyzed in the 8 and 10 Hz bands. For brain responses in the 8 Hz band, blue perception states are known as *perceptual dominance periods* and and red states as *non dominance periods*, each typically lasting a few seconds. For brain responses in the 10 Hz band, the opposite occurs; red states correspond to perceptual dominance and blue states to perceptual non dominance.

Similar to Richard Silberstein's SSVEP work (Section 6), scalp potentials are recorded, and coherence patterns over the scalp (at the 8 and 10 Hz stimulus frequencies) are determined for both the perceptual dominance and non dominance states. As indicated by the widths of the arrows in Figures 6–9 and 6–10 (greatly oversimplified), perceptual dominance periods are associated with increased coupling between cortical regions as measured by coherence at the frequency of the dominant color. When the subject perceives the red light (Fig. 6–9), the cross-hemispheric coherence at 8 Hz (blue light flicker frequency) is low. By contrast, when the subject perceives the blue light the cross-hemispheric coherence at 8 Hz is high (Fig. 6–10). The strongest changes tend to occur in frontal regions. In short, *a more integrated scalp coherence pattern at each frequency occurs with conscious perception of the stimulus flickering at the matching frequency.*

These studies of binocular rivalry are relatively new and await comprehensive interpretation. More generally, I have claimed that specific mental tasks typically occur with increased coherence in some frequency bands and decreased coherence in others, consistent with the formation of (possibly) overlapping networks. These data address the *binding problem* of brain science: How is the unity of conscious perception created by distinct neural systems processing different functions? Conscious perception, in Ramesh's experiments, occurs with enhanced dynamic "binding" of the brain hemispheres within narrow frequency bands. At the same time, dynamic processes occurring in other frequency bands can remain "unbound," allowing different parts of the

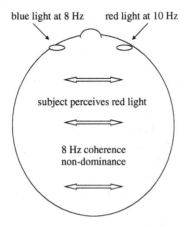

Figure 6–9 Binocular rivalry experiment carried out by Ramesh Srinivasan; the arrows indicate low cross-hemispheric coherence at 8 Hz when perceiving the red (10 Hz) flickering light.

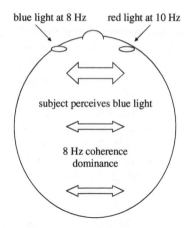

blue light at 8 Hz   red light at 10 Hz

subject perceives blue light

8 Hz coherence
dominance

Figure 6-10   Binocular rivalry experiment; the arrows indicate moderate- to high
cross-hemispheric coherence at 8 Hz when perceiving the blue (8 Hz) flickering light.

brain to engage in independent actions. Theoretical support for this general
picture is outlined in Chapter 7.

9. OBSTACLES TO PROGRESS: THE DEVIL AND HIS DAMN DETAILS

In order to make this book readable for a general audience, I have omitted
nearly all the technical details required to carry out genuine science. Readers
should not be misled into thinking that all one has to do is stick electrodes on
somebody, record EEG, and send data to a standard software program. Nearly
anyone off the street can record EEG, but producing good science is another
manner entirely. Each of the short summaries of experiments in this chapter
represents several papers published in reviewed scientific journals and years of
background work. My own book (with Ramesh as co-author), *Electric Fields of
the Brain: The Neurophysics of EEG* [8] includes a long chapter titled *Fallacies in
EEG*, demonstrating a feature that EEG has in common with all scientific fields;
namely, *the devil is in the details*.

As implied by the magic tablet fable of Section 4, the history of EEG is littered
with premature and ultimately futile attempts to adopt immature analyses to
enormously complicated aspects of brain function like *intelligence, schizophrenia*, and *more subtle brain dysfunction*. Consider intelligence—a number
of studies have reported plausible correlations between scores on IQ tests and
various EEG measures. On the other hand, individual subjects can adopt very
different "dynamic strategies," as measured with EEG, to perform identical
tasks, for example, when their brains operate with different frequency combinations. To adopt a football metaphor, some teams are better on offense, others
excel at defense; some are better at passing the ball, others have more success
running. A team's "intelligence" is best measured by its won/lost record; no

optimal strategy can apply across all teams since each team has a unique set of strengths and weaknesses. A similar metaphor for intelligence could involve nations at war. Given this picture, any attempt to measure (or much worse, *define*) human "intelligence" with EEG appears quite misguided. The discovery of robust EEG-IQ correlations still has substantial scientific value, but special care in judging the implications of such data is called for.

Despite its obvious shortcomings, EEG is an accepted and valuable tool for a restricted set of brain diseases and for certain cognitive studies as outlined in Chapters 5 and 6. Given this success, it is perhaps natural to ask how far EEG may be extended into other areas, but the sizeable graveyard of failed applications reminds us of the *fallacy of the easy first step*. It seems to me that much past failure originated from implicit (and perhaps unconscious) assumptions by both cognitive and physical neuroscientists that the brain is a simple system acting in accord with simple cognitive theories and producing relatively simple signals characterized as delta, alpha, and so forth. Unfortunately, MEG (magnetic field recording), first developed in the early 1980s, repeated many of EEG's mistakes.[9] I suspect that the more recent technologies, fMRI and PET, may also be guilty of oversimplifying their data from time to time, although I am not an expert in these areas. Simple models have quite a successful history in science but require progressive modifications as a scientific field matures. To again paraphrase Einstein, *things should be kept as simple as possible, but not simpler.* Explicit acknowledgment of brains as complex adaptive systems clearly requires sophisticated theoretical frameworks to guide experimental programs. In particular, the general idea of networks operating in multiple frequency bands and embedded in global synaptic fields suggests the importance of measuring EEG correlations between multiple cortical areas.

In 1990, when Mikhail Gorbachev was President of the Soviet Union and Francois Mitterrand was President of France, Gorbachev told the following joke after a Parliament session: "Bush has 100 body guards; one is a terrorist, but he doesn't know which one. Mitterrand has 100 lovers; one has AIDS, but he doesn't know which one. Gorbachev has 100 economists; one is smart, but he doesn't know which one!" EEG scientists certainly enjoy a higher percentage of smarts than Gorbachev's fanciful economists, but sorting out good EEG science from the bad is not always easy. EEG is a highly interdisciplinary field involving cognitive science, neuroscience, medicine, physics, engineering, mathematics, and computer science. No one person can be an expert in all these areas, so good cross-field communication is essential; unfortunately, for reasons that I can only guess, such communication in EEG has been woefully inadequate.

My guarded optimism for future progress is due partly to the fact that far fewer EEG failures seem to have involved the sophisticated experimental and analysis methods cited in this book. Nevertheless, I present the following potential EEG applications with some trepidation for fear of premature adulation. I do suggest, however, that the competent scientists cited in this book are candidates for one of Gorbachev's more accomplished economists; if appropriate solutions are possible, they may well find them.

I cited *SAM Technology* in Section 5 as an example of a semi commercial undertaking aimed more at securing financial support for scientific research than making investors wealthy. Here I list several additional applications of EEG based on years of basic research.

- *Epilepsy* is a disease affecting about 1% of the U.S. population. Despite treatments with antiepileptic drugs, about half of patients continue to experience seizures or severe side effects from the drugs. Epilepsy surgery is a viable option only when seizures originate in small, known tissue masses that can be safely removed. My former PhD student Brett Wingeier worked with me in Australia in 1998–2000 and upon graduation joined *NeuroPace*, a startup company funded by venture capitalists and focusing on implantable devices for the treatment of epilepsy. Their matchbox-sized device is implanted in the skull, records EEG, and contains software to recognize the EEG "signature" of a seizure onset. The device then delivers a mild electric stimulus to areas near the seizure focus, attempting to suppress the seizure. This is one of several practical examples of brain–computer interfaces. The device is now undergoing clinical trials to judge how well it works in real patients; preliminary reports are quite positive. Michael Crichton, the medical doctor better known as a fiction writer, anticipated this device in his 1971 novel *The Terminal Man*; hopefully *NeuroPace's* patients will enjoy more success than Crichton's fictional patient.
- Research on *brain–computer interfaces* is also directed to the task of establishing communication with locked-in patients.[10] As discussed in Chapter 2, patients in the fully locked-in state are unable to communicate with others even though they may possess near-normal levels of consciousness. They can understand what others are saying and doing, but they cannot respond either verbally or by moving body parts; in extreme cases, even eye blinks are not possible. For such patients, EEG (scalp) or ECoG (from implanted electrodes) are all that remain for communication. A patient viewing a computer monitor can "learn," by some unknown process, to modify his EEG to move a cursor toward target letters on the screen, eventually spelling out entire words. While this process is quite tedious, it represents vast improvement over the cruel state of complete isolation.
- *New drug development* is very time consuming and expensive; once developed, the best method of delivery to the appropriate organ system must also be found. Drugs must also be tested for safety and stability in the human body. Only about one new medicine enters the marketplace for every five thousand or so chemicals under initial study. *Neuropharmacology* is specifically concerned with drug action on the central nervous system. EEG covariance or coherence patterns can be strongly influenced by these drugs, suggesting a means of obtaining immediate quantitative feedback from the patient's brain. EEG tests, if

competently designed, appear to have enormous potential as a natural step in the testing of certain new drugs, for example, those used to treat ADHD, schizophrenia, or other neuropsychiatric disorders. As far as I am aware, no drug company has yet devoted serious funding to the kinds of sophisticated EEG studies most likely to achieve success.

- *Advertising* is another expensive business that may benefit from EEG. *Neuro-Insight*, a market research company started by Richard Silberstein in 2005, uses SSVEP together with patented technology to deliver insights into advertising effects, both rational and emotional, on its target audience (Disclaimer: I serve on the scientific board of *Neuro-Insight* but have no ownership or other financial interest). One goal is to predict which parts of an advertisement like a TV commercial are stored in long-term memory. At the time of this writing, several dozen trials with international companies like *Ford* and *Nestlé* have yielded promising results. Richard believes that commercial success in advertising can provide funding for future EEG applications in neuropharmacology and other medical areas.

10. SUMMARY

Early EEG science focused mainly on temporal patterns of scalp potential with emphasis on the frequency bands, delta, theta, alpha, and beta associated with distinct brain states. Early spatial analysis was severely limited by the electronic and computer technology available at the time. Some early success was achieved in locating cortical tumors and epileptic foci, but spatial analysis was mostly limited to distinguishing localized from global patterns. By contrast, modern systems typically record potentials at 64 to 130 or more electrode sites, and computer algorithms project scalp potentials to the cortical surface, a technology called *high-resolution EEG*.

The challenge of learning brain language involves the translation and interpretation of *spatial-temporal patterns* of scalp or cortical potentials, noting that spatial and temporal properties of cortical dynamics are interrelated. Cognitive processing involves widely distributed source constellations, parts of neural networks that form and dissolve on 100 millisecond or so time scales. Thinking brains have associated sources that can be anywhere and everywhere; localization of function is irrelevant in these cases.

Several experiments were outlined in which distinctive spatial correlation patterns are associated with specific mental tasks, suggesting the formation of underlying neural networks. These correlations may be estimated either with the time domain measure covariance or the frequency domain measure coherence. Correlations are observed in studies of ongoing EEG, transient evoked potentials, and steady-state evoked potentials (SSVEP). Specific mental tasks occur with increased correlations between some sites and decreased correlations between others, consistent with the quick formation and dissolution of networks needed for specific tasks. Furthermore, brains are often coherent in some frequency bands, and at the same time, incoherent in other bands. Task performance may be predicted by correlation patterns recorded during and, in some cases, even before the task is carried out.

A central question about any complex dynamic system is this: Is it composed of multiple subsystems with minimal communication, dominated by *functional isolation*? Or, is it more *globally coherent*, with all parts acting in almost the same manner? At various times, brains seem to operate over the entire range of this local–global range of dynamic brain states. The most complex brain states apparently occur between the extremes of fully localized and fully global behavior. Brainstem *neurotransmitter systems* may act generally to move the brain to different parts of the local–global range of dynamic behavior. Different neurotransmitters may alter coupling between distinct cortical areas by selective actions at different cortical depths. *A healthy consciousness is associated with a proper balance between local, regional, and global mechanisms.*

Chapter 7

Networks, Waves, and Resonant Binding

1. THE EASY PROBLEM

My first six chapters dealt mostly with selective aspects of mainstream neuroscience, and Chapters 5 and 6 translated a little of the brain's secret language into a more familiar dialect. The conceptual framework advocated in this book consists of neural networks embedded in global fields. This idea may be a little controversial, but it is mostly mainstream neuroscience, even if partly couched in nontraditional terms. Our minor departure from tradition is motivated by the central message—*the brain is not simple*; rather, it is a *complex adaptive system* requiring research methods appropriate for such systems. My central focus is directed to relationships between the cognitive and dynamic behaviors of brains, addressing the so-called *easy problem* of brain science as labeled by philosopher David Chalmers. The easy problem is not really so easy, but it is far easier than the *hard problem*, referring to the origins of our awareness, to be considered in Chapters 9–12.

This chapter's goal is to provide additional theoretical support for the general conceptual framework outlined in Chapter 4: topics include networks, small worlds, binding by resonance, standing waves, and boundary conditions. In order to minimize mathematical details, our discourse cites analog systems from several disparate scientific fields, extending the approach of earlier chapters. Neuroscientists are typically skeptical of brain analogs, often for good reason, thus I offer the following caveat to deflect such criticisms: I am *not* claiming that brains are actually like social systems, vibrating molecules, quantum structures, resonant cavities, hot plasmas, disordered solids, or chaotic fluids. Rather, I suggest that each of these systems may exhibit behavior similar to brain dynamics observed under restricted experimental conditions, including the spatial scale of observation. The multiple analogs then facilitate development of *complementary models of brain reality*. As suggested in Chapter 1, such "complementarity" is one of the keys to deeper understanding. Given that brains provide the pre-eminent examples of complex systems, perhaps we should not be too surprised if their dynamic behavior finds many analogs in the complex external world. In the context of theoretical brain models, *inside mathematics* can be similar to *outside mathematics*.

2. NETWORKS, SMALL WORLDS, AND NON-LOCAL INTERACTIONS

Interest in cell assemblies or neural networks leads us naturally to *graph theory*, a branch of mathematics concerned with the pattern of links between elements that compose the network (*graph*). Here I avoid most mathematics and adopt physical language with the corresponding mathematical labels in parentheses. The network (graph) shown in Figure 7–1 consists of 16 nodes (*vertices*) and 21 or 22 connections or links (*edges*). This might be a molecular model where the nodes and connecting links represent atoms and chemical bonds, respectively. Or it might represent a social system with links indicating friendships, one-time contacts, or any kind of paired human interactions. Graphs or networks are characterized by their connection density, expressed as the *clustering coefficient*, and the average number of steps (node crossings) between each node pair called the *path length*. The clustering coefficient is essentially the fraction of possible links that actually occur; it always falls between 0 and 1. Several kinds of graphs carry special labels. *Caveman graphs* consist of a number of fully connected clusters (*caves*) in which each node is connected to every other node in the same cave (*cliques*). If any cave in a graph is fully isolated, the path length for the whole graph is infinite. In *connected caveman graphs,* adjacent caves are connected; the clusters in this case are essentially supernodes (*metanodes*) or nodes defined at larger spatial scales. Neurons and cortical columns at several scales, with their intracortical and non-local (corticocortical) connections between local neurons, may be represented as graphs at different spatial scales.

A *small world network*[1] is a type of graph typically consisting of local clusters with dense interconnections. The label "small world" stems from the purported maximum of *six degrees of separation* between any two persons in the world. While cliques have full intraconnectivity, sub networks of the small world ilk may be near-cliques, having dense internal connections but sparse connections between different clusters, as in Figure 7–1. Small world networks typically have special nodes with large numbers of links (*hubs*), in the same sense that Atlanta

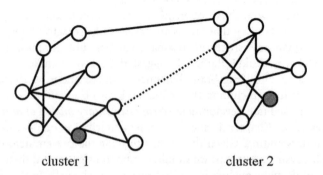

cluster 1   cluster 2

Figure 7–1   A network (graph) consisting of two clusters; the dashed line represents an optional link (edge).

is the hub for Delta Airlines. We anticipate correctly that increased clustering generally leads to shorter path lengths, but an interesting property of networks is how sharply this reduction in path length occurs. The addition of a small number of links between clusters can dramatically reduce path lengths even though the clustering coefficient exhibits only small changes. *The influence of non-local interactions is typically a critical feature of small world networks.*

The two gray nodes in Figure 7–1 have a path length of six links before addition of the new (dashed) connection; after this new link is added, the gray node pair's path length is reduced to three. For the whole graph, addition of the new connection only increases the clustering coefficient from 0.175 to 0.183 (+ 4.6%). By contrast, the graph path length (average over all node pairs) falls by a larger fraction, from 3.85 to 2.93 (−24%). Interactions in social networks, in which part of the population carries a communicable disease, provide practical examples. If the nodes are persons and the clusters are relatively isolated cities, disease spreads slowly or not at all between cities. But if travel volume increases beyond a critical point, sharp increases in intercity disease spread is expected. Ships carrying rats between Asia and Europe apparently provided such critical links to create a small world network facilitating spread of the Black Plague around the year 1400.

My first exposure to small world phenomena took place in 1964 in my first postgraduate job, although at the time I had never heard of graph theory or small worlds. My employer, a large defense contractor, operated under a fat government contract where profit was a fixed percentage of whatever money was spent; the more they spent, the more profit they made. As a result, our group had perhaps twice as many engineers as needed, so we were always thinking up interesting new projects. One guy in the next office spent several hundred thousand dollars of taxpayer money running computer simulations to find the optimum strategy for the casino game blackjack[2]. I labeled one of my side projects CAOS (computer analysis of scores), a program rating college football teams; to my knowledge no one had yet accomplished this. The nodes in my network were football teams; each game produced a link labeled by the point difference of the score.

Figure 7–2 is a graph with five clusters, a major hub (1) and four minor hubs (6, 11, 16, 21); the clustering coefficient is rather small (0.083), but the path length for the entire graph is only 2.94 links. If the four connections from the major hub to minor hubs are replaced by four connections between nodes on the outer boundary, the clustering coefficient remains unchanged, but the path length may more than double.

If Figure 7–2 were a football graph, each cluster would represent a conference and the connecting links would show which teams had played each other; the links would also be numbered to indicate margins of victory. Each college tends to play all or most other colleges in the same conference, forming near-cliques. I noted early on that my program only produced plausible ratings after some minimal number of interconference games were played, essentially when a small world network emerged abruptly from the more isolated clusters. In retrospect

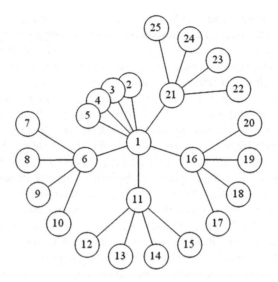

Figure 7–2   A network (graph) consisting of five clusters.

this seems obvious, but in 1964 very few people had ever used a computer, not even my engineering or physics professors. I mailed my ratings to 50 or so sports writers to judge their interest in adopting my services. Their defensive responses took me by surprise; many said essentially that *no computer can ever replace ME*. I did, however, receive a very positive reply from the sports editor of Playboy Magazine. Unfortunately, any fleeting fantasies of a new career with exotic fringe benefits were soon dashed when Playboy's editors rejected the idea based on technical deadline issues; it was time to return to graduate school. Only years later did football computer ratings become commonplace in daily newspapers.

The mathematics of graph theory is relatively clean and well defined (otherwise it wouldn't be called *mathematics*), but application to cortical anatomy involves several messy issues. The first question concerns spatial scale; which anatomical structures should serve as the appropriate nodes? While the single cell provides one likely choice, various neuroscientists have proposed minicolumns or corticocortical columns as basic functional units of cortex. As indicated in Figure 4–7, each cortical pyramidal cell sends local axons to the limits of its macrocolumn boundary. We don't know the actual fraction of local cells targeted by the central cell, but it is probably less than 1% of neurons in the macrocolumn, fewer than 10^4 links. The long-range axons provide non-local input to corticocortical columns, each containing about ten thousand neurons. The clustering coefficients at the single-cell and macrocolumn scales appear to be something like 10^{-7} to 10^{-6} and 10^{-2} to 10^{-1}, respectively, and the path lengths at both scales seem to be about three links. Although these estimates have very large error bounds, it appears that cortical/white matter fits in the class of small world networks over a range of spatial scales; the abundance of corticocortical fibers is mostly responsible for the short path lengths. Short path lengths generally suggest highly integrated dynamic behavior, but in cerebral cortex, such functional integration is mitigated by inhibitory synaptic action.

3. GRAPHS, RESONANCE, AND BUCKYBRAINS

Resonance is the tendency for systems to respond selectively to inputs in narrow frequency bands. Every cell phone has a private resonant frequency allowing it to select from thousands of simultaneous calls coded in the electromagnetic fields impacting every phone. TV and radio tuners are based on the same principle but allow control of local resonant frequencies by turning the dial to the frequency band matching the desired broadcast. Mechanical resonance of the basilar membrane in the cochlea enables us to distinguish different audio frequencies in voices. Mechanical structures like violins, pianos, bridges, power lines, and airplane wings display resonant responses; some resonance is good as in flute playing; some is bad as when earthquakes cause buildings to fall. Quartz watches use resonance to keep time; MRI is based on resonant absorption of electromagnetic energy by protons; atomic energy levels depend on a kind of quantum wavefunction resonance. Molecules have multiple resonant frequencies; various gases selectively absorb light or other electromagnetic fields at their resonant frequencies. Resonance is just about everywhere and, as argued below in Sections 4 and 5, it is also found in the brain.

If the two central links (solid and dashed lines) connecting the two clusters in Figure 7–1 are removed, the graph might represent two isolated oscillatory systems, perhaps molecules with links indicating chemical bonds or simply little balls connected by springs. If these balls (nodes) move in three dimensions, each cluster of N balls has 3N resonant frequencies called the system's *normal modes of oscillation*. Note that the two sets of resonant frequencies are holistic properties of each cluster; they cannot be identified with individual oscillators. The lowest mode is the *fundamental*; higher modes are the *overtones*. For purposes of relating these ideas to brain dynamics, the following features of a broad class of oscillatory systems are expected:

- When oscillating at the system's higher resonant frequencies, the entities (balls, carbon atoms, and so forth) tend to move in uncoordinated directions; their oscillations are asynchronous. By contrast, oscillations at the lower resonant frequencies are more in phase. Imagine a very low-frequency oscillation where all balls tend to move together—in and out in the radial direction from the cluster's center of mass. If the balls were stars and each cluster a galaxy, this motion is a standing wave called the *breathing mode*, a dynamic state of high functional integration.
- When the two clusters are joined by one or more connections, the combined system has same number of resonant frequencies as the sum from the separate clusters; however, all resonant frequencies are changed

by the new links. Again the set of resonances is a holistic (global) property of the full system. Consider an imagined tissue mass in the brain that produces narrow band oscillations when isolated, a so-called *pacemaker*. We expect its resonant frequency or frequencies to change should it lose its autonomy because of feedback from other tissue. The old (and mostly abandoned) idea of a thalamic pacemaker responsible for alpha oscillations can only make sense if some thalamic tissue mass receives negligible feedback from the cortex.

- As more and more balls are connected (increasing the clustering coefficient), the spectrum of resonant frequencies is expected to become compressed. We still have 3N resonances, but they will become more nearly equal and occur at low frequencies[3]. Genuine experimental measurements may have the additional complications of noise and non stationarity, say due to small variations in the properties of connecting springs. We may then be only able to identify the very lowest resonances experimentally.

A buckminsterfullerene (*buckyball*) is a molecule consisting of 60 carbon atoms connected by single and double bonds and forming a closed spherical cage with a soccer-ball-like surface; these bonds are normally modeled by classical mechanical springs of appropriate stiffness. Geometrical constraints prohibit six potential normal modes (resonances), so the buckyball has "only" 3N-6 or 174 resonances. The lowest (fundamental) frequency is the breathing mode where all carbon atoms oscillate together in and out from the center of the molecular structure, a radial standing wave, but here we are more interested in the buckyball's tangential standing waves, which are similar to the Schumann resonances discussed in Chapter 4.

Suppose the buckyball model is adjusted in a thought experiment to create a "buckybrain," a fanciful structure more similar to the cortical/white matter system. In this imagined system, the 60 carbon atoms are replaced by 52 "atoms" of different kinds analogous to structural differences between the 52 Brodmann areas: cortical regions at the scale of several centimeters, each containing a nested hierarchy of cortical columns. Each new atom is also connected to a new central structure representing the thalamus, providing both dynamic feedback and control of the strength of surface bonds. Several of the general dynamic properties discussed in Chapters 4 through 6 may be demonstrated with thought experiments on this buckybrain as indicated in the next section.

4. BINDING BY RESONANCE

In Section 3, resonance in selected mechanical and electromagnetic systems was emphasized. Here I argue that similar phenomena can occur in a much broader class of dynamic systems, including both neural networks and global fields of synaptic action. A famous account of functional resonance coupling is due to

Dutch mathematician and physicist Christian Huygens. In 1665 Huygens noticed that his two pendulum clocks hanging on the wall next to each other kept identical time and returned to synchrony even when one on them was disturbed. If, however, the clocks were placed on opposite sides of the room, they gradually drifted apart. He concluded that clocks hanging close together were coupled by small vibrations in the wall, but the coupling strength fell off with separation distance. This was evidently the earliest account of what brain scientists may choose to call *binding by resonance*, strong functional coupling of oscillatory systems with only weak physical connections due to "matching" resonance frequencies. As suggested by the quotation marks, the resonant frequencies *need not be equal* to be "matching"; rather, modern studies show that strong "binding" (dynamic coupling) can occur in weakly connected systems if the right *combinations* of resonant frequencies are matching as discussed below.

The next actors in our story are mathematicians Frank Hoppensteadt of the Courant Institute of Mathematical Sciences and Eugene Izhikevich of The Neurosciences Institute[4]. They studied a mathematical model consisting of an arbitrary number *of semiautonomous oscillators*; assumed to be *pairwise weakly connected* to themselves and to a "central" oscillator represented by the vector X_0, which may act to control other oscillators. The oscillator X_0 could represent a special thalamocortical network or it might be a global field. What exactly do they mean by the label "oscillator?" Our interest in their analysis arises from the broad class of systems, including many kinds of neural network models that fit their oscillator category.

The symbols X_n label distinct oscillators ($n = 1, 2, 3, \ldots$) of any kind—mechanical, electrical, chemical, global synaptic action field, or neural network, any system governed by a set of differential equations producing non chaotic dynamics as discussed in the Endnotes. When (mathematically) disconnected from the larger system in Figure 7–3, each oscillator X_n is assumed to produce non chaotic (that is, *quasi-periodic*) dynamics with a set of resonant frequencies $(f_{n1}, f_{n2}, f_{n3}, \ldots)$. If the governing oscillator equations are *strongly connected*, we expect strong dynamic interactions and new resonant frequencies to emerge in the larger system of coupled oscillators, but we are more interested here in the case of *weak connections*, as indicated by the dashed line in Figure 7–3. Typically,

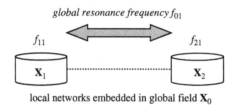

global resonance frequency f_{01}

f_{11} f_{21}

X_1 X_2

local networks embedded in global field X_0

Figure 7–3   Local networks X_1 and X_2 embedded in the global synaptic field X_0.

application of neural network models to genuine brain tissue is severely limited because of model dependence on unknown parameters, often with ambiguous or nonexistent physiological interpretations. The strength of this resonance theory lies in its independence from many of the unsupported assumptions of typical neural network models.

Eugene and Frank showed that *the individual, weakly connected oscillators interact strongly only if certain resonant relations exist between the characteristic frequencies of the autonomous (unconnected) oscillators.* Their oscillator category fits a large class of systems described by differential equations, linear or nonlinear. Suppose the vector X_0 represents a global field of synaptic action with a single (autonomous) resonant frequency f_{01}, and this global oscillator is weakly connected to two local oscillators (X_1, X_2) also weakly connected to each other, as indicated in Figure 7–3. X_1 and X_2 might represent cortical-thalamic networks, as long as the conditions of semi autonomy and non chaotic oscillations are satisfied. Assume that each local network has a single resonant frequency (f_{11} and f_{21}). In this example, the cortical-thalamic networks substantially interact only when the three frequencies (f_{01}, f_{11}, f_{21}) satisfy the resonant relation

$$m_0 f_{01} + m_1 f_{11} + m_2 f_{21} = 0 \tag{7.1}$$

Here (m_1, m_2) is any combination of non zero integers, and m_0 is any integer including zero. Two simple cases are

$$f_{11} = f_{21} \quad \text{and} \quad f_{01} = f_{11} - f_{21} \tag{7.2}$$

The first case is the well-known resonant interaction between two oscillators with equal resonant frequencies, demonstrated by Huygens' wall clocks, but many other resonant interactions are predicted for various combinations of the indices m's in Equation 7.1. Suppose two thalamocortical networks have the distinct gamma resonant frequencies $f_{21} = 37$ Hz and $f_{11} = 42$ Hz. The two networks may substantially interact, perhaps forming a temporary (functional) single network, when the global resonant frequency satisfies (Eq. 7.1); Table 7–1 lists several examples of the global frequency f_{01} needed to functionally couple the two networks. Section 5 outlines one model of the global field X_0 with resonant frequency under the control of neuromodulators.

The analysis of this section represents, at best, a huge oversimplification of genuine brain dynamic processes. No claim is made here that the exact relation (Eq. 7.1) applies to actual brains. Yet the model demonstrates unequivocally how the members of any semi-isolated tissue mass can act in concert in some frequency bands, while at the same time, act in isolation in other frequency bands. *Functional coupling between networks is then pictured as dynamic rather than hardwired; coupling strengths may easily change on short time scales.*

The so-called *binding problem* of brain science is concerned with how unity of consciousness is created by distinct neural systems processing vision, sound, memory, and so forth. Given both the small world nature of anatomical connections between cortex areas and the many possibilities for resonance-enhanced

Table 7–1 Binding of Two Gamma Oscillators (42, 37 Hz) by Global Resonance

m_0	m_1	m_2	Global frequency f_{01}
+1	+1	−1	5.00
+1	+2	−2	10.0
+2	+1	−1	2.50
+2	−1	+2	16.0
+3	+1	+0	14.0
+3	+0	+1	12.3
+3	+2	−2	3.33
+4	+0	+1	9.25
+4	+1	+0	10.5

coupling of weakly connected subsystems, brain science may actually have more of an *unbinding problem*—how can multiple subsystems retain the semi autonomy apparently needed to carry out specific functions? In this resonance model, cortical columns or cortical-thalamic networks may use rhythmic activity to communicate selectively. Such oscillating systems need not interact strongly even when they are directly connected. Or, the systems may interact through a global synaptic field effect, discussed in Section 5, even with no direct connections, provided the characteristic frequencies satisfy the appropriate resonance criteria.

*5. ARE BRAIN WAVES REALLY WAVES?

In this section I outline a model for the global (cortical-holistic) synaptic field producing the resonant frequency f_{01} considered in Section 4. The label "global" suggests dynamics dominated by long spatial wavelengths, implying large contributions to scalp-recorded potentials. As shown in Chapter 5, human alpha rhythms consist of long-wavelength (low spatial frequency) potentials plus more localized (apparent) network activity producing oscillatory activity with alpha band frequencies that may or may not closely match the global alpha frequencies (see the simulation in Figure 6–1). The model presented in this section is concerned *only* with global alpha rhythms, not with possible alpha or other oscillations generated in thalamocortical networks. As such, it is not an appropriate model for intracortical recordings, either in humans or lower mammals. More elaborate models that combine global fields with local networks are not developed here but are referenced in the Endnotes.

Standing and traveling waves and the critical importance of spatial scale of brain electrical recordings may be illustrated with an ocean wave metaphor. Ocean wave energy is distributed over more than four orders of magnitude of spatial and temporal frequencies. Similarly, experimental electrophysiology spans about five orders magnitude of spatial scale, depending mostly on the size and location of electrodes. Oscillations of the longest ocean waves, the tides and tsunamis, take hours to minutes; their characteristic frequencies are in the approximate range $10^{-5} < f < 10^{-3}$ Hz. Wind-driven waves of intermediate length have typical frequencies in the range $10^{-2} < f < 1$ Hz; ripples due to surface tension have even higher frequencies. The existence of a relationship between temporal frequency and spatial frequency (or spatial wavelength), called the *dispersion relation*, is a hallmark of wave phenomena.

EEG records potentials on the scalp, and, because of its poor spatial resolution, it "sees" only the longest spatial wavelengths that are actually contained in the full spectrum of cortical dynamics. The analogous ocean wave measurement is surface displacement averaged over ocean patches hundreds or even a few thousand miles in diameter; only the tides would be observed in such thought experiments. Intracranial recordings of brain potentials also "see" only a selected part of the cortical wave spectrum, depending on size and location of electrodes, and may miss the long-wavelength dynamics entirely. By analogy, wave height measurements taken from a ship or low-flying helicopter record mainly wave chop driven by local winds, missing tides and tsunamis entirely. Such small-scale ocean data would fail to provide an appropriate test of tide models. Similarly, intracranial recordings do not provide the appropriate test for global field models.

One group of clever neuroscientists has developed an algorithm that transforms MRI images of brain hemispheres from their usual wrinkled surfaces to smooth spheres as demonstrated in Figure 7–4.[5] The process is analogous to inflating a wrinkled balloon. One motivation for this computer transformation is to allow easy viewing of various kinds of activity in cortical folds. For our mathematical modeling purposes, it provides visual demonstration that the cortical/white matter systems of each hemisphere is topologically close to a spherical shell; corticocortical fibers relay action potentials around closed paths within this shell as suggested by Figure 4–13. Whereas some versions of brain wave modeling are based on this spherical shell as referenced in the

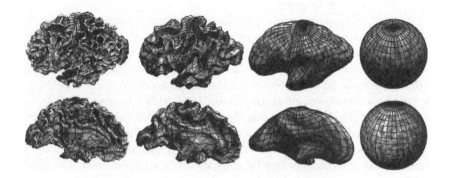

Figure 7–4   Each brain hemisphere image is progressively distorted to produce smooth surfaces and topologically equivalent spheres.[5]

Endnotes, I here outline the predictions of the simpler one-dimensional version, yielding predictions that are similar to those obtained for the spherical shell.[6]

The brain wave model is based mostly on the following idea. Scalp potentials (EEG) are generated by synaptic current sources at small scales; each cubic millimeter of cortical tissue contains more than a billion synapses. In contrast to this small-scale activity, EEG data are recorded at macroscopic (centimeter) scales, thereby presenting major problems for network models attempting connections to genuine large-scale data. I will have more to say about matching model scale to data scale in Section 6. The brain wave model follows the macroscopic dependent variables *action potential and synaptic potential densities*, for example, the number of excitatory synaptic events per square millimeter of cortical surface. All dependent variables are expressed as functions of time and cortical location. The basic approach ignores embedded network activity, although networks have been included (approximately) in more advanced models cited in the Endnotes.[6]

The gray lines in Figure 7–5 represent a vertical slice of cortical surface near the midline (*sagittal section*) with occipital and frontal areas on the left and right sides, respectively. The black lines represent standing waves of some variable, say excitatory synaptic action density, having a spatial wavelengths equal to cortical circumference divided by an integer n. With a smoothed cortex of effective circumference equal to 60 cm, the discrete wavelengths are 60 cm, 30 cm, 15 cm, and so forth. Local wave amplitude is indicated by the separation between the gray and black lines. The maximum inside and outside separations denote places where the synaptic action density is 180° out of phase, as in the occipital and frontal regions in the upper image ($n = 1$). The first overtone plot ($n = 2$) could also represent the ocean surface with the two high and two low tides on opposite sides of the Earth. Note that the spatial dependence of *any* dynamic variable may be *represented* as a linear combination of standing or traveling waves using the methods of Fourier analysis; interpreted this way, there can be no controversy about Figure 7–5. The proposed standing wave model goes further, however, suggesting that each of these standing waves is associated with a matching resonant frequency; spatial and temporal frequencies are purported to be related as in all *wave phenomena*. The upper half of the top image in Figure 7–5 (fundamental mode) matches approximately source simulation of Figure 6–1 and the EEG data shown in Figure 5–9 with front and back areas 180° out of phase.

Throughout this book, I have adopted a conceptual framework for cortical dynamic behavior consisting of networks embedded in global synaptic fields, the latter including standing and traveling waves. Up to this point, many of my arguments supporting this picture have been based on analogies to other dynamic systems. Whereas many genuine brain states probably reflect some mixture of global wave and network activity, the following summary of experimental implications is *based on the hypothesis that neocortical dynamics is partly composed of standing and traveling waves*. The brain wave model that I first

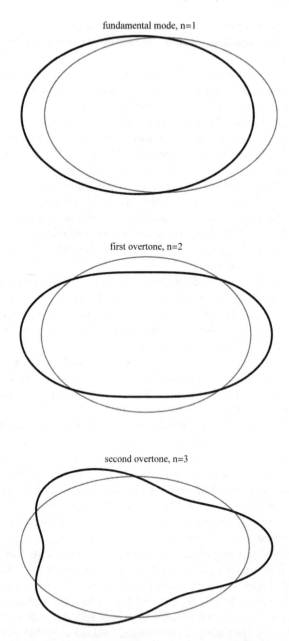

Figure 7–5 Theoretical one-dimensional standing waves in a closed, cortical-like one-dimensional structure, essentially the front-back circumference of one cortical hemisphere. The separation between the black and gray lines indicates the local positive or negative value of an excitatory synaptic action field. The fundamental mode (upper) indicates that the front and back regions are 180° out of phase. The 1st and 2nd overtones are also shown.

proposed in 1972 predicts the following approximate resonant frequencies for standing waves in cortex:

$$f_n \approx \frac{v}{L} \sqrt{n^2 - \left(\frac{\beta\lambda L}{2\pi}\right)^2} \qquad n = 1, 2, 3, \ldots \qquad (7.3)$$

The symbols and approximate values are:

v corticocortical propagation speed (600 – 900 cm/sec).

L effective front-to-back circumference of one cortical hemisphere after inflation to a smooth surface, roughly the shape of a prolate spheroidal shell or rugby ball as indicted by gray lines in Figure 7–5 (60 – 80 cm).

λ parameter indicating the fall-off in fiber density with cortical distance for the longest corticocortical fiber system (0.1 – 0.3 cm^{-1}).

β nondimensional parameter controlled by neuromodulators; parameter increases correspond to increased background excitability of cortex (stronger functional coupling); its value is unknown but believed to be of the order of 1.

f_n temporal frequency (Hz) of normal modes (standing waves), including the fundamental ($n = 1$) and overtones ($n > 1$). The spatial frequency (cycles/centimeter) of each standing wave is n/L; the fundamental wavelength ($n = 1$) is the long circumference of one unfolded cortical hemisphere.

Does the theoretical *dispersion relation* (Eq. 7.3) actually have any connection to a genuine cerebral cortex? As several cognitive scientist critics of mine have expressed, surely nothing so simple can do justice to any complex brain! But all I claim is this: At best it may enjoy some approximate connections to brains in their more globally dominated states—possibly coma, anesthesia, deep sleep, some generalized epileptic states, and the more globally dominant alpha rhythms. A few of the following experimental predictions rely on this equation, but others follow only from the more general idea of standing and traveling brain waves. Note that I claim only *relationships* not *comprehensive explanations* to complex physiological processes!

- *Temporal Frequency Range.* From the value ranges given above, $v/L \sim 7\text{–}15$ Hz; the lowest oscillatory mode apparently occurs for $n = 1$ or 2, yielding oscillations in the general range of alpha frequencies.

- *Tuning the Brain.* As the parameter β (cortical excitability) increases in Equation 7.3, each mode (resonant) frequency and the corresponding mode damping are also reduced and ultimately become non oscillatory. At the same time, new high-frequency modes occur; similar behavior has been observed in the halothane anesthesia rhythm; deeper anesthesia results in lower frequencies. We may tentatively anticipate an inverse relationship between amplitude and frequency, although such prediction requires one of the nonlinear versions of the crude linear model discussed here (see Endnotes[6]).

- *Effect of Propagation Speed. The faster the propagation, the faster the global mode frequencies.* If all parameters except corticocortical propagation speed v are fixed, brains with faster velocities should produce higher global frequencies. Axon velocity depends on axon diameter and myelination, which increases in the developing brain. A posterior rhythm of about 4 Hz develops in babies in the first few months; it attenuates with eye closure and is believed to be the precursor of the global adult alpha rhythm. Frequency gradually increases until an adult-like 10 Hz rhythm is achieved at about age 10.
- *Effect of Size. The larger the cortex, the slower the global mode frequencies.* This prediction requires several assumptions—that the longest corticocortical fiber tracts scale approximately with cortical size (the product λL approximately constant), and axon diameters and myelination remain constant with brain size changes (no change in axon velocity v). In this idealized case, each global mode frequency f_n would be inversely proportional to characteristic cortical size L. As discussed in Chapter 5 (note 3), the only two studies of the putative relationship between head size and alpha frequency of which I am aware have confirmed the predicted weak negative correlation. These studies excluded children because maturation of axon myelination provides a much larger influence than the small size changes in the developing brain.
- *Traveling Waves.* Cortical inputs at multiple locations are expected to act as epicenters for wave propagation as illustrated in Figure 4–14. From an experimental viewpoint, we expect to see short periods when waves travel in some consistent direction and other periods when standing waves are more evident. Numerous experimental studies based on measurement of relative phases across the scalp have found traveling waves in both spontaneous EEG and SSVEP (steady-state visually evoked potentials). Most observed propagation speeds (*phase and group velocities*) are in the general range of corticocortical axon speeds, although the speed issue is partly clouded by technical factors.
- *Standing Waves.* When traveling waves meet, interference occurs due to partial canceling of excitatory and inhibitory mass action, thereby producing standing waves and associated resonant frequencies as demonstrated in Figure 4–14. Some experimental support for standing waves of alpha rhythm is provided in Figures 5–9 through 5–12. Even more convincing data is provided by sinusoidal visual input (SSVEP), which most obviously activates primary visual cortex. Various locations over the upper scalp respond selectively in the alpha band when the stimulus frequency is varied as one would expect in a resonant system. Furthermore, the spatial patterns of SSVEP, well away from visual cortex, are sensitive to small (of the order of 1 Hz) changes in frequency, suggesting global rather than local (primary visual system) resonance. Most convincingly, frontal responses are easily recorded only near the

peak alpha frequency, apparently revealing a standing wave with peaks in occipital and frontal cortex, or about one-half wavelength separation if the standing wave has a fundamental wavelength equal to (front-back) cortical circumference as shown in the upper image of Figure 7–5 and the source simulation of Figure 6–1. I know of no better explanation for this experimental observation.

- *Relationship of Temporal and Spatial Frequencies. Higher temporal frequencies are associated with higher spatial frequencies above the fundamental mode.* This is a fundamental feature of nearly all wave phenomena, one of the defining properties, at least of linear "waves." The specific relationship, called the dispersion relation, is a property only of the wave medium; Equation 7.3 is the simplest version for brain waves with the index n identifying spatial frequency. Such a relationship has been demonstrated in EEG for frequencies between roughly 10 and 40 Hz in several studies at three different laboratories. Generally the procedure involves Fourier transforms in both time and surface spatial coordinates, essentially picking out the spatial modes in Figure 7–5 and estimating their temporal frequencies (see Endnotes[6]).

- *Comparison of Scalp and Cortical Recordings. The ECoG should contain more high frequency content above the low end of the alpha band than the corresponding EEG.* While this observation has been verified in studies of natural rhythms, scalp amplitudes generated by implanted (artificial) dipole sources are unaltered by implanted source frequency. How can we reconcile these two observations? The partial answer is that higher temporal frequency cortical potentials tend to be asynchronous over moderate to large areas; essentially they contain relatively more high spatial frequencies, as in the lower images in Figure 7–5. Volume conduction causes *low-pass spatial filtering* of potentials passing from cortex to scalp, thus *temporal filtering is a byproduct of spatial filtering.* But, why should higher temporal cortical frequencies occur with higher spatial frequencies in the first place? One answer is this is just what waves do; the relationship is indicated by the dispersion relation (Eq. 7.3).

Some colleagues have questioned whether my proposed conceptual framework, consisting of networks embedded in global fields, including standing waves, simply represents a novel way of looking at familiar processes, rather than suggesting more profound implications for brain science. In response, I contend that the experimental predictions listed above (and mostly confirmed) have substantial implication for future studies. My central hypothesis is that local and regional networks can coexist naturally with widely distributed sources that we characterize in terms of global synaptic fields. Either of these overlapping and interacting processes may be selectively emphasized with different experimental strategies. Conventional EEG and evoked potentials are most sensitive to global fields. High-resolution EEG acts as a spatial band-pass filter of cortical potentials, thereby reducing the contribution of global fields relative to network activity in smooth (gyral) surfaces. The magnetic field (MEG) is mainly sensitive to isolated sources in cortical folds (sulcal walls); thus, MEG is relatively insensitive to global fields, except (potentially) at the edges of large synchronous source regions. Intracortical recordings are perhaps dominated by local network dynamics.

The differences in spatial sensitivity of these measures imply that different temporal dynamics will be recorded in different experiments. Even the global fields alone can be expected to show different dynamics at different spatial scales as implied by the underlying dispersion relation. Local and regional networks in different parts of cortex are generally expected to produce distinct dynamic behavior; however, such network dynamics may partly reflect the common (top-down) influence of global fields, as in the example of the global–local resonant interactions depicted in Figure 7–3. These interpretations should impact the experimental designs of future studies.

*6. BOUNDARY CONDITIONS IN COMPLEX SYSTEMS: WHY SIZE AND SHAPE COUNT

In this section I aim to clear up several misconceptions about relationships between simplified models of complex systems and the actual systems themselves. Simple models often eliminate a system's inherent dependence on spatial coordinates, potentially neglecting important dynamic spatial structure facilitated by the system's *boundary conditions*, the boundary values forced on dependent variables by system "containers" or boundaries. For example, piano string displacement is forced to be zero at its fixed ends, the velocity of a fluid is zero at confining walls, the population of land animals goes to zero at the water's edge, and so forth. In a closed shell with no tangential boundaries, all dependent variables must be continuous around the shell circumference (*periodic boundary conditions*) as in the Schumann resonances of Figure 4–12 and my putative brain waves in Figure 7–5. Boundary conditions are partly determined by system size and shape. The issue of brain size and boundary conditions is well off the radar screens of most neuroscientists when considering EEG dynamic behavior. I suggest here that this omission is likely to be an error. Just to mention one example, boundary conditions can often impose spatial structure that inhibits temporal chaos.

The size influence and other boundary conditions in a complex system may be demonstrated with the convection tank shown in Figure 7–6; this might just be a heated pot of chicken soup. The heated fluid rises to the top in *convection cells* (the fat arrows), moves to the side, and then descends back to the bottom. Convection occurs in the atmosphere, the ocean above underwater volcanoes, and the sun; convection cells in soup are more easily observed if it contains little particles like rice. Mathematical models of this process employ the complicated mathematics of coupled nonlinear partial differential equations; limited solutions are obtained only with computer-intensive brute force. The mathematical and physical issues are outlined in the Endnotes.[7] In the 1960s, atmospheric

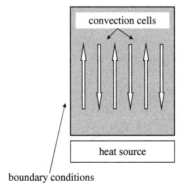

Figure 7–6 A convection tank (perhaps a pot of soup) with arrows showing fluid flow.

scientist Edward Lorenz aimed for a better intuitive understanding of convection by employing a very crude and, as he was well aware, physically inaccurate approximation to the complicated mathematics—the three simple ordinary differential equations now known as the *Lorenz equations*.

The Lorenz equations enjoy only a tentative relationship to genuine convection processes; any chef or housewife knows that heated soup can produce turbulent dynamics, essentially *spatial-temporal chaos*. Rather, the big surprise discovered by Lorenz was that very simple systems can exhibit *low-dimensional chaos*, meaning extreme sensitivity to initial conditions and system parameters in seemingly simple systems with only a few dependent variables. Mathematical modelers have now published numerous papers on chaos in all kinds of systems; my Google Scholar search generated more than a million hits on *chaos* and about twenty-five thousand hits on the much narrower topic, *Lorenz equations*. Some of this work has close experimental ties, but much more consists of mathematical exercises with no obvious connection to physical reality. The important lesson of the Lorenz work is that bona fide simple systems (genuine convection is *not* in this category) can exhibit essentially unpredictable dynamic behavior, even when perfectly accurate system models are known: the so-called *deterministic chaos* to be found again in Chapter 8.

What do brains have to do with pots of soup? Fluid convection systems are governed by a set of known equations. Even though no analytic solution is apparently possible, the unsolved equations provide substantial guidelines for the design of experiments (see Endnotes[7]). By contrast, we are unlikely to have a comprehensive brain equation in the foreseeable future to guide analogous neuroscience. As a thought experiment, let us pretend that you don't have a clue as to the governing equations; nothing beyond direct observation is known about heated pots of soup. What dynamic behavior are you likely to see if many such pots of different sizes are studied experimentally? Since in this little fable I am a minor god (it's my fantasy), I actually know the fundamental equations and can predict how the frequency spectra of the oscillations in fluid motion

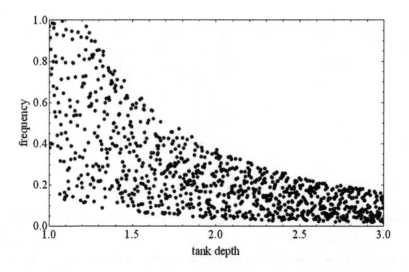

Figure 7–7 A simulation showing the dominant oscillation frequency (center of spectrum) for the velocity of a fluid particle in convection tanks with constant shapes but varying sizes; lower frequencies tend to occur in larger tanks.

change with pot size and fluid properties. Figure 7–7 shows my simulation of the overall frequency spectra of rice oscillations in a thousand soup pots whose shapes remain constant while their sizes vary by a factor of 3. The frequency spectra from any single pot can be relatively simple (quasi-periodic) or chaotic; all I have estimated is the variation of the "centers" of these generally complicated spectra with pot size. The other feature determining frequency is thermal conductivity, the ease of heat transfer through the fluid; I let this vary randomly by a factor of 10 to simulate chicken soup, salt water, olive oil, or any other fluid.

Other features being equal, larger pots tend to produce slower frequencies. The time taken for a grain of rice to complete a closed loop tends to increase (lower frequencies) in larger pots, but this effect may be partly offset by faster rice speeds in larger pots near the right side of Figure 7–7. The main point is this—a mathematician or theoretical physicist sets up equations expressed in nondimensional variables, including time. Once this is accomplished, he can forget (temporarily) about the actual physical system. By contrast, the experimental scientist must deal with actual pots and temporal and spatial variables expressed in dimensional measures like seconds and centimeters with corresponding frequency spectra in Hz. The lesson is this: *For the experimentalist, system size and shape count, even in chaotic systems.*

In addition to overall size, the boundary shape of complex systems can have large impacts on dynamic behavior. Around 1900, physicist Lord Rayleigh essentially predicted that convection cells are expected to form only when the depth of soup lies in a certain range compared to pot width. Modern studies of other systems have shown that spatial structure imposed by boundary conditions can inhibit temporal chaos. Or, spatial coherence facilitated by boundary conditions can be maintained even when the temporal behavior becomes chaotic. These studies imply that the size and shape of the cortical/white matter system should be expected to provide important influences on global field dynamic behavior. The standing wave model of Section 5 provides one simple example, but the influence of boundary conditions on system dynamics, especially at large scales, seems to be much more general.

7. THEORY, MODELS, AND POPPER'S FALSIFIABILITY

Like many scientists, I often adopt careless language by mixing up the scientific categories *model* and *theory*. The appropriate distinctions are debated by philosophers; no surprise here, philosophers debate just about everything. Much of Chapters 4–6 is based on a *conceptual framework* consisting of cortical networks embedded in synaptic action fields. This framework is neither theory nor model and is unlikely ever to be falsified because it is based entirely on well-established neurophysiology. The essential question is whether the proposed framework is scientifically useful. My answer to this question is "yes"; the framework encourages the design of specific experiments to look for synaptic field behavior like standing or traveling waves and other experiments to estimate network activity by measuring EEG correlation structure; that is, coherence, covariance, and so forth, as discussed in Chapter 6. The cognitive studies outlined in Chapters 5 and 6 affirm the framework's utility.

For physical scientists, a "theory" is normally expressible in mathematical language and makes predictions in a broad class of experiments. In this view, most so-called "cognitive theories" are better described as "models" or "conceptual frameworks." A "model" is more restricted to specific systems and carries less status. Maxwell's equations constitute a theory of electromagnetic fields; electric network models are derived from the theory as special cases. In other instances, models replace theories that are too complicated to apply. The chemical bonds of the buckyball must ultimately be governed by the theory of quantum mechanics, but application of Schrödinger's equation to find resonant frequencies is far beyond the power of any computer likely to be developed in the foreseeable future as will be argued in Chapter 8. The buckyball is, however, nicely represented for many purposes by a *model* in which chemical bonds are treated like little mechanical springs.

Models employ *Aristotelian idealizations* where all properties of the genuine system that are deemed irrelevant to the problem at hand are neglected. When I wrote software in 1965 for a future Venus probe, planets were naturally modeled as point masses. But, every small piece of a planet is attracted by gravitation to every other piece of other planets, making orbital mechanics problems potentially very complicated. However, gravitational theory shows that when separated objects interact, full accuracy is achieved if all mass is assumed to be concentrated at the objects' centers of mass.

Models also employ *Galilean idealizations* in which essential properties of genuine systems are deliberately neglected in order to create models simple enough to be useful. Galileo modeled falling bodies with no air resistance even though he lacked the technology to make the air go away. Modern economic, ecological, and network models idealize populations and networks as existing in isolation. In some cases, more accurate models evolve progressively from simpler models. Weather systems provide one such example; weather models are developed progressively by integrating the theory of fluid mechanics with new experimental data. I recently proposed an economic mathematical model of price inflation in a simple fictitious society that I called Oz.[8] Since no such society exists outside of our fantasies, the model's only possible value is in providing new, if highly oversimplified, insights into the workings of genuine economies. The Oz model may then be called a *toy model* of inflation, as the Lorenz set of equations is a toy model of convection. There is, of course, a vast difference. The Lorenz model has had major impacts well beyond its original purpose, leading to genuine model and theory development in many disparate chaotic systems previously assumed to behave simply.

The famous Austrian and British philosopher of science Karl Popper is known for his proposition that falsifiability is the critical test that distinguishes genuine science from non science. In this view, any claim that is impossible to disprove is outside the scientific realm; several of his targets in the mid–20th century were psychoanalysis, Marxism, and the Copenhagen interpretation of quantum mechanics. Quantum physicist Wolfgang Pauli famously applied Popper's philosophy when shown a paper by another physicist. "That's not right, it's not even wrong," was his devastating condemnation. Much can be said in favor of Popper's proposition, although its application to real-world models and theory is often ambiguous.

Many mathematical brain models run counter to Popper's proposition by adopting variables, perhaps with vague labels like *activity*, having no apparent connection to any genuine experiment. Typically, these models are not right; they are not even wrong. Even if the aim is more focused, say to model electrical events, the modeler may appear blissfully unaware of the issues of spatial and temporal scale, avoiding critical issues of sensor size and location in any related experiment. If the so-called "activity" can never be measured, the model cannot be falsified; it is just computation, not science. Some such efforts may demonstrate mathematical and computer methods adopted later by others with genuine theoretical skills, as opposed to strictly mathematical or computational skills, but I suspect this occurs only rarely.

The brain wave model outlined Section 6 employs both Aristotelian and Galilean idealizations, especially the neglect of local network effects. Thus, the model is easily falsified in brain states with cortical dynamics dominated by local networks. But it was never claimed to be anything but a crude model of globally dominated states in which network dynamics is suppressed. Once in a fit of uncharacteristic humility, I applied the adjective "toy" to the model, but its half dozen or so successes with experimental predictions justify the label "tool model," meaning that it may represent a genuine view of brain dynamics, but one only observable in very limited experimental conditions.

8. SUMMARY

The mathematical field of graph theory is outlined and related to several kinds of networks consisting of nodes and connecting links. Networks are characterized by their clustering coefficients and path lengths. Clustering coefficients lie in the range 0 to 1, indicating the extremes of no connections or fully connected. A network's path length is the average number of steps between each node pair. Small world networks are typically sparsely connected with small clustering coefficients but have relatively short path lengths. Cortical tissue appears to fit this small world category largely as a consequence of the non-local corticocortical fibers

Resonance is the tendency for systems to respond selectively to inputs in narrow frequency bands. Weakly coupled oscillators may interact strongly when, as autonomous (unconnected) oscillators, they produce certain special combinations of resonant frequencies, a phenomenon labeled here as *binding by resonance*. Either central (thalamic) oscillators or global fields can control interactions between local networks using resonant interactions. It is speculated that these general mathematical relations may apply, in some very approximate sense, to real brains such that functional coupling between systems is dynamic rather than hardwired.

A dispersion relation, relating spatial and temporal frequencies, is proposed as part of a brain wave (global field) model. In this view, some global (holistic cortical) fields are best described as standing waves of synaptic action. The model makes a half-dozen or so disparate experimental predictions of globally dominant alpha and SSVEP properties that have been approximately verified, including alpha frequencies, standing waves, traveling waves, and the relationship between temporal and spatial frequencies. The model is consistent with networks embedded in the global field; wavelike properties are evident experimentally only when network activity is sufficiently suppressed. Practical distinctions between conceptual frameworks, models, and theories are considered in the context of models and theories from several fields, including the proposed brain wave model. The important influence of boundary conditions on dynamic behavior, including *temporal chaos* with coherent spatial structure and *spatial-temporal chaos* (turbulence), is discussed.

Chapter 8

The Limits of Science: What Do
We Really Know?

1. THINKING THE IMPOSSIBLE

Scientific books tread very carefully over speculative issues, mostly for good reason. But, we are faced here with the formidable puzzle of the mind, the most profound of human enigmas, presenting high barriers to genuine scientific inquiry. Plausible attempts to illuminate this so-called *hard problem* will demand much wider speculation than is normally comfortable, otherwise this book would end with Chapter 7. No apology is offered here for speculation; rather, my aim is first to distinguish speculative ideas from more reliable knowledge domains. Secondly, metrics are needed to distinguish the really wild ideas from those that are only a little crazy. In this and in the following chapters, I consider a spectrum of speculative ideas, with probability identified as an important measure of human ignorance.

One goal for this chapter is to ease the transition from our normal worldviews based on everyday experience and common sense to the quantum world and its relatives in Chapters 10–12. The formidable challenge of the hard problem leads us into areas where many ideas seem counterintuitive or even fantastic, fully outside of common experiences. As a result, our normal option of falling back on common sense or gut instincts fails us. Needless to say, I will not solve the hard problem here, nor is any comprehensive solution likely to surface in the foreseeable future. Our consciousness is perhaps the most amazing of the many fantastic features known about our universe. We humans may take consciousness for granted, but our fanciful friend, the black cloud of Chapter 3, might be quite shocked that such small creatures, made mostly of little bags of water, could be conscious. In Chapters 9–12, I will address fantastic ideas that may cast just a little light on the hard problem and try to sort out the serious ideas from the fantastic nonsense.

My transition begins with some issues in practical probability, emphasizing events with such small probabilities that some may consider them miracles, the statistical realm of black swans and fat tails. This will hopefully ease our transition to the metaphorical Land of Oz or world beyond mathematician Charles Dodgson's looking glass:

> I can't believe that, said Alice to the White Queen. Try again, take a long breath and shut your eyes, she replied. There's no use trying, one can't believe impossible

things, said Alice. Why, sometimes I've believed as many as six impossible things before breakfast, replied the Queen.

2. PROBABILITY: A MEASURE OF HUMAN IGNORANCE

Cal Tech professor Leonard Mlodinow tells how randomness influences our lives in *The Drunkard's Walk*.[1] Suppose the state of California made the following offer: A random drawing is to be held to choose one winner and one loser among those who enroll; the winner is to receive several million dollars, but the loser will be taken to death row and executed the next day. Would anyone play such a macabre game? Actually, people enroll with enthusiasm, although California does not promote its lottery quite this way. Based on highway fatality and lottery statistics, Mlodinow estimates that the probability of winning the lottery is roughly equal to the chance of being killed in an auto accident while driving to purchase a ticket. But few people look at lotteries this way; our brains are not very adept at distinguishing ordinary long shots from near miracles.

The future is uncertain, yet every day we make decisions based on gut instincts, unconscious memories, or conscious estimates of future events. To paraphrase Niels Bohr: "It's difficult to make predictions, especially about the future." Or pondering Yogi Berra's unhelpful advice, "When you come to a fork in the road, take it." Our predictions typically rely on the implicit assumption that the future will be much like the past. Most hurricanes in the Gulf of Mexico have missed New Orleans; many, including your author, erroneously assumed that Katrina would repeat this history. This error demonstrates the *problem of induction*, another of philosopher Karl Popper's interests. Popper suggested psychological causes for inductive thinking, citing a human bias toward expecting events to repeat just because they have occurred reliably in the past.

Despite its potential for error, inductive reasoning is often the most effective cognitive tool at our disposal, as illustrated by the fable of three scientists walking in an unfamiliar countryside. The astronomer, noting an apparent black sheep far in the distance, remarks—"it seems sheep in this part of the world are black." The physicist corrects him—"We have seen only one sheep; the sample size is much too small to come to that conclusion." The mathematician has the final word—"You are both wrong, all we can say with certainty is that one-half of one sheep is black." For some, the mathematician may be the hero in this story, but in the real world with only a little reliable information at hand and with serious consequences for being wrong, I would probably place my bet on the physicist.

Our reliance on the past to predict the future may be expressed formally with experimental probability. Consider a range of possible outcomes x_k of some arbitrary process repeated N times. N might be the number of Gulf hurricanes in the past 20 years, with x_1, x_2, and x_3 indicating the number that have crossed the Florida, Louisiana, and Texas coastlines, respectively. Past experience with hurricanes then provides *estimates of the probabilities* of each outcome expressed by

$$\hat{P}_N(x_k) = \frac{x_k}{N} \qquad (8.1)$$

The little hat sign on $\hat{P}_N(x_k)$ indicates that these are just *estimates* of the probabilities; the subscript N indicates the number of hurricanes on which the estimates are based. Estimates based on, say the past 50 years, will differ from those based on 20 years. Failure to appreciate the critical distinction between the *actual* (with no hat) probability $P(x_k)$, which we can never know with certainty, and the estimated probability (Eq. 8.1, with hat) lies at the root of the induction problem.

While Equation 8.1 provides experimental estimates of probability, the symmetries of simple system outcomes often provide theoretical estimates. If a coin is tossed and no cause favoring either heads or tails is apparent, we postulate that each outcome has a probability of 0.5. Theoretical probability is also illustrated by throwing dice. If each die in a pair has six sides, the theoretical probability of obtaining any result (the sum of two up-faces) is obtained by identifying all possible outcomes (called the *sample space*), 1+1, 1+2, and so forth, a total of 36 possible outcomes. Only one combination adds to 2 (snake eyes), but six combinations add to 7, and so on. Assuming all numbers are equally likely to land face up (fair dice), the probabilities of rolling a 2 or a 7 are then 1/36 or 1/6, respectively. If the dice are fair, the relative frequencies of each number are expected to approach the theoretical frequencies predicted from the sample space. This histogram, shown in Figure 8–1, is called the *discrete probability density function*, which roughly approximates a continuous bell curve or *normal distribution*.

More interesting issues arise when we don't actually know if the dice are fair. Dice have a long history; professional gamblers and loaded dice even

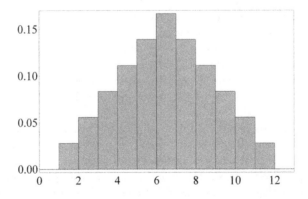

Figure 8–1   Histogram showing the probability of obtaining each of the numbers 2–12 in one toss of a pair of dice.[10]

populated the Roman Empire. An experimental histogram with suspect dice provides *estimates of the probabilities* of each roll expressed by Equation 8.1; x_k is the number of times that some number (say, $k = 7$) is rolled. Again we distinguish the actual probability $P(x_k)$, which we can never know, from the estimated probability (Eq. 8.1). The *expected value* of an event in any random process is the "center of mass" of the probability density function; the expected value of a dice roll is 7. This does not mean we really expect to obtain a 7 on each roll; the probability of rolling a 7 is only 1/6. The expected value for the roll of a single die is 3.5, which never occurs.

I often flip a coin in my university classes and ask my students for estimates of the probability of heads, obtaining the near unanimous answer 0.5, excepting a few students who remain silent because they suspect some trick like a two-headed coin. I then take an obvious peek at the coin and repeat the question. The majority answer is still 0.5, but this time their responses come only after a noticeable delay. Once I have looked at the coin, the probably of heads for me is either 0 or 1, while the estimated probability from my student's perspective remains 0.5. This little exercise demonstrates a critical difference between probability theory and genuine mathematics—the "truth" about probability is observer dependent. Experimental probability is a measure of observer ignorance while mathematics is concerned with absolute truths. We will encounter an entity closely related to probability, information, and observer ignorance in Chapter 12 called *entropy*.

3. SWANS WITH FAT TAILS: FOOLED BY RANDOMNESS

I borrowed the title of this section from two books by options trader Nassim Taleb; *black swan* is his term for a rare event with the following attributes[2]: *(1)* highly improbable; past experience cannot convincingly point to its likelihood, *(2)* carries substantial impact, *(3)* human nature causes explanations to be concocted after the fact, making the event seem predictable when it was not. In the following chapters, I consider several classes of events: Some satisfy *(1)* and *(2)*, but plausible explanations are eventually obtained, violating *(3)*. We might call these latter events *gray swans*, but other events are genuine black swans. In Chapters 9–12, we will ponder events that, based on common intuition, seem not only improbable, but completely impossible. Still other strange events are so ambiguous that we just cannot interpret them or even be sure they have actually occurred.

Suppose a coin is tossed 100 times; what are the probabilities of obtaining a certain number of heads? If the coin is fair, we may again consider the sample space to find the probability of obtaining, let's say, 55 or more heads. The theoretical probability density function for this coin-tossing process is shown in the upper part of Figure 8–2, a *normal distribution* (the so-called bell curve) with a mean and expected value of 50 heads and a *standard deviation* of 5 heads, the latter providing a measure of the spread (width) of the normal distribution. The extreme ends of probability density functions, called their *tails*, are of special

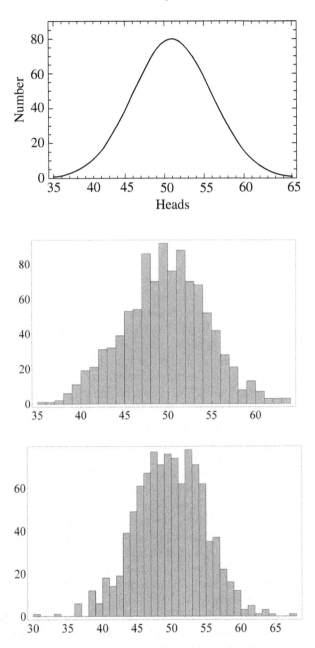

Figure 8–2   (Upper) The normal distribution with total area under the curve equal to 1,000. (Middle and Lower) Histograms based on two computer simulations of coin tosses: 1,000 blocks, each consisting of 100 tosses. The vertical coordinate shows the number of times that a certain number of heads (horizontal axis) was obtained.[10]

Table 8–1   Probability of Obtaining X +1 or More Heads When Tossing a Coin 100 Times If the Single Toss Probability Is *p*

X heads	p = 0.5	p = 0.6
50	0.460	0.973
55	0.136	0.821
60	0.018	0.462
70	1.6×10^{-5}	0.015
80	1.4×10^{-10}	5.9×10^{-6}
90	1.7×10^{-18}	3.8×10^{-12}
95	3.2×10^{-24}	5.4×10^{-17}

interest to us. The theoretical probability of obtaining X or more heads is equal to the area under the curve to the right of the X coordinate, divided by the area under the entire curve. Technically, the area under any probability density curve should equal 1, indicating *some* outcome must occur, but here I have multiplied probabilities (vertical axis) by 1,000 to match the following computer simulations. The two lower images are histograms based on two computer experiments, in each case tossing a "coin" 100,000 times and counting the number of heads in 1,000 batches of 100 tosses each.

As we are especially interested in rare events, I include Table 8–1, showing the theoretical probability of obtaining more than a certain number of heads for a fair coin (2nd column) and a loaded coin having a 0.6 chance of coming up heads on each throw (3rd column). For a fair coin, the probability of obtaining more than 60 heads (61 or more heads) in 100 tosses is 1.8%. But if the single toss probability is just a little higher, say 0.6, the probability of 61 or more heads improves dramatically to 46.2%.

The mathematical probability and psychology of rare events can be demonstrated with the coin toss metaphor. Imagine gambling in a private home or casino; you place bets on coin tosses but win less than 40% of the time after a large number of bets. How do you interpret this outcome? Maybe you decide that it's just a case of bad luck. But suppose your winning rate is only 30%; with 100 bets the likelihood of luck this bad is around 1 in 100,000. Maybe it's time to become suspicious; the gambling environment may not be what it seems. Your original theoretical probability estimates may be worse than useless, providing far too much false confidence. This little story illustrates the *fat tail fallacy*, caused by placing too much confidence in the skinny tails of the normal distribution, located at several standard deviations from the mean. Genuine (as opposed to model) processes often follow distributions with much fatter tails, a feature not always appreciated until the unexpected appearance of black or gray swans. In the financial markets, option pricing employs the normal distribution with standard deviations (called *implied volatility* in Wall Street lingo) based on option prices paid in free markets; fat tails can provide special money-making (and losing) opportunities.

Rare events happen all the time. Shuffle a deck of cards and deal all 52, obtaining an unremarkable sequence like 8♣, 4♦, Q♦, K♥, A♣, ... I call this ordering "unremarkable," but the probability of obtaining this or any other particular sequence of all 52 cards is actually 10^{-68}, a fantastically rare occurrence. Suppose, on the other hand, that a friend deals A♥, 2♥, 3♥, ...K♥...with the other suits also in order, a sequence apparently having the same small probability of 10^{-68}. Your likely explanation would be that your friend forgot to shuffle a brand new deck, or perhaps he purposely switched decks while you were distracted, the magician's trick. Both sequences have the same apparent probability, but only the second, involving something very special about the sequence pattern, is deemed unusual. We will run into similar arguments when considering the small probability of a universe coming into existence that is able to produce carbon-based life in Chapter 9. A burning question for cosmologists as well as the rest of us is: *Did something or someone stack the deck?*

In my first full-time postgraduate job, I was pressured to join a lunchtime bridge game when the engineering group's fanatical bridge cabal was desperate for a fourth player. Early on, to my astonishment, I obtained a hand with 11 hearts out of 13 cards. Note that the probability of obtaining 11 or more cards of the same suit in a bridge hand is about one in ten million. My crazy bidding (from one spade directly to six hearts) elicited much eye rolling and open disgust among the crusty bridge veterans—until someone caustically pointed out that I had mistakenly picked up the discards from an earlier hand. The idealized probability estimate was shown to be way off the mark once this critical information was revealed; a gray swan event had occurred. Evidently I was branded an incompetent bridge player; I was not invited back to the game.

4. DETERMINISM AND CHANCE

Accurate estimates of future events often rely on scientific knowledge. Every year in La Jolla, California, a "watermelon queen" drops a watermelon from the seventh floor of UCSD's Urey Hall, a tradition initiated by a physics professor in 1965 while I was a graduate student. Students hope to break the "splat record" for the horizontal extent of debris created in the plaza below. How accurately can one predict the watermelon's future? Impact speed can be predicted quite accurately. If the watermelon were dropped from a height of 50 feet, the probability of its impact velocity lying between 50 and 57 feet per second is high; the main uncertainty being air resistance effects, especially if spinning about different watermelon axes occurs. Rare (black swan) events like watermelon-on-swan air collisions have not been reported. Estimating the probability that the diameter of the splat is, let's say, in the range of 150 to 200 feet is much more difficult, but still well within the province of physics. But, as the time interval from the initial drop of the watermelon increases, more uncertainty becomes evident. What, for example, is the probability that more than 50 seeds will be eaten by birds within 20 minutes of the drop? Such questions bring in issues of environmental boundary conditions, say the numbers of birds and humans nearby, ignored for earlier stages of this process. But even with perfect knowledge of boundary and initial conditions, our ability to predict the watermelon's future, even in controlled experiments, is quite limited.

Useful predictions in complex systems are likely to be statistical in nature. The interrelation of theory and practice is illustrated by attempts to make money in a casino by predicting the final state of a roulette system, given the initial position and velocity of the ball relative to the spinning wheel. This problem is evidently too complex and/or chaotic for prediction of the exact slot in which the ball will fall. Full accuracy is not required to earn money, however. A statistical prediction that some slots are better bets than others will do the job, for example by eliminating just one-quarter of the slots as bad bets on each run. In his book *The Eudemonic Pie. Or Why Would Anyone Play Roulette Without a Computer in His Shoe?*, Thomas Bass tells of a group of hippie graduate students living in a commune in Santa Cruz, California in the 1970s who developed small computers designed to fit a player's shoe.[3] Many members of this "chaos cabal" worked on this project for no pay, receiving only a share of putative future profits, a slice of the so-called "eudemonic pie." The ball's initial conditions were signaled to the player with the special shoe by a second player. The computer was apparently moderately successful, although beset by technical problems in the casino environment. Several members of the group later became prominent in complex systems and chaos theory; apparently some also made money on Wall Street.

The interrelated concepts of *determinism* and *reductionism* require special scrutiny in our consciousness studies. Determinism applied to physical or biological systems refers to the position that every event is causally determined by a chain of prior events, implying that at any instant there is exactly one physically possible future. Classical physics is sometimes interpreted this way, but this interpretation is highly misleading. All physical, biological, and social systems have boundaries. The rectangular box on the left side of Figure 8–3

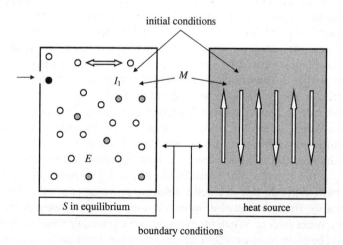

Figure 8–3   Small-scale entities E interact according to rules I_n within a confined boundary to produce macroscopic properties M at molecular (left) and fluid (right) scales.

might represent a living cell; the behaviors of its complex molecules depend on the interaction rules I as well as the properties of the membrane forming the cell boundary. If the box represents a microwave oven, the cooking process depends partly on the interactions of the electromagnetic field with inner walls. To analyze any system, *boundary conditions* must be specified. System dynamics also depends on *initial conditions*; in the molecular example, this includes the locations and velocities of each molecule when the analysis begins.

The rules of interaction between system elements might be simply modeled but could actually be quite complicated, especially if the "elements" themselves consist of complex subsystems, say, structures forming a nested hierarchy. For example, the box might represent a chicken coop, with the different shaded circles indicating the resident chickens and several kinds of feed available from holes in the wall. For purposes of simplifying the argument, suppose the chicken interaction rules I are well known; chicken dynamics still depends of where the chickens are placed when the food is first introduced, the time since their last feeding, and so forth, the initial conditions. Chicken behavior also depends on wall locations of the feed sources, the boundary conditions. The issues of boundary and initial conditions resurface several times in our various approaches to consciousness as in the example of fluid convection in the tank shown on the right side of Figure 8–3.

Consider a room full of air containing oxygen and nitrogen molecules (white and gray circles) as indicated on the left side of Figure 8–3. Suppose a single molecule of ammonia (black circle) is injected into the room. Let's make the idealized, but unrealistic, assumption of near perfect knowledge of all rules of interaction between the different molecules, I_1, I_2, and so forth for each interaction. Whereas typical *models* of molecular interaction may be relatively simple, genuine interactions are quite complicated. Consider the following fundamental question of determinism. Using our fastest computer, what can we say about the location of the ammonia molecule several seconds after injection in the upper left corner? The answer is essentially *nothing* except that it is still inside the room if the hole is closed immediately after injection.

The reason for our ignorance of the molecule's location is that with so many collisions between molecules, the trajectory errors in each collision accumulate very quickly, leading to exquisite *sensitivity to initial conditions*. This phrase means that tracking the black ball (the ammonia molecule) would require *exact* knowledge of the initial locations and velocities of all molecules, as well as their internal vibrational states.[4] In addition, we would require perfect knowledge of the rules of interaction for collisions between the air or ammonia molecules and the vibrating molecules forming the room walls (the boundary conditions), also a practical impossibility. Accuracy to a hundred decimal places will not do; our knowledge must be exact, again a practical impossibility. *Contrary to the belief of some, the classical behavior of complex systems is not predictable.* We cannot track the motion of the ammonia molecule, not even "in principle," if we limit this label to natural (not supernatural) scientists and their computers.

This failure of determinism at microscopic scales does not prevent us from explaining important macroscopic properties M of the air system S in terms of molecular dynamics. Our science (classical statistical mechanics and the kinetic theory of gases) predicts that, if the system is in equilibrium, molecular speeds will follow a *normal distribution*, as shown in Figure 8–2. From this curve we can estimate the number of molecules moving in any direction between any range of speeds, say between 900 and 1,000 miles per hour in the horizontal direction. If the gas is in *equilibrium*, this number does not change with time or location in the room, even though each individual molecule undergoes rapid ongoing changes in both velocity and location. But, the system's statistical properties do not require that we know anything about the location of any particular molecule E. An important caveat is that statistical theory may make erroneous predictions, for example, that some molecules are moving faster than light speed (in non relativistic theory) or that velocity distributions for molecules near the walls are unaltered by wall effects. Our statistical theory is only an approximation, albeit a very good one in many applications. We can, for example, gain a deeper understanding of macroscopic air properties M—pressure, temperature, sound speed, and viscosity—in terms of the statistical properties of the molecules E.

The exquisite sensitivity to initial conditions, boundary conditions, and interaction rules I demonstrated in Figure 8–3 were known features of *complex systems* long before the relatively recent interest in *chaos*, even if this sensitivity was not fully appreciated by all scientists and philosophers.[4] Although several overlapping definitions are found in the literature, here I define a complex system simply as one with many interactions I between many components E (*many degrees of freedom* or *high dimensional*). Some may complain that I have omitted the requirement of nonlinearity; my response is that this adjective is typically redundant since nearly all genuine systems are ultimately nonlinear if treated with sufficient accuracy. Sensitivity to initial conditions has more recently come to be popularly known as the *butterfly effect*, so called because of a presentation given by meteorologist Edward Lorenz entitled *Predictability: Does the Flap of a Butterfly's Wings in Brazil set off a Tornado in Texas?*[5]

Chaos, often referred to as *deterministic chaos*, refers to the generation of (initially) unpredictable behavior from simple nonlinear interaction rules, typically expressed in terms of mathematical equations. The rules have no built-in noise or randomness; however, repeated application of the rules can lead to rich emergent patterns or structures in time, space, or both. The adjective "deterministic" tells us something about the mind-sets of the mathematicians who favor it. Deterministic chaos is perfectly repeatable in computer simulations if the computer is provided *perfect* knowledge of the initial conditions, boundary conditions, and interaction rules. The rich patterns of chaos that are unpredictable on in the first computer run are perfectly predictable on all subsequent runs. But wait! Perfect initial conditions and so forth are impossible in genuine systems. Thus, in genuine science so-called "deterministic chaos" must refer to systems that exhibit non deterministic behavior in genuine experiments. But when *simulated* with perfect initial conditions, boundary conditions, and interaction rules, computer solutions of the same systems exhibit deterministic chaos. This confusing terminology evidently reflects the mathematician's tendency to downplay the critical distinction between genuine physical systems and mathematical models of these systems. In my humble opinion, this kind of thinking lies at the core of much sloppy engineering and science. One way to look at the difference between a computer simulation with perfect initial conditions and a genuine experiment is that the former assumes a *supernatural observer* of the physical system. But here we are interested in real systems like the chicken soup with convection cells in Figure 8–3, heated and consumed by humans, rather than esoteric equations of soup consumed only by the gods.

Complex systems can sometimes act in a manner that is directly opposite that of simple (*low-dimensional*) chaotic systems. Complex systems containing many elements E may produce surprisingly simple patterns of organized macroscopic behavior M. By contrast, chaotic systems consisting of only a few elements E can produce unexpectedly rich and complicated dynamic behavior. Both kinds of systems exhibit sensitivity to initial conditions, but with complex systems we are often able to ignore initial conditions due to our focus on statistical and large-scale behavior. Brains, as highly complex systems, can be expected to cover a wide spectrum of dynamic behavior, ranging from the relatively simple to the very complex in various brain states, at different scales of observation, or both. Fractal-like dynamics, in which each spatial scale exhibits its own characteristic behavior, is discussed in Chapters 4, 7, and 12.

5. TWO EXAMPLES OF OUR LIMITED KNOWLEDGE: VITAMIN C AND PARAPSYCHOLOGY

Here I consider two areas that lie within the province of scientific study but are nevertheless sufficiently problematic to demonstrate classical limits on our understanding of complex systems. Such limits have superficial similarities to but also deep fundamental differences from the quantum ignorance discussed in Chapters 10–12. The so-called *common cold* refers to contagious infections caused by any of several hundred different viruses. Vitamin C has long been promoted in its prevention and treatment, notably by Linus Pauling in a long war with mainstream medical science. Several dozen clinical trials over the past 30 years have mostly failed to show clear vitamin C benefits; for many scientists, the war is over and Pauling has lost. From a broader perspective, however, we must not forget that genuine science approaches truth as a series of successive approximations, never claiming that final and complete accuracy has been achieved. This view is especially pertinent to (notoriously complex) living systems, suggesting possible undiscovered nuanced effects of vitamin C. The probability of benefits from large doses of vitamin C may be low, but it is certainly not identically zero. Given this background, I address a basic practical choice based on limited information: *When I get a scratchy throat, should I take vitamin C?* Consider a conceptual framework based on the following information.

- Through natural selection, the *simians* (higher primates, including humans) have lost their ability to synthesize vitamin C, which must be consumed in diets to avoid the serious disease *scurvy*.

- Most simians consume vitamin C in amounts at least 10 times higher than the 50 to 100 milligrams normally recommended by governments for humans.
- Goats, as vitamin C–producing animals, reportedly synthesize more than 13 grams per day in normal conditions and more under stress. Trauma, including smoking, has also been reported to deplete vitamin C in humans.
- Toxic effects of vitamin C below 2 grams per day (or even much higher) are very rare in humans.

Next consider possible experimental limitations of the clinical trials.

- Individuals may respond differently; vitamin C may help Joe but not Bill.
- Different cold viruses may respond differently.
- Vitamin C might inhibit progression from viral to bacterial infections, but this may occur too infrequently to show up in trials.
- Some other effects may occur that no one has thought of.

With these ideas in mind, when I get a scratchy throat, I take one or two grams of vitamin C per day until I feel well again. Large, regular doses of vitamin C may cause slightly increased health risks, say for development of kidney stones, so I limit extra doses to short periods. The critical factor is this—there seems to be no known downside to short periods of high dosage; even a 1% chance of benefit seems justified since the risk–reward ratio is apparently near zero. Sometimes I get full-blown cold symptoms, but sometimes I am well by the next day. Was the extra vitamin C beneficial to me in any of these scratchy throat events? I don't expect ever to know the answer; I just keep my vitamin C in a little jar marked *placebos* as a reminder of my ignorance. *When dealing with complex systems, even good science has substantial limitations.*

Now I am going to open a huge (and ugly for many) can of worms by raising the issue of parapsychology (*psi*) research. A possible psi definition might refer to anomalous processes of energy or information transfer that are currently unexplained in terms of known scientific processes. But this definition seems inadequate as it could have been construed to include chaotic events before their scientific basis was discovered. Engineers have long been familiar with manifestations of chaos known in the trade as *glitches*, causing *factors of safety* or *fudge factors* to be adopted in system design. Historically, however, psi refers to phenomena lying well outside the normal boundaries of science, areas like extrasensory perception or telepathy. Subjective judgment is in play here; when does a glitch become a potential psi event? Only controlled and repeatable experiments can address this question.

Right at this moment, I am experiencing "precognition"—*my mental crystal ball shows a slice of the future—scientific colleagues gnashing their teeth as they read this.* I introduce parapsychology to this book with some reluctance, but my avowed aim of quantifying speculative ideas demands at least a cursory look. Let me first say unequivocally that I don't take psi-related accounts in the popular press seriously; they seem to consist of unwarranted conclusions, wishful thinking, or outright fraud, the antithesis of good science or rational thinking. But I am also skeptical of scientists or non scientists who make brash public statements that no scientific evidence for psi exists or absurd claims that psi is impossible. How do the skeptics know? Have they studied the literature or participated in every psi experiment? Just what scientific principle prohibits psi? I *can* say that *I* know of no unequivocal evidence for psi, but then I have never attempted a comprehensive review of the field. A few additional psi observations are thus:

- Repeatability of experiments is the hallmark of good science, but this ideal is often difficult to achieve in complex systems. As more experiments are repeated, confidence in the outcome increases in a series of successive approximations. If this is exceptionally difficult or even impossible to achieve in psi experiments, it doesn't prove that psi is not real, just much less likely to be real.
- Good experimental design is typically very difficult in the absence of a solid conceptual framework supporting the phenomenon to be observed. While quantum effects have been proposed, they provide, at best, only vague hints of possible theoretical bases for psi.
- The mainstream science literature includes many poorly designed experiments, so guilt by association with poorly designed psi studies should not automatically disqualify *all* psi studies.
- If psi were proved to exist, I would find it no more astounding than several established features of relativity and quantum mechanics. No known scientific principle prohibits most psi.
- Scientists "brave" (foolhardy?) enough to engage in psi research risk having their credibility destroyed, especially if their psi reports are positive.
- Unequivocal validation of psi might open the door for a whole host of nonsense to gain even more credibility, potentially a substantial setback, not only for legitimate science, but for all rational thinking. This fear probably accounts for much of the scientific hostility to psi research.

I neither endorse nor disclaim large-dose vitamin C usage or psi phenomena; rather, my goal is brutal honesty about just what we know and don't know and what we may never know. The experimental design and repeatability issues raised in the first two bullet points above are interrelated with the falsifiability issue raised in Chapter 7 and warrant further discussion in a general context. My own experience with experimental EEG has surely been duplicated widely in many studies of complex systems, especially our human subjects who are rarely simpletons. Suppose result X_A is obtained at laboratory A, but a different result X_B is found at laboratory B in the (apparently) identical experiment. Genuine experiments require many little trade-offs dictated by practical considerations like limited financial resources, disparate skills of laboratory personnel, and so forth. Experimental scientists attempt to finesse such trade-offs so that critical results are independent of such compromises. But when experiments are not repeatable across laboratories, closer examination of the trade-offs is required.

At this critical step, some conceptual framework (whether explicit or implicit) must be employed to identify offending methods so that modified designs may yield repeatable experiments. Thus, in genuine experimental science, repeatability and falsifiability are not absolute. Rather, they are idealized goals; the closer the ideals are approached, the stronger our belief in the ideas being tested. Science advances most rapidly through a happy marriage of experiment to theory. With just a few parts of a tentative theory or conceptual framework in place, better experiments are carried out, followed by additions to or modifications of the original framework, and so forth. Science progresses through a series of successive approximations in this manner; at no point can we say that final and complete accuracy has been achieved.

6. REDUCTIONISM

Consider the reductionist idea that chemistry is just applied physics, biology is just applied chemistry, and so forth. Figure 8–4 shows part of the *nested hierarchy of matter*. *Electrons* and *quarks* are fundamental particles; as far as is known, they cannot be broken down into smaller units, but I will have more to say on this in Chapter 10. The word "particle" is somewhat misleading here; electrons are shadowy entities that behave like waves in some experiments and particles in others, and they have no macroscopic analogs in the world of human observers. Also, it appears that quarks cannot be isolated, and they come only in groups of two or three. *Neutrons* consist of two *down quarks* and one *up quark*; *protons* of two up quarks and one down quark, where the adjectives "up" and "down" are just labels for a fundamental microscopic property with no macroscopic analogs.

All ordinary matter is composed of *elements*, substances consisting of one kind of *atom*. Atoms are composed of protons and neutrons in a central nucleus

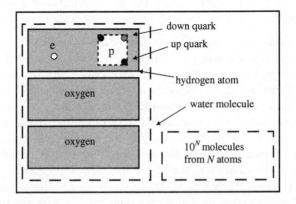

Figure 8–4   The nested hierarchy of matter at several small scales.

surrounded by electrons in outer shells. Different elements are distinguished by their number of protons; hydrogen has one proton, helium has two, gold has 64, uranium has 92, up to the last known stable element number 101. The atoms of a single element having different numbers of neutrons are called *isotopes*; for example, common hydrogen has no neutrons; its isotopes deuterium and tritium have one and two neutrons, respectively.

Figure 8–4 depicts the nested hierarchy of matter on four levels of elementary particles, atoms, and molecules. Mathematician and neuroscientist Al Scott has estimated the number of theoretically possible distinct molecules[6]. The number of atoms is 95, excluding the noble gases that rarely react with other atoms; *valence* is a measure of the number of chemical bonds that may be formed by each atom. Al's estimate of the maximum possible number of distinct molecules formed from N atoms is $95^{N/2}$, or roughly 10^N for our purposes. The molecules of living cells, the proteins, DNA, and so forth may contain thousands of atoms, but even if N is limited to a relatively small number of atoms, say 100, the number of possible distinct molecules is more than 10^{100}. To get a feeling for the enormity of this number, imagine a mass containing just a single molecule of each kind; this mass could barely be squeezed into the volume of the known universe (after borrowing molecules from other universes). By contrast, the number of known distinct molecules is only about 10^7. A mass consisting of just one molecule of each kind would fit on the head of a pin. By contrast to provocative phrases like "end of science" and "theory of everything" sometimes appearing in the science press, we can expect that chemistry will exist as a separate and developing field as long as there is intelligent life to study it.

Scientists know of nothing in chemistry that is inconsistent with quantum mechanics and have recruited selected aspects of quantum theory to better understand chemical bonds. But the rules governing chemical behavior were developed at the same level (spatial scale) as human observations of these phenomena. We should also not forget the critical roles of boundary and initial conditions in any dynamic system including chemicals in solution. One can say that the laws of quantum mechanics are more "fundamental" than those of chemistry, but this may be a rather a hollow sentiment for a practicing chemical engineer. Once a molecular property is known, scientists can rationalize this property in terms of quantum theory; however, we have no realistic chance of accurately simulating, let's say, protein molecules bottom-up from fundamental quantum mechanics, not in practice, apparently not even in principle.

As the higher levels of nested hierarchy are crossed from molecule to cell, organ system, human, and social system, arguments of increasing complexity apply. Consider the human brain containing about 10^{11} or so nerve cells or *neurons*. Each neuron contains perhaps 10^5 distinct protein molecules and numerous copies of each kind, a total of something like 10^{10} protein molecules. As discussed in Chapter 4, the brain's outer wrapping, the *cerebral cortex*, has roughly the thickness of a five-cent coin (3 mm) and contains about 10^{10} neurons. Up several levels in the cortex's nested hierarchy are the cortical *macrocolumns*; each one contains 10^5 to 10^6 neurons. At the macrocolumn scale, the cortex is interconnected by both nearest neighbor and non-local fibers. On average, each macrocolumn is connected to perhaps 10^4 other macrocolumns; that is, 10% of full interconnectedness. If for purposes of argument, we make the (wildly oversimplified) assumption that different humans are distinguished only by their macrocolumn connection patterns, we can estimate the total number of humans possible having this basic brain structure. Using the binomial theorem of statistics, the estimate is $10^{14,115}$, enough to fill many, many universes with sane and crazy people.

Some supporters of strong (autistic) reductionism imply that computer technology will eventually solve the enormous barriers of crossing hierarchical levels from the bottom up. One way to address this issue is to estimate fundamental limits on future computer technology. Computer speeds are measured in *floating point operations per second* (*FLOPS*). A hand calculator may operate at 10 *FLOPS*; your desktop computer may operate a billion times faster at 10^{10} FLOPS. Today's fastest supercomputers operate near 10^{15} FLOPS. The physics literature contains several ideas about fundamental limits on computer speed, including esoteric quantum computation using black holes. With such arguments, MIT professor and self-described "quantum mechanic" Seth Lloyd has suggested a limit of 10^{105} FLOPS, presented as a fundamental barrier based on an imagined ultimate computer composed of all the energy and matter in the universe. If we imagine this "computer-verse" computing continuously from the origin of the big bang to the present day, the computer will have performed "only" 10^{122} operations. While I haven't attempted estimates of required computational power, Lloyd's ideas suggest to me that crossing even one major level in the hierarchy of matter using "bottom-up" brute force computer calculations can probably never be accomplished, not *in practice*, not even *in principle*. Again, we are interested in "principles" that govern natural processes observed by humans, not magic created by supernatural beings. This limitation does not, however, prevent science from establishing properties at some macroscopic level (based on experiments at the same level) and later obtaining a deeper understanding of the origins of these properties at lower levels, as in the example of chemical bonds based on quantum mechanics.

7. ARE CONSCIOUS COMPUTERS DESTINED FOR OUR FUTURE?

During the Second World War, mathematician Alan Turing, often described as the father of modern computer science, contributed to the breaking of German codes for British intelligence, an accomplishment of enormous military significance. After the war, British authorities rewarded Turing with a prize: criminal prosecution for homosexual acts with his partner (illegal at the time in both Britain and the US), forcing him to undergo estrogen treatments to avoid prison. He died shortly after, apparently of self-inflicted cyanide poisoning.

The so-called *Turing Test* employs two sealed rooms, one occupied by a human and the other by a computer. Typed questions are sent to both rooms and answers received on a monitor. If, after a very large number of answers have been received from both rooms, the scientist cannot tell which room holds the computer, Turing proposed that the computer should be regarded as having "human-level intelligence." Although some have interpreted this as a consciousness test, this was apparently not Turing's view, nor is it mine. Attributes that Turing and his contemporaries cited as distinguishing computer zombies from genuinely conscious computers include: appreciation of music based on emotions felt, writing papers and understanding what was written, feeling pleasure with success, being made miserable by failures, friendliness with humans (or at least computer peers), making moral judgments, falling in love, and generally exhibiting a wide diversity of human-like behavior.

Some think that conscious computers are just around the corner, basing arguments partly on the rapid growth of computer accomplishments, duplicating human expertise in many areas—prescribing drugs, diagnosing equipment malfunctions, recognizing speech, and so forth. Some scientists and philosophers support a so-called *computational theory of the mind* in which brains process symbols, and thought is a kind of computation. In this view, objections to techno-optimistic predictions reflect mere "tissue chauvinism," perhaps a mistaken belief that only living tissue, not electronics, can operate the "software" necessary to produce consciousness. My first problem with this so-called "theory" is that "computation" seems quite ill defined. An analog computer is just a dynamic system with controlled inputs and the means to read outputs. Many physicists view the evolution of the universe as a giant computation best described in terms of ongoing information exchange. If "computation" is generally defined in terms of information exchange, then the *computational theory of the mind* may be trivially true, a tautology. One problem with such "mind theory" is that the labels "information" and "computer" can mask critical hidden assumptions about the nature of consciousness. We will return to this topic in Chapter 12, where I adopt the labels *ordinary information* and *ordinary computer* to indicate the everyday use of these terms, normal entities viewed as subsets of proposed broader categories, *Ultra-Information* and *Ultra-Computer*.

My colleague Lester Ingber has developed a genuine multiscale computational brain model based on real physiology and anatomy. In this view, small-scale dynamic patterns of local neural activity might be viewed as "symbols" associated with digital processing, while at the same time, larger (columnar) scale dynamics can be thought of as analog processing.[7] Lester's work is consistent with the general conceptual framework advocated in this book: the large-scale brain dynamics recorded as EEG is viewed in terms of local "networks" (cell assemblies) *embedded* in global (holistic-cortical) synaptic action fields. Of course, the issue of whether any of this constitutes a genuine description of *mind* remains quite open.

Arguments concerning the computational theory of mind and physicalist views generally are presented in extensive writings by philosopher John Searle.[8] My colleague Ed Kelly (with coauthor Emily Kelly) provides a comprehensive review of mind/brain issues in the context of scientific psychology in *Irreducible*

Mind, beginning with the early works of F. W. H. Myers and William James.[9] Ed argues the case for a dualist-interactionist mind, in which brain structure and function support and interact with mind but are insufficient to *create* mind. In this view, an appropriate brain metaphor is a kind of antenna/filter system that selectively interacts with some sort of external entity. I will return to this issue in Chapter 12 to speculate on the possible existence of an entity called *Mind*, one of the proposed subcategories of *Ultra-Information*.

I have repeatedly characterized the brain as a complex adaptive system in which interactions across spatial scales constitute an essential feature. Some assume (implicitly or otherwise) that matching this complexity with an artificial system can be accomplished in a robot with perhaps 10^{11} interacting elements mimicking the number of brain neurons in some way. Yet as discussed in Section 6, each neuron is itself a very complex system with 10^{10} or so interacting molecules, and each molecule is a smaller-scale complex system. Scientists produce physical or computer models of complex systems, but these models may be only hollow representations of genuine systems. It is not even clear that science will soon be able to produce a fully accurate electronic model of the pot of soup with convection cells in Figure 8–3, much less a primitive brain. So when it is implied that brains can be replaced by "equivalent" electronic structures, I would challenge the assumption of equivalency, which seems to be largely unsupported. I pose the following alternate conjecture—creation of artificial consciousness may require FULLY *accurate* simulations of tissue, including cross-scale interactions, possibly even down to sub electron scales as discussed in Chapters 10–12. If this is so and the fundamental limits on computer power discussed in Section 6 are valid, *creation of artificial consciousness may not be physically possible, even if the computational theory of mind is (in some sense) correct.*

The world's first general-purpose computer was tagged ENIAC for *electronic numerical integrator and calculator*. Completed in 1945, it weighed 30 tons and filled a large room. In a widely circulated joke of the day, engineers posed a question to the computer, *Is there a God?* After several tense minutes, a card was ejected that read, *There is NOW!* Computer algorithms able to convince many observers that they are indeed conscious may be close to development, but perhaps we should employ the same skepticism as we do with ENIAC's fanciful claim. Zombies may soon be among us! As technology advances, *x-zombies* could become progressively more persuasive with their *zombie denials*, challenging our (perhaps) very primitive ideas about the actual origins of consciousness.

8. THE SPECIAL ROLE OF MATHEMATICS IN SCIENCE

What has mathematics to do with consciousness? Several answers are apparent—mathematical models can provide tentative explanations for experimental brain electric field patterns closely associated with the conscious state. Mathematics is also central to building imaging machines and the analysis of data. But, in this section I aim to discuss the special place of mathematics in science generally, especially its role in building bridges between scientific minds that would otherwise be far more isolated.

My attempts to settle on a suitable definition that encompasses all of "mathematics" have not succeeded too well, which is not surprising based on my interactions with mathematician colleagues over the years. A common response to questions about something that might qualify as genuine mathematics is a statement like, "Oh no, that's not mathematics, its just X" (fill in the blank here with arithmetic, statistics, physics, or some other field of implied lower status). Perhaps *non mathematics* is like pornography as viewed by former U.S. Supreme Court Justice Potter Stewart, "It's hard to define, but I know it when I see it." Such views originate with the aesthetics and elegance of mathematics; it has both artistic and scientific features. If pornography is sex without love, perhaps non mathematics consists of organized symbols without beauty. Physics involves statements that are simultaneously true and false as emphasized by complementarity; mathematics consists of statements that are considered absolutely true. Regardless of the definition, even an outsider like me can appreciate the deep beauty of genuine mathematics.

For our purposes, one clarifying feature is the distinction between pure and applied mathematics. Pure mathematics is an end in itself; applied mathematics is used as a tool. The designer of a fancy power saw finds fulfillment with his creation. The carpenter may also appreciate the saw's aesthetics but is more interested in how well it cuts lumber. Applied mathematics is the principal language of the physical sciences and engineering and its most powerful tool. In 1960, the physicist Eugene Wigner wrote his famous essay *The Unreasonable Success of Mathematics in the Natural Sciences*. To resolve part of the mystery of this success, Wigner emphasizes that mathematics allows us to string together a series of logical steps without adding cumulative errors along the way.

The success of mathematics in science also has much to do with efficiency of communication between scientists. If I express a subtle idea to a colleague in English or another non mathematical language, there is excellent potential for misinterpretation. My colleague's brain is likely to add or subtract something important based on his past experiences, and as a result, we may develop only a fuzzy *mind meld*. By contrast, mathematical steps have precise meanings; we mostly avoid questions analogous to "Is your experience of the color red different from mine?" I have observed several humorous interactions between scientists in disparate fields, in which both sides appear clueless that identical words have quite different meanings to the two sides. Perhaps interactions between mathematicians and medical scientists provide the best examples of this kind of farce, which Shakespeare would have appreciated immensely.

Mathematics opens wide the communication channels to both living and dead, and the dead have many good stories to tell us. We can learn much by looking deep into the minds of dead mathematicians. Philosophers argue extensively over the precise meaning of language; much discussion is directed to the published writings of historical figures. In the legal field, new court decisions are often based on the perceived intent in the minds of judges long dead. What did America's founding fathers really mean by "involuntary servitude" in the U.S. Constitution, and how does their intent influence the constitutionality of a military draft? Consider the non mathematical publications of Newton's contemporaries on the topics "energy," "momentum," and "force." I have found it nearly impossible to make sense of this material; it not only lacks beauty, it's truly messy. But, between the time of Newton and the late 19th century time of Maxwell and his famous equations, much of ugliness of earlier physics was transformed into mathematical beauty. Our modern understanding of the works of mathematicians and physicists from the latter part of this period is excellent.

The precision of mathematics allows us to combine distinct scientific ideas in a strikingly efficient and practical way, as demonstrated by a simple equation. Note to readers—don't freak out on me here—if you don't speak mathematics, don't worry; you can easily follow the essentials of the argument. The basic *conservation equation* is

$$\nabla \cdot \mathbf{J} + \frac{\partial \rho}{\partial t} = 0 \tag{8.2}$$

This equation says "del dot $\mathbf{J}$ plus the partial derivative of rho (ρ) with respect to t equals zero". The two symbols $\nabla \cdot$ form a mathematical operator, which is simply a *rule* to be applied to the symbol just to its right (in this case, $\mathbf{J}$). This operation involves rates of change in space of the vector $\mathbf{J}$, while the term following the plus sign is a time rate of change of the scalar variable ρ. The equation is expressed in terms of the vectors ∇ and $\mathbf{J}$ (as indicated by the boldface) rather than their components along the axes of some coordinate system. This vector feature is critical because natural laws must be independent of human choices of coordinate system; any proposed new coordinate-dependent law would be rejected immediately.

To see what this equation means physically, consider Figure 8–5 showing, let's say, a 1 cubic centimeter box containing a bunch of tiny (sub millimeter scale) balls that go in and out of the box through all six faces by some process that need not concern us. We apply the basic idea of calculus to shrink the box (and balls) to an arbitrarily small size. In this case, ρ is the density of balls inside the box at any time, measured in, let's say, balls per cubic centimeter. The symbol $\mathbf{J}$ stands for the net *flux* of balls through the six faces of the box, typically measured in balls per square centimeter per second. The conservation equation then tells us that by counting all the balls that go into and out of the box every second, we can determine the resulting increase or decrease of ball density inside the box. If more balls are going in than are going out, there will be an inevitable build-up of balls in the box. But, this result is trivially obvious! Why do we need an equation at all; why not just use the words to describe this intuitively obvious process? The answer is that Equation 8.2 may be conveniently modified to describe cases where balls are not conserved, combined with other equations to produce a robust conceptual framework, suggest new experiments, and predict experimental results.

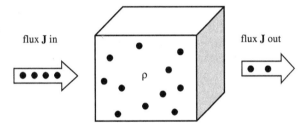

Figure 8–5   The net flux **J** of some entity into a "box" with instantaneous entity density ρ.

Equation 8.2 restricts the behavior of anything that is "conserved," anything that cannot be created or destroyed inside the box. When ρ is charge density and **J** is current density, this equation says that charge must be conserved. When ρ is radiation energy density and **J** is radiation flux, we have a statement of the conservation of radiation energy in empty space. Both of these relations are implicit within Maxwell's famous equations of electrodynamics. When ρ is mass density, and **J** is the flux of mass, for example in the case of air flow, the flux is just given by $\mathbf{J} = \rho\mathbf{v}$, where **v** is air velocity, and we have a statement of the law of mass conservation.

Our basic conservation equation (Eq. 8.2) may be conveniently modified to describe systems in which the "balls" (mass, charge, energy, and so forth) are not conserved. Consider, for example, cooking a potato in a microwave oven. Although total energy is conserved, radiation energy is not conserved inside the oven because some radiation energy is converted in the potato to heat. Equation 8.2 may then be modified to read

$$\nabla \cdot \mathbf{J} + \frac{\partial \rho}{\partial t} + potato\ heating\ term = 0 \qquad (8.3)$$

This same conservation equation also occurs in quantum mechanics; the "balls" conserved in this case consist of a probability density function that predicts where a particle is most likely to be found at any particular time, to be discussed in Chapter 11.

9. THE "AS IF" CAVEAT

The discussion in Section 8 serves as a reminder that ordinary non mathematical language can be loaded with hidden assumptions and biases. I have attempted to expose some of this "mokita-like" (things we don't like to talk about) concealed bias inherent in labels like "in principle" and "deterministic chaos." In preparation for Chapters 9–12, I here add the "as if" caveat to this list.

A radio or TV transmitting station at some location X uses a voltage source to generate (coded) alternating current in a structural pattern of conductors called an *antenna*, thereby generating an electromagnetic field that becomes "detached" from X and propagates away in all unblocked directions. At a second location Y, this electromagnetic field induces current in the local antenna in the same frequency band(s). You jiggle your electrons at X, and my electrons at Y jiggle a little later in a predictable manner, even in empty space. If my radio, TV, or cell phone is tuned in, information is received. Einstein once described it thus—

> A wire telegraph is a kind of a very, very long cat. You pull his tail in New York and his head is meowing in Los Angeles... Radio operates exactly the same way: you send signals here, they receive them there. The only difference is there is no cat.

Einstein might have added that radio waves seemed to behave *as if* there really were a "cat" (a medium supporting the waves) until focused "cat searches" concluded that the cat is just space itself.

My antenna description implies that electromagnetic fields enjoy a genuine physical existence; otherwise I might have said that receiving antenna at Y behaves *as if* it were exposed to electromagnetic fields, leaving the issue open. This important distinction has its roots in 19th century physics, which focused for several decades on finding an underlying structure for electromagnetic fields. Many attempts were made to find the *ether*, the putative supporting structure; after all, sound waves, water waves, seismic waves, and so forth involve physical structures in motion, but experiments failed to reveal evidence for the ether. This outcome together with Einstein's special theory of relativity (1905) eventually forced the abandonment of the idea that electromagnetic fields require a physical medium in which to propagate. Science now regards electromagnetic fields as something much more profound than did the early physicists. Nevertheless, electromagnetic fields retain an abstract quality—*the fields are defined only in terms of the observable effects that they produce on charges and currents.* Such effects are accurately predicted by Maxwell's equations; furthermore, electromagnetic fields have energy, an *energy contained in the field itself.*

Practicing engineers normally regard the electromagnetic field as a real physical entity based largely on the incredible accuracy of Maxwell's equations in predicting the behavior of charges and currents in macroscopic systems. But this view can run up against serious barriers at microscopic scales. Einstein reaffirmed the validity of Maxwell's *wave* equations in his 1905 paper on special relativity. Paradoxically in the same year, he also published a paper offering a very *antiwave* explanation for the *photoelectric effect*: shine a light on a metal surface and electrons are emitted. Based on the wave nature of light, one would expect the kinetic energy of emitted electrons to depend on the *intensity* of light, which is proportional to the squared magnitude of the electromagnetic field, but this prediction is dead wrong. Einstein showed that the experimental observations of emitted electrons could be explained only if light were assumed to be composed of little packets of energy (now called *photons*), and that photon and emitted electron energies are proportional to wave *frequency*. Einstein's Nobel Prize in 1921 was awarded for this work on the photoelectric effect, not his works on relativity, which were more controversial at the time.

The photoelectric effect led scientists to adopt the concept of *wave–particle duality*, initially only with great reluctance, in which light and (later) particles with mass simultaneously possess the macroscopic properties of both waves and particles, each property manifested according to the experimental circumstances. Light and other electromagnetic fields can behave *as if* they are waves, or they can act *as if* they are particles; the wave and particle descriptions are complementary models of physical reality. How can this possibly be? If you find this idea difficult to grasp, take comfort in what Einstein said in 1954—

> All these fifty years of conscious brooding have brought me no nearer to the answer to the question, "What are light quanta?" Nowadays every Tom, Dick and Harry thinks he knows it, but he is mistaken.

In Chapters 9–12, we will encounter ghostlike fields and particles and "as if" caveats down just about every rabbit hole, and plenty of disagreement about just when this disclaimer is appropriate.

10. SUMMARY

In preparation for the strange ideas presented in Chapters 9–12, a spectrum of speculative ideas is considered here, employing probability as a measure of human ignorance. Failure to appreciate the critical distinction between the actual probability of an event, which we can never know, and the estimated probability based on past experience lies at the root of the *induction problem*. Rare events are labeled *gray* or *black swans* depending on whether or not accurate explanations are available after the events have occurred. The *fat tail fallacy* is due to placing too much confidence in the overskinny tails of probability distributions far from the mean. Genuine processes may follow distributions with much fatter tails, a feature not always appreciated until the unexpected appearance of black or gray swans. The benefits of vitamin C and paranormal phenomena are areas lying within the province of science but are sufficiently problematic to demonstrate our classical ignorance in preparation for the quantum ignorance of later chapters.

Science provides methods to predict the future, but predictions are severely limited in *complex systems* due to system sensitivity to initial conditions, boundary conditions, and interaction rules. This sensitivity was known long before the relatively recent interest in *chaos*, even if not fully appreciated by all scientists and philosophers. *Deterministic chaos* is perfectly repeatable in computer simulations if computers are provided perfect knowledge of all conditions, but perfect conditions are impossible in genuine systems. Thus, in science as opposed to mathematics, the tag "deterministic chaos" must refer to systems that actually exhibit non deterministic behavior in genuine experiments. In other words the so-called "determinism" can be experienced only by supernatural observers.

Crossing even one major level in the hierarchy of matter using "bottom-up" brute force computer calculations can probably never be accomplished, not *in practice*, not even *in principle*. If consciousness requires fully accurate simulations of tissue, including all cross-scale interactions, fundamental limits on computer power may forever preclude the creation of artificial consciousness even if, as assumed by many scientists, the brain actually does create the mind.

Mathematics consists of statements that are absolutely true; physics involves statements that are simultaneously both true and false. Mathematics allows stringing together logical steps without adding cumulative errors along the way. The success of mathematics in science also has much to do with efficiency of communication between scientists. Subtle ideas expressed in non mathematical languages are easily distorted or misinterpreted altogether.

Charge and mass are entities that act as "antennas" revealing the presence of electromagnetic and gravitational fields, respectively. Other kinds of fields, say the quantum wavefunction, also carry information but are not afforded the same physical status. Rather, some may say that quantum particles behave "as if" they were guided by the quantum field. For several kinds of fields, there is plenty of disagreement about whether or not the "as if" caveat is appropriate.

Chapter 9

Modern Physics, Cosmology, and Consciousness

1. WHAT HAS MODERN PHYSICS TO DO WITH CONSCIOUSNESS?

In the following chapters, I will characterize the mind/brain (hard) problem in rather stark terms: *Either the brain creates the mind, or the brain acts as kind of antenna that interacts selectively with some external entity,* the dualistic conjecture suggested on the right side of Figure 9–1. Many scientists reject dualism out of hand. As a scientist having spent his career studying relationships between EEG dynamics and mental states, my intuition also leans strongly towards the anti dualism position. Yet I also favor a frank admission of our profound ignorance of the origin of conscious awareness. It seems to me that this state of ignorance demands that dualism be accorded a close look using our best scientific tools. Chapters 9–12 will focus on my claim that serious attempts to address the profound enigma of consciousness must employ the full arsenal of modern scientific knowledge, including cosmology, relativity, quantum mechanics, and thermodynamics. Any one of these subjects is far too big for any one book; my modest goal here is to provide some of the flavor of the new ways of thinking demanded by modern physical science and their possible relevance to the hard problem of consciousness.

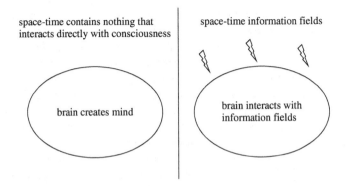

Figure 9–1   Two opposing views of the origins of consciousness.

The central question to be addressed in Chapters 9–12 is whether modern physics can shed light on the deep fundamental challenge of consciousness in a manner that is impossible using only classical concepts. For purposes of our discussion, I label the putative deep connection between relativity, quantum mechanics, thermodynamics, and consciousness, *the RQTC conjecture*, independent of the actual nature of any proposed connection. Many scientists and non scientists alike are quite skeptical of RQTC for compelling reasons; I fully appreciate the skeptical position, as it was my own view until a few years ago. Foremost to this skepticism is the fact that unequivocal empirical evidence for RQTC is lacking. Skeptics may suspect that the central motivation for RQTC is some vague notion that since quantum mechanics and consciousness are both mysterious, perhaps they are somehow related.[1]

Another suspicion of skeptics is that RQTC proponents are searching for ideas to support ingrained religious views. The skeptics raise valid points, but recent thoughts have moved me from RQTC skeptic to RQTC agnostic. Why I have I devoted four chapters to a topic on which I adopt an equivocal position? My reason is unequivocal—*If consciousness studies lie within the purview of legitimate scientific enquiry, RQTC must be considered seriously if only because classical physics cannot even begin to explain consciousness.* In broader terms, I have come to believe that the study of consciousness must be essentially a study of the nature of reality, and no serious thinker should doubt that modern physics deals with important aspects of physical reality. A number of scientists, notably Berkeley physicist Henry Stapp,[2] have long pointed to the following irony: Anti dualism is often promoted as the most "scientific" position, yet its supporting arguments are often mired in a world view based on 19th century science. A genuine scientific position is that serious studies of consciousness should be prepared employ a full complement of scientific tools, including relativity, quantum mechanics, and thermodynamics. This approach does not prejudge the relevance of such modern tools; it says only that we should give them a test run.

Cosmology is the study of the universe (or multiverse) and humanity's place within it, embracing the entire nested hierarchy of matter–elementary particles, atoms, molecules, living cells, brains, and social systems. As the universe aged, more complex structures evolved, including the huge furnaces known as *stars* that cooked the heavy elements required for life as we know it. Thus, one may argue that cosmology is every bit as relevant to the consciousness challenge as Darwinian evolution; it just addresses the dynamic processes leading to awareness on a longer time scale. To be more specific, physical cosmology is based on the three pillars of modern physics–relativity, quantum mechanics, and thermodynamics, but do these fields have anything to do with consciousness? In one sense the quantum connection is obvious–chemical bonds are rooted in the quantum wavefunction and uncertainty principle, neurotransmitters are chemicals essential for brain state control, and so forth. Quantum atomic processes provide the basis for larger-scale properties like chemical bonds, action potentials, and so on, but these phenomena have alternate, albeit very approximate, classical descriptions at large scales. In Chapter 12 we will consider a thought experiment in which we imagine the construction of an artificial brain and ask if a purely classical brain can be expected to experience awareness.

The thermodynamic connection is also clear as living systems operate with ongoing energy transfers in accordance with energy conservation, *the first law of thermodynamics*. In the context of the *second law of thermodynamics*, living systems emerge with decreased local *entropy* (disorder) that must be offset by increased entropy elsewhere. Entropy is also related to information, observer ignorance, and the deep riddle of *time* as discussed in Chapter 12.

2. RELIGIOUS AND PHILOSOPHICAL IMPLICATIONS

Any evaluation of possible religious implications of modern physics and physical cosmology must account for the ever present human biases; here I outline several obvious examples:

As I see it, the "job" of religious fundamentalists is to search for evidence supporting a God possessing attributes acceptable to their followers. Fundamentalists apparently strive to avoid any lessening of their faith, essentially following the commandment: *thou shall not entertain the idea that the God of your religion may be false.* God is also prohibited from taking on an impersonal image like *Nature* or from becoming a human-like super being as the Greek gods of old. Over the past century, many Christian fundamentalists have focused on the monumental (and seemingly self-defeating) task of trying to disprove Darwinian evolution in favor of the so-called *intelligent design* of living systems. But to most scientists, this effort seems hardly more credible than claims that the Earth is flat. Even the Catholic Church now considers Darwin, evolution, natural selection, and God to be compatible bed partners.

The more progressively faithful have turned to an altogether different interpretation of intelligent design, in which the universe itself is created to produce life and human consciousness. In this religious view, no conflict with evolution need occur. As outlined in this chapter, this position is far stronger than the anti evolution version of intelligent design. Thus, a substantial movement away from the anti evolutionary effort to the much more plausible position of *Cosmological Intelligent Design* may pick up speed. I expect proponents of this more progressive view to adopt some mixture of valid and exaggerated or extrapolated cosmological interpretations, the latter inducing substantial heartburn in professional cosmologists deploring misinterpretation of their life's work.

In sharp contrast to religious fundamentalists, the job of physical cosmologists is to explain observations of our universe within the context of scientific inquiry, without reference to supernatural interventions, including gods or God. Cosmologists do not aim to *disprove* the existence of God or gods; to paraphrase Laplace's famous reply to Napoleon, *They have no need for that hypothesis.* In fact, a number of religious physicists and cosmologists inhabit our scientific culture, and in any case, proof of the nonexistence of God is apparently not possible, not even in principle. Among the formidable barriers to such "proof" is the infinite regress problem: Perhaps one can explain properties of our universe in terms of the multiverse, but this just creates the question of who or what created the multiverse, and so forth, following progressive levels up some grand nested hierarchy of ultimate existence. In any case, God images existing outside of time and space are well protected from human erasers. God and science remain nicely compatible if science is seen as revealing God's works; conflicts arise when religious spokespeople promote antiscience views overlapping areas of scientific purview.

Most readers of this book are unlikely to be either cosmologists or religious fundamentalists, thus, our job is to search for truths possibly related to consciousness and to evaluate our ignorance levels in different areas. This may seem to imply that we should proceed in the manner of professional cosmologists or quantum physicists, but that is not quite what I have in mind. First, the hallmark of good science is attention to detail; here we mostly gloss over technical detail, relying instead on the competence of established physicists and astronomers to tell us what their science actually reveals. Second, we are perhaps a bit freer to speculate in areas that, while not violating known physical laws, are not promising for genuine scientific study in the foreseeable future due mainly to formidable experimental barriers. We shall be entirely free to irritate both scientists and religious fundamentalists on a case-by-case basis.

The astounding view of the world provided by quantum mechanics, in particular, has inspired numerous claims of connections to various mystical teachings, Eastern religions, and so forth. These putative connections run the whole gamut from the semi plausible to the ridiculous, the latter including claims that quantum mechanics can improve your health, financial condition, or love life, the modern version of snake oil sales. In the midrange of this spectrum of putative mystical connections are some interesting metaphors that may or may not find deeper meanings in future scientific work. I adhere to the view that going too far in speculative directions cheapens the discourse; the well-established experiments and their weird implications require no embellishment to be entertaining. Rather, we will see that some weird event A is "explained" provided the universe behaves *as if* it possesses some weird feature B, C, . . .and so forth. We will search for the most plausible explanations, but none will fit comfortably into our everyday intuitive views of reality.

Today, we are fortunate to have at our disposal a number of excellent books presenting the philosophical conundrums of modern physics in non technical language, making these fascinating ideas available to anyone who is truly interested. I will make full use of these writings in Chapters 9–12. Still, many laymen and non physical scientists alike are only vaguely aware of these revolutionary new concepts. Even those who are aware of the new ideas face the challenge of distinguishing genuine from the "flaky" physics; I will try hard here to avoid the "flaky," but we cannot escape from the "weird."

The environment for communication of modern physics underpinnings to non experts has not always been so friendly. Only in the past 20 years or so have the philosophical underpinnings of quantum mechanics (and the study of consciousness for that matter) been widely considered to fall within the purview of genuine scientific inquiry. This represents an important attitude shift as senior faculty make the critical hiring and tenure decisions at universities, but we must remember to tread carefully in order to distinguish the genuine from the irresponsibly speculative. In Chapter 11 we will meet physicist John Bell and his famous theorem leading to experiments showing an unexpected nonlocal connectedness in the universe. While we must speculate only with great care, we also note Bell's caution to avoid falling into the so-called FAPP ("for all practical purposes") trap in which genuine scientific enigmas are explained away with tautology or FAPP explanations. Bell's warning is closely related to both the Copenhagen interpretation of quantum mechanics and the *as if* caveat introduced in Chapter 8.

3. WHY APPEAL TO MODERN PHYSICS?

The following is a summary of my justifications for proposing the RQTC conjecture; the discussion will be expanded in Chapters 10–12.

- Empirical data show unequivocally that mind and brain processes are correlated. Classical brain models may successfully explain several computer-like properties, sensory information processing, memory storage, motor commands, and so forth, but no understanding of *conscious awareness* seems possible in the context of classical thinking. Imagine a computer as powerful as you wish; we have no idea what attributes it would require to achieve awareness, or even if this is possible in principle. I know of no unequivocal evidence showing that relativity, quantum mechanics, and thermodynamics can do any better, but these fields do provide a number of intriguing *hints* for the RQTC connection. Unless we are prepared to give up scientific consciousness studies entirely, modern physics obviously belongs in our intellectual toolbox.

- In the past century, our view of the structure of reality has undergone a major revolution. An astounding view of the universe has emerged from developments in relativity and quantum mechanics. The new ideas run so counter to intuition based on everyday experiences that they seem more aligned with witchcraft than science. Quantum mechanics exhibits a (nonlocal) holistic nature that is entirely foreign to classical thinking. The observer and the observed are joined in new and intimate ways governed by the quantum wavefunction. Electrons regularly jump between locations, evidently without ever occupying the space in between, *as if* reality itself consists of successive frames of a motion picture. The grand conceptual leap required by the transition from classical to quantum systems provides some feeling for how far brain science may eventually stray from current thinking. The resulting humility may make us especially skeptical of attempts to "explain away" (with tautology or FAPP solutions) observations that fail to merge easily with common notions of consciousness: multiple consciousnesses in single brains, group consciousness, the role of the unconscious, hypnosis, and so forth. If nothing else, relativity and quantum mechanics provide important epistemological lessons for brain science and philosophy.

- The majority, if not near-universal, scientific view is that the brain creates the mind. Perhaps conscious awareness is nothing but a byproduct of sensory, motor, and memory information processing. Philosopher Daniel Dennett advances an extreme view: *Consciousness appears to be the last bastion of occult properties, epiphenomena, and immeasurable subjective states.* Who knows? Dennett may be right, but I see a woeful lack of evidence for his position. Furthermore, this position strikes me as essentially saying: *The problem is too hard so let's pretend there is no problem.* An opposing view elevates consciousness, perhaps above physical theory, to a built-in property of our universe. Perhaps rather than creating mind, the brain acts more like an antenna that interacts with some sort of *information field* or "Ultra-Information" (defined in Chapter 12). The latter view, seemingly preposterous or even occult-like in the context of classical thinking, appears much more credible when viewed in the context of modern physical theories. In particular, the quantum wavefunction acts *as if* it is a spatially extended information field influencing the tendency of small particles to act in certain ways. The origin and structure of the universe, including undiscovered fields of energy and information, could be central to the consciousness challenge, motivating the discussions of cosmology in this chapter.

- Each human brain is a massive information processing system; organized information density in the 1000 cm^3 space occupied by each human brain is large. Science has established that brain structure and large-scale dynamics (as measured by EEG and other methods) are strongly correlated with behavior and conscious experience. Given this background in modern neuroscience, perhaps the most likely explanation for consciousness is that the brain creates the mind. However, given our very limited understanding of consciousness, it seems prudent to cast a wide net to capture data that might suggest a quite different view. Modern physical theories may be cast in the form of fundamental information barriers. *Relativity, quantum mechanics, and the second law of thermodynamics are all limitations on the speed, quantity, or quality of information transfer.* Humans apparently remain individuals only by limiting information transfer with other humans.

- The mystery of consciousness may be related to the *mystery of time.* Relativity, verified in many experiments, says that we live in a four-dimensional space-time. Intelligent beings living in different parts of the universe are expected to experience time in different ways; their time intervals are relative. Suppose events A and B occur simultaneously in some location X. Observers Y moving with respect to X and/or experiencing a different gravitational field may see event A occur before B. Still others in location Z may say that event B happened first. One man's future can be an alien creature's past. Relativity rejects the idea that time *flows*; rather, past, future, and present seem to exist as a unified whole. Our universe seems like a full motion picture in which we are aware only of progressive frames, *as if* consciousness itself moves through-four dimensional space-time along the time axis.

4. IN THE BEGINNING

Scientific cosmology is the study of the universe, its origins, and evolution. Modern cosmology depends on astronomical data obtained with telescopic systems sensitive to light, radio waves, and other parts of the electromagnetic spectrum. It also entails theoretical studies involving quantum mechanics, general relativity, and thermodynamics. By contrast to this science, religious cosmology typically depends on creation myths. Christianity and Judaism teach that the universe and humans were created at some beginning time by God. Buddhism and Hinduism picture a universe that passes through endless cycles of creation and destruction. The long history of conflict between scientific and religious cosmology is well evidenced by historical figures like Copernicus and Galileo; however, the modern Catholic Church and most other mainstream religions have embraced important tenants of scientific cosmology, for example, that the universe began roughly 14 billion years ago with the *big bang*.

So our universe apparently began with a bang. But this was not an explosion into an existing space like a firecracker or bomb in which matter expands into empty space, as sometimes imagined. Rather, space itself expanded from an infinitesimal point, called a *singularity*. If you find this hard to picture, rest assured, you are not alone. Our familiar space is three-dimensional, making it seemingly impossible to picture space itself expanding; only four-dimensional creatures could be expected to visualize expanding 3D space. The standard metaphorical description asks us to imagine two-dimensional creatures living on the surface of an expanding balloon. Such creatures would notice that distances between all objects in their world were continually increasing. Their surface universe would have no center, no special place of origin, analogous to the apparent lack of any center in our universe of three spatial dimensions. Of course, a spherical balloon has a center, but the center lies in the third dimension, forever inaccessible to two-dimensional creatures just like a fourth spatial dimension would be inaccessible to us, except through our imaginations and fancy mathematics.

The ability of space to stretch and become curved or warped is fundamental to Einstein's *general theory of relativity*. Thus, the expansion of the universe need not involve the migration of galaxies through space, although such migration also occurs. Rather, the space between galaxies is continually stretching. Because of the finite speed of light and accelerating expansion of the universe, we cannot see or know of anything beyond a horizon currently estimated at 47 billion light years; we call the sphere surrounding us with this radius the *observable universe* as represented by the dashed boundary line in

Figure 9–2. Earth is located at the center of our observable universe; alien creatures must be located at the centers of their own observable universes that may or may not overlap ours. We only see the most distant galaxies as they existed 14 billion years in the past; these same galaxies are believed to be now located at about 47 billion light years due to the accelerated expansion of the universe, as represented by the dashed boundary line in Figure 9–2. Shortly after the big bang, these galaxies emitted the light that we now see. The *entire universe* is probably larger yet; it may even be infinite, but it's hard to see how this question can ever be settled unequivocally. Note that the galaxy in Figure 9–2 is not drawn to scale; a typical spiral galaxy like ours is about 100,000 light years across or roughly 1/100,000 of the diameter of the observable universe.

Despite past success of the big bang theory in explaining observations about our current universe, discrepancies remained, especially with regard to the observed uniformity of our universe and its apparent lack of overall curvature (warp). Current cosmology explains these discrepancies by the *inflation theory*, in which the initial universe expanded from the size of a proton to that of a grapefruit in less than 10^{-35} seconds and then settled down to a more moderate expansion rate. The imagined inflation rate is much faster than light velocity, but there is no violation of relativity, which only limits light (and other signal) transmission through our existing space.

Thus far, we have avoided the issue of time, but Einstein's theory says that we live in a four-dimensional space-time, three space dimensions and one time dimension. Essentially, relativity says that space cannot exist without time and time cannot exist without space. If we imagine following the big bang backward in time to its origin at the singularity, we conclude that time itself originated with the big bang. If this picture is correct, it seems that no time and no place existed before the big bang, thus questions about the origin of the big bang

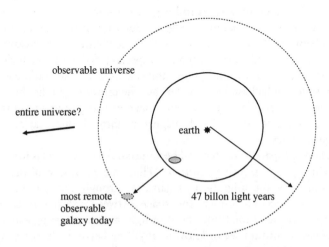

Figure 9–2 The observable universe may be only a small part of the entire universe.

appear meaningless. In contrast to this picture, a more recent viewpoint is that our universe may be just one "bubble" of expanding space among many universes that emerge spontaneously because of fundamental quantum processes. This postulated collection of universes is known as the *multiverse.* Physical laws may or may not differ between universes or between our universe and the multiverse. Thus, the question of the origin of time remains quite open.

5. LIFE IN OUR UNIVERSE

Life as we know it required a series of intricate steps in the evolution of our universe. Physicist Paul Davies lists three apparent requirements for life to develop:[3] *(1)* Physical laws must allow for the formation of stable complex structures. *(2)* The universe must posses substances required for life, carbon atoms or alternate substances that can combine to form complex structures. *(3)* The universe's physical environment must allow the essential substances to combine in the appropriate manner.

Most ordinary matter in the universe is hydrogen and helium, the latter made in the first few minutes after the big bang. The first stars formed after gravitational forces caused hydrogen and helium atoms to condense into dense clouds. When the clouds became sufficiently dense such that their centers reached temperatures of several million degrees, nuclear reactions were triggered. The same *nuclear fusion* is the basis for hydrogen bombs in contrast to the *nuclear fission* in atomic bombs and today's nuclear power plans generating electricity. Stars are nuclear fusion reactors that synthesize heavier elements from lighter ones; after several steps involving intricate nuclear reactions, carbon and other heavy elements are formed. When the inner core of a star runs out of nuclear fuel, it can no longer sustain the enormous pressure required to oppose the gravitational forces of the star's outer regions. The core collapses inward forming either a *neutron star* or a *black hole* depending on the star mass. The outer material also plunges inward but rebounds in a stellar explosion called a *supernova.* Supernovae typically occur a few times per century in each galaxy and seed their galaxies with the carbon and other heavy elements required for life; we humans are made from star stuff like that shown on this book's cover.

I have avoided most details in this picture of the origin of heavy elements, but many intricate steps are involved in their production. These steps depend critically on the masses and charges of elementary particles and on the strengths of nature's four known forces. These forces (or fields) include the two that are obvious in our everyday experience, the *gravitational* and *electromagnetic* forces. The usual mechanical pushing and pulling forces of one object on another are just due to electromagnetic forces operating at small scales. The other two fundamental forces are the *weak* and *strong nuclear forces* that hold nuclei together and govern nuclear reactions. In the 19th century, electric and magnetic forces (together with light) were discovered to be different aspects of the same underlying phenomenon, that is, electric and magnetic forces were "unified." Thus, we now speak of the electromagnetic force (or field). The electromagnetic and weak nuclear forces have now also been unified so we may speak of the *electroweak force*, although this later unification is rightly ignored by electrical engineers and others working on practical problems at macroscopic scales.

Most physicists believe that all four basic forces will eventually be unified, that is, seen as different manifestations of some underlying process, but this step has proved quite elusive. Currently, *string theory* and its extension *M theory* together with *loop quantum gravity* are considered by most physicists as the more promising avenues to a so-called (unified) "theory of everything." In string theory,[4] elementary particles are treated as vibrating strings with different resonant frequencies corresponding to different particles, analogous to violin strings producing different notes. But, the strings move in nine or ten space dimensions and one time dimension with the unobserved space dimensions "rolled up" in complicated shapes. To imagine this, think of long hose with a progressively smaller cross-sectional radius; when the hose circumference gets very small, its radial dimension is essentially lost. If we accept this picture, it is perhaps not so surprising that electrons can behave very differently from the so-called "particle" electron that we often imagine based on our macroscopic experiences with marbles and baseballs.

6. ANTHROPIC REASONING: IS OUR UNIVERSE FINELY TUNED FOR LIFE?

A number of physicists have emphasized the idea that our universe appears to be very finely tuned for the production of heavy elements and ultimately for life to evolve as we know it. This has come to be known as the *anthropic principle*, although no established principle is involved. I will refer instead to *anthropic reasoning*, which says that if the laws of physics and the structure of the universe were just a little different, many processes apparently necessary for life could not occur. To take one example, gravitational forces between masses are proportional to a parameter G called the gravitational constant. If G were larger, stars would burn faster and die sooner, possibly too soon for life to involve on their planets. If G were too small, stars could not form in the first place, and carbon and the other heavy elements would never be created. Another example is the electromagnetic force. If the electric force between charged particles were stronger, repulsion between protons might overcome the attractive nuclear force preventing the formation of atomic nuclei. It turns out that there are many other examples where very small changes in the parameters that determine fundamental forces or masses of elementary particles appear to result in universes where no life is possible.

In Chapter 2, I cited Richard Dawkins' computer simulations of synthetic "life forms" discussed in his book, *The Blind Watchmaker*. He was able to create complex forms by a simple rule for producing stick figures composed of branched lines. Dawkins' drawing rule was based on nine parameter choices or "genes" that determined features like length and angle of branch and number of successive generations. After 50 or so generations, many of his creations looked a bit like living things. He didn't plan the "animals" that evolved; the shapes emerged in the absence of his active direction. His simulations demonstrated that complex shapes may emerge from simple one-step processes and no active designer of specific animals is required. However, intelligence of the creators of the computer and program is, in fact, required for the ultimate production of Dawkins' little animals. So whether or not the watchmaker is actually "blind" depends on one's definition of the "watch."

Consider the following thought experiment: Imagine replacing Dawkins' computer program with a sophisticated program encompassing all of known physics. The *Standard Model* and general relativity have proved very successful in explaining particle physics and gravitational attractions, respectively. Taken together, these theories contain roughly 30 parameters that must be set in playing our imagined new computer game, "Create Your Own Universe." Future unified theories may show that these parameters are not all independent, but for now we ignore this complication. *When playing this game, our goal is to produce a virtual universe containing virtual conscious beings, or at least virtual life of some sort.* Our central question is this: Suppose we choose some arbitrary set of parameter settings for our game, the fundamental constants of the new universe. What is the likelihood that our new virtual universe will contain virtual life? John Barrow and Frank Tipler's 1986 classic, *The Anthropic Cosmological Principle*[5], addresses this question in technical detail, but even a superficial study suggests that some of the parameters must be set to an accuracy of better than 1% for life to be possible.

The required fine tuning appears to be much sharper than this. Physicist Lee Smolin approaches this issue by estimating the probability that a "random" universe will contain stars that last for at least five billion years, that is, if the universe is created by randomly choosing the gravitational constant, particle masses, and other parameters in the Standard Model.[6] Smolin's "miracle of the stars" calculation yields the extremely small probability of 10^{-229}. This is much smaller than the probability of picking out a single electron from the observable universe. It seems that no human is likely ever to win the computer game "Create Your Own Universe." In this analysis, our universe containing life, and even conscious beings, would seem to qualify easily as a miracle, at least in the absence of information to the contrary.

7. ANTHROPIC IMPLICATIONS

How might we interpret the fact that our universe appears to be so finely tuned for life? The following (overlapping) explanations for our strange universe are based mainly on the writings of Davies,[3] but with contribution from physicists Smolin, Barrow, Tippler, John Wheeler, and Leonard Susskind, and a few minor ideas of my own thrown in.

- *The Absurd Universe.* We were very lucky; the universe just happens to be the way it is. If had been a little different, we would not be here to argue about it. There is no designer and no purpose. Life developed as the result of extraordinary accidents, and there is no connection between consciousness and the physical world. Life and consciousness are just artifacts of this universe.

- *The Unique Universe.* The universe is governed by single fundamental theory that forces the theory's parameters to take on their observed values. It could be some variant of string theory, loop quantum gravity, or something quite different. All laws of physics and the parameters of these laws follow from this final theory of everything. As in the first example, life and consciousness are just accidental outcomes.

- *The Multiverse.* In one version, an infinite number of bubble universes originate in big bangs; our universe is just one of many in the multiverse. Perhaps some laws of physics hold true across the entire multiverse, but parameters like masses and charges of elementary particles vary. Or perhaps, the physical laws themselves vary across universes. Conscious observers only arise in a small fraction of universes; we happen to inhabit one such universe.

- *The Naturally Selective Universe.* Some sort of Darwinian-like natural selection occurs that favors universes that are life friendly. The inside of black holes involves the physics of quantum gravity, for which no theory has been developed; we have little idea of what happens inside. Smolin suggests that new universes may be created inside black holes[6]. Each universe able to produce stars and black holes then sires many new black holes that produce still more universes analogous to never-ending tree branches. This idea apparently assumes that the physical laws of mother universes remain intact in daughter universes. The parameters of physical laws have their observed values because these have made star and black hole production much more likely than other choices. Susskind[7] proposes an alternate version of the naturally selective universe that I won't attempt to describe here.

- *The Informational Universe.* Some sort of fundamental information or large-scale intelligence is responsible for physical laws and/or their parameters. One possibility is *Cosmological Intelligent Design*; however, this politically charged label may or may not suggest the God(s) of mainstream religions. The so-called Designer might be an architect from a super civilization in another universe, analogous to Richard Dawkins' relationship to his Biomorphs. Or, perhaps the structure of the multiverse is governed by *Ultra-Information*, an entity defined in Chapter 12, which determines the properties of all universes. By contrast to our first four choices, this picture might elevate consciousness to a central position in the cosmos.

- *The Participatory Universe.* Space-time is closed; if an observer were able to wait a sufficiently long time, he would re-experience the big bang. To varying degrees, earlier descriptions suffer from the problem of infinite regression; predictions of any universe require that we specify initial and boundary conditions. If we choose the Multiverse or Designer options, we are left with the question of how or who created the Multiverse or Designer in the first place. With this new option, space-time is closed, and future descendents of humans or other conscious beings may develop methods to alter the structure of our universe so that it becomes life-friendly before the time loop is again closed. Or, perhaps backward-in-time influences allow the universe to create itself. Perhaps humans and other conscious creatures eventually evolve into a single universal intelligence, *Mind*, an entity currently existing only in primitive form as a subset of *Ultra-Information*. Again, consciousness occupies a central position in this universe in this speculation.

- *None of the Above.* The nature of our universe, including consciousness, involves entirely new concepts of space, time, and information that are currently beyond human ability to comprehend, but the new concepts may involve selected aspects of the other six imagined universes.

Davies includes another choice, *The Fake Universe*, in which we are living in a grand simulation. I consider this part of *The Informational Universe* because it seems to me that the question of what is "real" and what is "fake" is observer dependent. A Designer running a computer simulation of our universe considers himself real and us fake, but the Designer himself may be part of a simulation run by a Super Designer, and so forth.

Choice among the above options appears to be mostly a matter of individual preference; universal beauty is in the eye of the beholder. As I write this on a Sunday, I tend to assign the highest probability to *None of the Above*, with *The Informational Universe* in second place. But, if I were to repeat this futile, but nevertheless intriguing, guessing game on a Wednesday or after several glasses of wine, my preferences might easily change. I put most weight on *None of the Above* based only on the fact that our fundamental views of the nature of time and space have changed so drastically in just one century. It seems likely that the scientific view from, let's say, 1,000 years in the future will involve concepts that are entirely foreign to our current ways of thinking.

Some physicists like Roger Penrose support Plato's view that fundamental physical laws have a real existence in a so-called *Platonic World* that transcends physical reality. The proposed *Ultra-Information* of Chapter 12 employs similar ideas. Taking this general view, we might expect some fundamental laws to hold throughout the multiverse; call them *multiversal laws*. An even more expansive view would retain mathematics but remove physics from the Platonic World. All possible physical laws that are expressible in self-consistent mathematics would govern different parts of the multiverse. Some universes would have three space dimensions, others would have more. Some laws might be regular, some inherently random, and so forth. This extreme view really opens up unlimited possibilities for virtual travel and mathematical exploration, taking speculation to new and lofty heights but perhaps leaving genuine science well behind in its wake.

8. RELATIVITY

My discussions of modern physics avoid most technical details so as to encourage a wider readership; in any case, the finer details are unnecessary for our approach to the consciousness challenge. Nevertheless, some details are both easy to understand and quite illuminating of nature's physical reality; of course, "easy to understand" does not mean "easy to believe."

Here we enter the strange Alice in Wonderland world of *special relativity*, aiming to provide a gentle transition from the "common sense" intuitive thinking of our everyday lives to the strangeness emerging from physics over the past century. Special relativity is concerned with observers moving at constant relative velocity; it requires no mathematics beyond high school algebra. *General relativity*, which requires the advanced mathematics of tensor calculus, is concerned with observers moving with accelerated motion or experiencing substantial gravitational fields. Many professional physicists now consider the relativistic view of space-time to be rather mundane, going so far as to include relativity under the rubric of "classical physics." I do not embrace this lofty position. Rather, I adopt the descriptors "strange" for relativity and "weird" for quantum mechanics, indicating that the latter takes us even deeper down the proverbial rabbit holes from our surface views of reality.

Einstein's relativity makes substantial use of the *thought experiment*, an imagined experiment that may be impossible to perform because of practical limitations, used to test a theory. For example, the physics principle that objects with different masses fall at the same velocity is valid only in a vacuum with no air resistance. Galileo lacked the technology to carry out the ideal experiments in a vacuum but was able to formulate the principle with a combination of thought experiment and actual experiments with air present.

Our first thought experiment is pictured in Figure 9–3, indicating the top view of a train traveling at velocity V_T past a stationary platform. A gun,

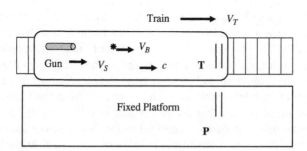

Figure 9–3   A gun mounted on the top of a moving train produces a bullet (V_B), a sound wave (V_S), and a light flash (c). When the sensors systems on the platform and train (each indicated by two parallel lines) line up, six relative velocities are measured. The correct relativistic velocities are listed in Table 9–2.

Table 9-1 Speeds in Train Experiment If Light Were a Particle or Classical Wave with Ether Fixed to the Platform

	Bullet	Sound	Light is particle	Light is wave
Platform observer, **P**	$V_T + V_B$	V_S	$V_T + c$	c
Train observer, **T**	V_B	$V_S - V_T$	c	$c - V_T$

mounted on top and to the rear of the train, fires a bullet with muzzle velocity V_B, the bullet velocity with respect to the moving train. The gun simultaneously emits three things: a bullet, a sound, and a light flash. The heavy parallel lines near the front of the train and (directly opposite) on the fixed platform indicate sensors to measure bullet, sound, and light velocity relative to their positions. When the train reaches the location shown, six speeds are measured simultaneously: three by a moving observer **T** on the train and three by a fixed observer **P** on the platform.

The expected classical results of these measurements (based on ideas in place before 1905) are shown in Table 9–1. Observer **T** on the moving train records the gun's muzzle velocity V_B. However, platform observer **P** finds that the train motion adds to the bullet velocity, so he records a bullet velocity $V_T + V_B$ with respect to his fixed platform. The results for sound velocity are just the opposite. The gun sound produces a local disturbance in the air outside the train car, a sound wave packet that travels with a velocity V_S(with respect to local air and fixed platform) proportional to the average velocity of air molecules or air temperature. Familiar wave propagation involves disturbances of material media. Wave velocity depends on the properties of this medium and not on the velocity of the sound source; motion of the source will change the sound's pitch (the Doppler effect) but not its propagation speed. Platform observer **P** records the gun sound velocity V_S, whereas train observer **T** records the lower gun sound velocity $V_S - V_T$ because his measuring apparatus at the front of the train is essentially running away from the sound wave. If the train velocity exceeds the local velocity of sound, train observer **T** will never hear the gun. A supersonic bullet or airplane also produces a continuous sound, a wake that cannot be heard in front of its location. An analogous example is provided by a boat's bow wake, a water wave that spreads to the sides and rear of the boat but not upstream.

In Table 9–1, I have included two columns for the expected classical speeds of the light (pre-1905), depending on whether light was assumed to behave like a wave or particle. Since many 19th century experiments revealed the (apparently) unequivocal wave nature of light, scientists at that time expected light waves to behave similarly to sound waves—to propagate in some supporting medium (the so-called *ether*) analogous to air. The air in our experiment is stationary with respect to the platform; observations of sound speeds would, of course, differ if the gun were located inside the train where the internal air is carried forward with the train.

Table 9–2   Correct Relativistic Speeds in Train Experiment

	Bullet	Sound	Light
Platform observer, **P**	$\dfrac{V_T + V_B}{1 + (V_T V_B / c^2)}$	V_S	c
Train observer, **T**	V_B	$\dfrac{V_S - V_T}{1 - (V_T V_S / c^2)}$	c

The entries in the fifth column of Table 9–1 are based on an imagined *ether* fixed to the platform, making the "classical" light velocities analogous to observed sound velocities. But, more realistically one might expect the ether to be fixed with respect to some reference like the distant stars such that the platform would be moving with respect to the ether. In this case, light traveling parallel to the platform would be expected to register a different speed than light traveling perpendicular to the platform. But, all attempts by 19th century scientists to find this speed difference failed; scientists eventually concluded that no material medium is needed to support light propagation. We now know that light (and other electromagnetic waves) travels through empty space without any known physical medium to carry the disturbance. *Empty space itself exhibits definite physical properties.* Light energy is contained in the electric and magnetic fields themselves, rather than in a material medium as in the case of mechanical waves like sound and water waves.

The six velocities predicted by special relativity are shown in Table 9–2. Note that actual light velocities differ from both bullet and classical wave behavior; light acts *as if* it is something quite different. Both the moving and stationary observer measure the same velocity of light c. Another interesting result concerns the velocity of the bullet experienced by the platform observer. Even though the muzzle velocity of the bullet adds to the train velocity at low velocities (from the viewpoint of the fixed platform), **P** can never observe a bullet exceeding the velocity of light c. For example, if train and muzzle velocities are both equal to $0.8c$, the platform observer **P** measures a bullet velocity of $0.976c$ rather than the superlight speed of $1.6c$ expected with pre-relativistic thinking.

9. EPISTEMOLOGICAL LESSONS OF RELATIVITY

I have listed the velocities in Table 9–2 without showing how they were obtained; such derivations are widely published in physics texts. Rather, I here emphasize *epistemology*, concerned with questions like: What do we know about speeding systems and how do we know it? or How do we know what we know? In this section, I strive to provide some flavor for the reasoning behind special relativity and to discuss briefly some of its major implications.

Einstein developed special relativity based on two simple postulates. The first, originally due to Galileo, is that identical physical laws are experienced by different observers moving at constant velocity with respect to each other. Any scientific experiment carried out on the fixed train platform must yield the identical result if performed inside the moving train, provided the train moves with perfectly constant velocity (no bumps or jerks allowed). Thus, an observer with knowledge obtained only from inside the train, whether human or a perfectly sensitive scientific instrument, is unable, even in principle, ever to know if the train is moving or stationary. Obviously, the train windows must be closed, the train walls insulated, and so forth to block access to all external information in this thought experiment.

Another way to look at this issue is to ponder the implications if fixed and moving observers were actually to experience different physical laws. In this case, one must ask which observer is ever fixed? Our "fixed" train platform rotates on the Earth's surface; the Earth rotates around the sun, which rotates around a galaxy that moves with respect to other galaxies. If our universe had a known, fixed boundary, we could express motion with respect to this boundary, but no such boundary is known. An *inertial frame of reference* is defined as a space (coordinate system or spaceship or train car) in which bodies initially at rest remain at rest if not acted on by forces, that is, a frame moving with constant velocity. In Einstein's words, *all inertial frames are completely equivalent.* We can speak just as easily of the platform moving at velocity $-V_T$ with respect to the train as we can say the train moves with velocity $+V_T$ with respect to the platform.

This first postulate of special relativity will seem quite plausible to most. The TGV is the fast train connecting Paris to other French cities; in commercial use, its usual top speed is about 200 mph, although it is capable of exceeding 350 mph in test runs. When I rode the TGV, I was unable to appreciate the fast velocity even by looking out the window without knowing reference distances like separations between telephone poles. My French colleagues who switched from a slow train to the fast train experienced no psychological difference; they just reached their destinations in about half the original time. While riding in commercial airlines, we cover a distance equal to three football fields every second, but this high speed fails to register on our consciousness.

Einstein's second postulate is far bolder: the velocity of light is independent of the motion of its source; the equal values of c in the third column of Table 9–2 demonstrate this postulate. It turns out that if one accepts the validity of Maxwell's equations governing electromagnetic field behavior, this second postulate is unnecessary since it is implied by the first postulate; however, most physicists (including Einstein) prefer to retain the postulate of constant c, thereby allowing special relativity to provide an independent check of Maxwell's equations and vice versa. Many publications provide derivations of the velocities in Table 9–2 and the other even more astounding consequences of special relativity. I will not repeat such analyses here but just emphasize that they follow from taking Einstein's two fundamental postulates very seriously and following them to logical conclusions using high school algebra and some subtle reasoning.

I will, however, outline two of the most famous consequences of special relativity, *time dilation* and *mass-energy equivalence*. According to Einstein's original derivation, the interval Δt_M between clock times experienced by an observer moving with speed v with respect to a stationary observer is related to the corresponding clock tick interval Δt_S of the stationary observer by

$$\Delta t_S = \frac{\Delta t_M}{\sqrt{1 - \dfrac{v^2}{c^2}}} \qquad (9.1)$$

This relation was derived from a consideration of light beams passing between mirrors as experienced by the moving and stationary observers; time intervals are defined in terms of the different observed spatial separations between light source and receiver. This is the famous expression for time dilation indicating that the stationary time interval Δt_S is longer than the moving interval Δt_M, leading to the so-called *twin paradox* discussed below.

An immediate question concerns the apparent symmetry of the two observers: Why can't the roles of the moving and stationary observers be interchanged? When our train in Figure 9–3 moves with velocity $v = V_T$ with respect to the platform, it just means that the platform is moving with velocity $-V_T$ with respect to the train. The answer is, they can indeed be interchanged if no acceleration is involved, leading to an outcome that is quite strange: the observers **P** (Pat) and **T** (Tom) disagree about whose clock is running slower.

To see that Pat and Tom's perceptions of temporal reality differ, suppose four clock intervals are measured when the two sensors (parallel lines) in Figure 9–3 line up as the train passes the platform. Platform observer Pat measures his own interval Δt_{SP} and the interval on the train Δt_{MP} (the *SP* and *MP* subscripts indicate "stationary" and "moving" from Pat's perspective). Similarly, moving train observer Tom measures his own interval Δt_{ST} and the interval on the platform Δt_{MT}; keep in mind that from Tom's viewpoint, he is stationary and the platform is moving. If the distance between the platform and train sensors is zero when the measurements are made, Equation 9.1 provides the correct time intervals for each observer. Thus, Pat and Tom both conclude that the other guy's clock is running too slow, an outcome perhaps seeming to imply the existence of two distinct branches of physical reality! But according to relativity, all observers in the universe moving with respect to each other or experiencing different gravitational fields perceive different time intervals between identical events as viewed from their own reference frames (planets or spaceships). If humans were to observe simultaneous cosmic events, say supernovas, in galaxies A and B, aliens would generally not agree that events A and B occurred at the same time; some aliens might say event A preceded B, others that B preceded A.

What happens if our train traveler Tom gets off at the next train station and takes another train in the opposite direction to compare clocks with Pat who has remained on his platform? Now the thought experiment is no longer symmetric. Tom has deaccelerated on his train back to zero velocity with respect to Pat, accelerated in the opposite direction, and finally deaccelerated to stop at platform P. When they compare watches, they *agree* that Tom's watch is running slower than Pat's. We are quite relieved; there is only one branch of reality after all! But note the following caveat: Einstein's original arguments in 1905 never mentioned acceleration; consideration of accelerating bodies had to wait for his publication of general relativity in 1915. But Einstein's 1905 derivation has been studied extensively, and his answers turn out to be correct.

Real trains travel much too slowly to produce appreciable time differences between stationary and fixed observers. The famous twin paradox is illustrated for twins Tom and Pat by replacing the fast train by a much faster spaceship. Suppose Tom at age 30 enters the spaceship that accelerates to a large velocity, later deaccelerates, and lands on Earth after experiencing an internal flight time of 1 year. Tom would then emerge from the spaceship as a 31-year-old, but his Earth-bound twin Pat could easily be much older. In fact, Tom might find that even Pat's grandson was an old man, depending on the actual velocities achieved by the spaceship.

The basic idea of relativity is that the *velocity of light* c *is a fundamental property of our universe*, which limits the velocity of any kind of ordinary information exchange between spatially separated locations, whether "observed" by humans, scientific sensors, or biological tissue. Special relativity says that all physical (and by implication) biological laws must be consistent with this *limitation on information transfer*. Time dilation is a direct result of this constancy of light velocity. Suppose we have two watches with identical properties when are both at rest. Let one watch be worn by Tom moving at 80% of light velocity for 6 years. While Tom notices no changes in his watch consistent with Einstein's first postulate, his clock tick interval is related to that of the stationary observer Pat by Equation (1), yielding

$$\Delta t_M = 0.6\Delta t_S \qquad (9.2)$$

To keep things simple, I have ignored effects of acceleration in obtaining Equation 9.2, but this simplification does not alter the essential outcome. Although clock comparisons may be impractical while the spaceship is in motion, the end result will become apparent when the ship returns to Earth. While Tom has experienced a trip of 6 years, Pat and his fellow Earth-bound humans insist that 10 years have actually elapsed. Tom and Pat's different psychological experiences are consistent with a single objective reality; we apparently live in a well-regulated four-dimensional space-time.

You may find this identification of clock times with altered speeds of biological processes like human aging to involve a substantial conceptual leap beyond Einstein's two fundamental postulates. If so, you are not alone. That said, time dilation and many other consequences of special relativity have now been verified to precise accuracy in experiments involving elementary particles.

Atomic clocks have been placed in jet airplanes or spacecraft orbits; their slowed clock speeds are in close agreement with special relativity. GPS satellite clocks tick more slowly by roughly 7 microseconds per day due to the velocity effect of special relativity. But, they also tick more rapidly by about 46 microseconds per day due to the weaker gravitational field at large distances from the Earth, as predicted by general relativity. The difference is about 39 microseconds per day; this discrepancy is corrected by altering the onboard clock frequency before launch, demonstrating that relativity has practical engineering applications in everyday life.

Perhaps you remain skeptical that time dilation is a genuine phenomenon. If so, remember that this idea emerges from a self-consistent theory in close agreement with many disparate experiments and has no known disagreements. The most dramatic demonstration of special relativity is the equivalence of mass and energy; Einstein's famous equation is

$$E = mc^2 \tag{9.3}$$

How is this relationship obtained in special relativity? I will not derive it here but just point out that Newton's third law of motion is altered by special relativity such that the mass of a moving body, as observed by a stationary observer, increases with its velocity. In classical mechanics, a body at rest with zero potential energy has zero total energy. By contrast, such body has total energy given by Equation 9.3, with $m = m_0$, where m_0 is called the *rest mass*. Equation 9.3 provides a basis for nuclear reactions in which elementary particles react in a manner that reduces their total mass and energy is released. Thus, Einstein revealed mass in an entirely new light; *mass is essentially stored energy*. A pound of any kind of mass, if fully converted to energy by nuclear reactions, yields about 20 megatons, the energy equivalent of 20 million tons of TNT exploding by means of conventional chemical reactions.

10. SUMMARY

The possibility of deep connections between modern physics (relativity, quantum mechanics, and thermodynamics) and consciousness is labeled here as *the RQTC conjecture*, independent of the actual nature of any such connection. While many are quite skeptical of this idea, it is raised here partly because classical physics apparently cannot even begin to explain consciousness. I claim that the study of consciousness must be essentially a study of the nature of reality, and modern physics deals with important aspects of physical reality. I know of no unequivocal evidence supporting the RQTC conjecture, but modern physics provides a number of intriguing *hints* of possible connections. Such hints will be discussed in more detail in Chapters 10–12.

Our universe appears to be very finely tuned for the production of heavy elements and ultimately life as we know it. If the laws of physics and the structure of the universe were just a little different, many processes apparently necessary for life could not occur, a demonstration of the so-called *anthropic principle*. How do we interpret this? Several kinds of theoretical universes are proposed that might be consistent with known properties of our universe. Some imagined life-friendly universes are accidental, some occur as a consequence of some sort of cosmic natural selection, and some contain some sort of fundamental information/intelligence field that I call *Mind*, a subcategory of another entity *Ultra-Information*, defined in Chapter 12.

This overview of *special relativity* aims to provide a gentle transition from the intuitive thinking of our everyday lives to the strangeness of modern physics. Special relativity involves observers moving at constant relative velocity, whereas *general relativity* is concerned with observers moving with accelerated motion or experiencing substantial gravitational fields. The "observer" in these thought experiments can be a human being or a scientific instrument; however, only *natural* (not *supernatural*) observers are allowed. In other words, the measuring instruments themselves must conform to physical laws, a requirement critical to interpretations of quantum mechanics in Chapters 10 and 11.

A thought experiment involving a train passing a fixed platform is adopted to illustrate the tenets of special relativity. *Empty space itself is found to exhibit definite physical properties, limiting the transfer speed of all ordinary information to the fixed speed of light.* Two of the most famous consequences of special relativity are time dilation and the equivalence of mass and energy. In Chapter 12, I will speculate on the possible existence of an entity called *Ultra-Information* involved with nonlocal influences not limited by finite light speed.

The time interval between events experienced by a moving observer differs from those experienced by a stationary observer, leading to the so-called *twin paradox*: a space traveler ages more slowly than his Earth-bound twin. Cosmic events A and B that appear simultaneous to one creature can occur at different times from another creature's perspective. Mass can be viewed as stored energy; a pound of mass represents an enormous quantity of energy as demonstrated with nuclear weapons and nuclear power reactors.

Chapter 10

The Weird Behavior of Quantum Systems

1. QUANTUM WEIRDNESS AND HINTS OF A LINK TO CONSCIOUSNESS

Several prominent scientists have proposed deep connections between quantum mechanics and consciousness. On the other hand, many skeptics view such speculative links as simply vague and unsupported notions that since both topics are mysterious, perhaps they are somehow related. I do *not* claim here that quantum mechanics provides a "proven" basis for conscious awareness or even that such connection is likely to be firmly embraced by many scientists anytime soon. Rather, I propose that the well-established and widespread experimental verifications of weird quantum effects provide a number of intriguing *hints* of possible quantum connections to mind, suggesting that the idea be taken seriously if, as proposed here, the hard problem of consciousness lies within scientific purview. A genuine interest in fires suggests looking long and hard in smoky places even if the fire is not obvious.

Chapters 10–11 will outline several features of quantum weirdness; most sections are aimed at readers unfamiliar with the essential ideas embodied by quantum mechanics. I will attempt to provide some flavor of the astounding world view that has emerged in the past century. Quantum concepts remain largely unappreciated by most non physicists, including many scientists, and run quite counter to everyday experiences, seeming more like magic than science. But for many, quantum mechanics seems so abstract and remote from their daily lives that they have hardly given it a second thought. Nevertheless, quantum mechanical footprints can be found nearly everywhere, quite evident in the natural world as well as in human technology, touching our lives on a regular basis.

Quantum mechanics reveals a holistic character of the universe entirely foreign to classical thinking. The scientific observer and the observed system are joined in intimate ways governed by an "information field" called the *quantum wavefunction*, hinting at possible links to consciousness. Elementary particles appear to be influenced from distant parts of the universe with no time delay (*nonlocal influences*); they also may reside in a kind of quantum limbo or alternate realm of reality with undefined properties until observed with scientific instruments. Particles may jump between locations, evidently without ever occupying the space in between, *as if* reality itself consists of successive frames of a motion picture. As argued here and in Chapters 11 and 12, a central concept that may help to unify various ontological interpretations of weird quantum effects is that of *information*. This suggests a possible link to the hard problem if consciousness is viewed as a special, expanded category of information processing.

The field of quantum mechanics is too large and dependent on mathematics to be appropriate for comprehensive treatment in this book; no such ambitious attempt will be pursued here. Fortunately, however, detailed treatment is not required for our purposes as the most essential concepts can be demonstrated with a few simple experiments and carefully chosen metaphors. But any such quantum metaphor must be coupled with appropriate caveats to indicate where analogs are not meant to be taken too seriously. Adoption of inappropriate metaphors or metaphors lacking appropriate caveats could easily reduce this chapter to nothing more than a *quantum cartoon* characterized by minimal distinctions between fantasy and reality. With this warning in mind, I will attempt to walk the fine line between technical fundamentals of quantum mechanics and a trivialized quantum cartoon.

While the mathematical framework of quantum mechanics is mostly absent from our discussion, mathematics plays an essential role behind the scenes by supporting the appropriate metaphors and their caveats. The central variable in any system of particles is the quantum wavefunction, governed by a deceptively simple-looking linear wave equation (*Schrödinger's equation*). Thus, the most obvious metaphors involve familiar wave phenomena, the sounds produced by musical instruments, for example. As both sound waves and the quantum wavefunction are governed by similar wave equations, the resulting dynamic behaviors are also quite similar, thereby allowing close analogies between familiar musical sounds and quantum wavefunction behavior.

This convenient wave correspondence is, however, substantially complicated in the actual practice of quantum mechanics, which is carried forward in two distinct stages. One stage involves quantum wavefunction solutions; the second stage concerns the actual experimental system (including both preparation and measurement) involving, in traditional terms, a strange process called *collapse of the wavefunction*. To adopt still another metaphor, the "easy problem" of quantum mechanics involves wavefunction calculations, whereas the "hard problem," commonly known as the *measurement problem*, involves ontological interpretations of quantum observations. Recall that in Chapter 1, I proposed relative complexities and depths of understanding for several areas of human knowledge with the field of mathematics (shown in Figure 1–4) identified as both the simplest and the best-understood field. Consistent with this idea, the easy problem of quantum mechanics involves solutions of Schrödinger's equation, which provide unambiguous statistical information about the wavefunction associated with a collection of particles. We have no such convenient mathematical framework at our disposal to address the hard (measurement) problem.

The cozy links between classical and quantum waves apply only to the wavefunction stage; other, more forced, metaphors are adopted here to describe the experimental measurement stage. My chosen metaphors for the experimental stage involve the magic balls of Section 2 and the cosmic orchestra of Section 6. Unfortunately, these "magic" metaphors require much more of a reality stretch than the analog musical instruments and can be criticized as excessively cartoonish. Professionals in quantum mechanics can become quite irritated by quantum cartoons; nevertheless, the cartoons chosen here seem to capture the essential flavor of the weird properties of our world revealed in genuine quantum experiments. My defense of these cartoons is based on the proposition that even a superficial knowledge of quantum mechanics is better than abysmal ignorance. But when viewing these cartoons, one should keep in mind a well-worn caveat, *a little knowledge can be a dangerous thing.* Unsupported leaps of faith between quantum cartoons and putative "explanations" of consciousness would be strictly forbidden if I were in charge of the universe.

2. MOSES PRESENTS HIS QUANTUM BALLS

In Chapter 6, I related a fable of an alien named Moses who provides humans with a magic tablet showing dynamic patterns to be deciphered. In my new fable, Moses returns to Earth with what appears to be a much simpler system, a bucket of magic balls and a blueprint for a *ball machine* to be human-made. Gray balls are injected into the top of the ball machine (Fig. 10–1), which has no apparent magic properties.[1] The quantum balls, however, behave in weird ways, as demonstrated by the following series of observations. In the first experiment, the right leg of the ball machine is closed by Michael and Lisa, chief scientists in the government's top secret *Moses Project*. All balls injected into the top of the ball machine end up in the box on the left side as expected. Similarly, when the

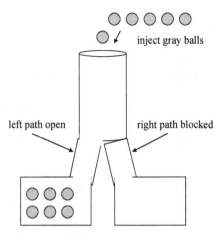

Figure 10–1   Magic ball machine with left path open.

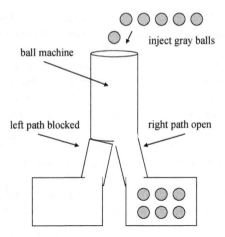

Figure 10–2   Magic ball machine with right path open.

left leg is blocked, all balls end up on the right side as indicated in Figure 10–2. No surprises occur in the first two experiments.

The first surprise occurs when scientists open both legs of the magic box as indicated in Figure 10–3. Rather than finding the expected approximately equal number of gray balls in each box, both boxes actually contain mixtures of black and white balls. This observation suggests that perhaps each gray ball is actually composed of a white and a black ball. Lisa postulates that these balls behave like little blobs of paint as indicated by the equation with a question mark in Figure 10–3. But since the ball machine itself is quite ordinary, the apparent separation of gray balls into composite black and white balls is mysterious. How could the simple forked path in the ball machine, leading to separate legs and boxes, trigger the putative ball transformations? Remember, the ball machine is human-made. Further investigations by Michael show that experimental results are insensitive to ball machine design, provided its legs are identical. The ball machine can be made of metal, cardboard, plastic, bubblegum, or just about anything else; the legs can be any length. It must, however, have one essential feature: it must block direct observation of ball paths; *it must control information available to observers.*

The standard scientific approach to unresolved questions is to design new experiments to establish the answers. One obvious approach is to create a little observation window in one of the legs as indicated in Figure 10–4. When a gray ball is dropped into the top of the ball machine, the scientists may see a shadow pass the window (the balls fall too fast to determine their color before landing in one of the boxes). About half the time, a shadow is observed, indicating a ball passage through the left leg as expected. But, now the mystery really deepens: the two boxes are found to contain only gray balls! How has opening the observation window (Fig. 10–4) prevented the gray balls from being transformed into white and black balls as in Figure 10–3? Michael thinks he knows the answer:

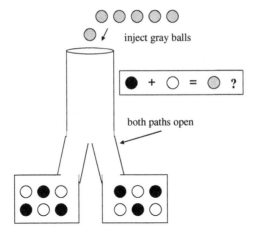

Figure 10–3 Magic ball machine with both paths open.

When the observation window is opened, light enters the left leg; maybe the black and white balls are transformed back to gray when exposed to light. But wait, says Lisa, balls (apparently) passing through the right leg where there is no light also accumulate as gray balls in the right box. (The ball machine is sufficiently refined to insure that no light from the observation window at left reaches the right leg.) This kind of experiment is known in quantum mechanics as a *Renninger negative-result measurement,* in which information is gained about a system through the *absence* of a detection event.

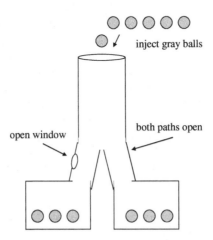

Figure 10–4 Magic ball machine with both paths open and an observation window also open.

When both legs are open and the window closed so that no *information* about ball passage through the left leg is available, mixtures of black and white balls are again found in the boxes as in Figure 10–3. The time of ball passage from the top of the machine to the boxes is known from observation; this gives Michael another idea: Inject each ball with both legs open and the window closed; then wait long enough so that each ball must have passed the fork into one of the legs. Then quickly open the window before the ball has had a chance to pass the window. This experimental modification is not difficult to accomplish because the legs of the ball machine can be made arbitrarily long. If a gray ball "decides" whether or not to split into two balls at the fork, we expect each gray ball to produce one white and one black ball in the boxes (as the window is closed when the ball passes the fork). But no, we again get all gray balls in the boxes!

This latter test is known in the field of quantum mechanics as a *delayed choice experiment*. Let me summarize the major mysteries:

- When both paths are open and the observation window is closed, each gray ball appears to split at the fork into a black ball and white ball. When the window is open, however, no split occurs. How does opening the window prevent the gray balls from splitting?

- Opening the window after a single ball has apparently passed the fork (when both paths are open) results in an unsplit gray ball in one of the boxes. But in the earlier experiment with both paths open and the window closed, each gray ball apparently split into black and white balls at the fork. If this interpretation is correct, how can the act of opening the window possibly reverse a split that occurred earlier? On the other hand, if the "split at the fork interpretation" is not correct, where did the earlier splits shown in Figure 10–3 occur?

OK, we ask Moses, "So what's the trick?" Moses adopts a magician posture and Mona Lisa–like face to frame his reply, "That, dear humans, is for you to figure out." Over the past century, scientists and philosophers have enjoyed only very minimal success in finding the "trick." Some say the balls themselves do not really exist until they are observed; the combined system consisting of both balls and ball machine, with paths and windows in specific open or closed states, form the "real" observed system. Others imply that the balls contain internal structures consisting of "computer" and "antenna" that receives information about open paths and windows, allowing the balls to behave as observed. Some even claim that ball behavior is partly due to interactions with similar balls and scientists in other universes. Still others offer explanations based on influences that act backward in time.

3. THE TWO-SLIT EXPERIMENT

The machine processing magic balls in Figures 10–1 through 10–4 is not real; it is just a metaphor presented in preparation for our discussion of real

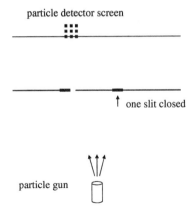

Figure 10–5 The famous two–slit experiment with the right slit closed.

experiments with small particles. The widely documented *double slit experiments* of Figures 10–5 through 10–8 are quite real, however. Small particles (electrons, photons, or atoms) are fired at a barrier containing two small openings (slits) pictured here as having little sliding doors. The gun can either fire rapidly so that many particles reach the barrier at nearly the same time, or it can fire slowly so that each particle hits the screen before the next particle is fired. The experiment can be performed with the doors open or closed, and a particle sensor behind the door at left can be either on or off. A screen at the top records the arrival of particles at various horizontal locations; the more particles hitting a particular location, the blacker the screen becomes at that location. The experiments follow closely those of the magic ball metaphor as follows:

- When one door is closed as shown in Figure 10–5, particles accumulate behind the open slit just like the gray balls landing in a single box of the metaphorical experiment shown Figures 10–1 and 10–2. The upper plot in Figure 10–6 shows a more detailed picture of the distribution of particles hitting the screen. When only the left slit is open (horizontal coordinate = −2), particles are distributed according to the dashed curve, which peaks directly behind the open slit. Similarly, when only the right slit is open, the particle distribution is given by the solid curve, which peaks directly behind the open slit at horizontal coordinate +2. This behavior is just what is expected if many particles pass through the slits at small random angles.

- When both doors are open and the sensor is off, we expect a particle distribution to consist of the sum of the two plots in the upper part of Figure 10–6 as shown in the middle plot. However, an entirely different (non particle-like) pattern appears on the detector screen; this pattern corresponds to the black/white ball mixture of our metaphorical experiment indicated in Figure 10–3. In the actual experiment of

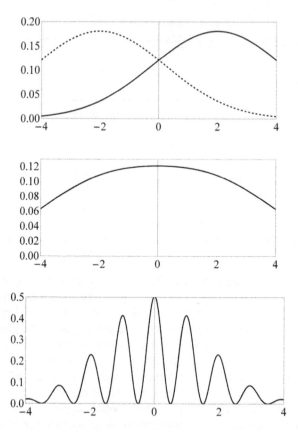

Figure 10–6. (Upper) The two patterns on the sensor screens obtained when either the left (dashed line) or right (solid line) slits are open. (Middle) The expected particle pattern when both slits are open is shown as the sum of the two (rescaled) traces in the upper figure. (Lower) A classic interference pattern expected if waves (not particles) pass through both slits.

Figure 10–7, an extended pattern is created on the screen, consisting of alternating bands with and without particle hits; this is the classic *wave interference pattern* shown in more detail as the lower plot in Figure 10–6.

• Could the interference pattern be somehow caused by interactions between particles? To check this idea, we reduce the gun's firing rate so that each particle reaches the screen before the next particle is fired. We find that a single particle's hit location on the screen is largely unpredictable, but after a large number of particles have been fired, the interference pattern in Figure 10–6 (lower) again appears. In other words, this experimental interference pattern is found to be a measure of *the probability that the particle will hit the screen at a particular location.* The interference pattern is, in fact, an experimental *probability density function.* By definition, the area under each curve (fully extended on both sides) in

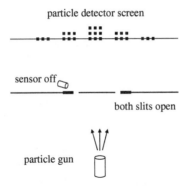

Figure 10–7 The two-slit experiment with both slits open yields the interference pattern.

Figure 10–6 must be equal to 1; meaning any particle passing through one of the slits must hit the screen somewhere. Since this pattern was created one particle at a time, it evidently could not have occurred as a result of interactions between gun particles (at least not in just one universe).

• When the sensor is turned on with both slit doors open (Fig. 10–8), we are able to determine if any single particle passes through the left slit. This sensor corresponds to the window in the magic ball experiment of Figure 10–4. If the sensor records a passing particle, we know it passed through the left slit; we then determine where it hits the screen. If no particle is sensed at the left slit but one is recorded by the screen, we assume it must have passed through the right slit. In this experiment, to our great surprise (if this phenomenon were new to us), the interference pattern is eliminated; the particles accumulate directly behind both slits. The probability density function produced when both slits are open and the

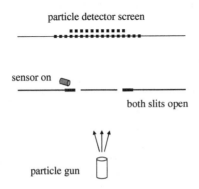

Figure 10–8 The two-slit experiment with both slits open, but the sensor turned on, yields the particle pattern.

sensor turned on (middle plot of Fig. 10–6) is just the sum of the probability density functions produced when one slit is open at a time (upper plot of Fig. 10–6). This is, of course, just the behavior expected of classical particles, but the intuitive classical behavior vanishes and the interference pattern returns if the sensor near the left slit is turned off.

In summary, the act of gaining *information* about the particle's path changes the screen hit pattern from the alternating bands characteristic of the wave interference phenomenon (lower trace of Fig. 10–6) to the lumped pattern characteristic of particles passing through two holes (middle trace of Fig. 10–6). This genuine experimental outcome is very similar to that produced in the metaphorical magic ball experiment with the black and white ball mixture analogous to the interference pattern. How is this possible? This question has been addressed by many prominent scientists over the past 80 years or so. We are now confident that whatever the answer to this mystery, it will not conform to our everyday intuitive ideas about macroscopic objects. No Moses will be coming down from some mountaintop to reveal that the whole thing is just some simple parlor trick. Since we cannot escape from the depths of this rabbit hole, we may as well have a look around to see what other weird things occur in this holey environment.

4. THE PARTICLE INTERFEROMETER EXPERIMENT

The famous two-slit experiment demonstrates quantum weirdness: under certain conditions, small "particles" like electrons, atoms, and photons exhibit wavelike behavior. These same issues may be addressed with a device called a particle interferometer shown in Figure 10–9. A beam of particles produced by a particle gun enters the interferometer at the left and is apparently divided into two separate beams that pass through the two arms. The arms merge on the right side, and the particles impact on a sensor screen that records the output particles as a function of location. A second sensor system on the upper arm involves a window that may be either open or closed. When the window is

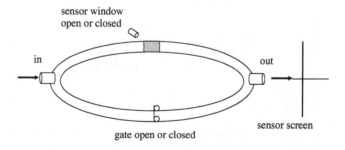

Figure 10–9   An interferometer allowing particles to pass through the upper and lower arms.

closed, the sensor is essentially turned off. The lower arm contains a gate that may be open or closed to block the passage of particles.

Figure 10–6 again represents (approximately) the distinct patterns that may appear on the output sensor screen. We need not be concerned with the exact pattern, which depends on details like interferometer geometry and wavelength of interfering waves; the bands in the interference pattern may consist of concentric circles, for example. The main point is that the series of bands separating regions of large and small particle impact density is actually the appropriate interference pattern consistent with quantum theory. The pattern is apparently due to the interference of separate waves passing through each arm of the interferometer and cannot be explained by classical notions of particle behavior. The output sensor screen on the right side will reveal either particle-like or wavelike behavior depending on the experimental conditions.

Now consider several experiments with beams of atoms (or electrons or photons) used as inputs to the interferometer. First, suppose that both the lower gate and upper sensor window are closed. As expected, the output recorded on the sensor screen is the characteristic particle pattern (or its two-dimensional equivalent) shown as a dashed line in the upper plot of Figure 10–6. Particles only pass through the upper arm because the closed gate blocks their passage through the lower arm. In the second experiment, the gate remains closed, but the sensor window is opened so that the passage of particles in the upper arm may be observed directly. Opening the window produces no apparent change; the characteristic particle pattern is again obtained as expected.

In the third experiment, the sensor window is closed, but the lower gate is opened. Classical thinking predicts the particle pattern given by the middle plot of Figure 10–6, reflecting passage of particles through both arms of the interferometer. But, such classical thinking is again found to be spectacularly wrong; the actual output is a wave interference pattern. How can this be? When the lower gate is closed, particles collect on the screen directly in line with the output tube. By opening the gate, we expect particles moving through the lower arm to simply add to those moving through the upper arm. But somehow, opening the lower gate alters the fundamental nature of particle flux in *both* arms. Our particle beam now seems to be a wave that splits into two waves at the input end of the interferometer and recombines at the output end.

Suppose we attempt to fool these tricky "particle wave creatures" into revealing their true nature. In Experiment 4, we repeat Experiment 3 with the gate open but turn down the intensity of the particle beam such that only one particle at a time can pass through the interferometer. Surely a single particle cannot be a wave? At first, the particles appear to form a random pattern on the screen; however, when a large number have passed through the interferometer, they tend to fall on locations consistent with the interference pattern shown in the lower plot of Figure 10–6. The wave interference pattern is again observed; it just takes longer to produce. How then does an atom, which leaves the gun as a localized particle, "know" how to adjust its motion so as to contribute to a statistical wave interference pattern?

The craziness gets worse. In Experiment 5, the lower gate remains open so that particles remain free to pass through both arms of the interferometer as in Experiment 4. The difference is that the upper sensor window is opened, and a light source is used to detect particles passing through the upper arm. Light reflected off passing particles produces little flashes that may be observed visually or recorded with some instrument. In this case, the interference pattern disappears, and the particle pattern is again obtained! You may wonder about the interaction of the light sensor on the particles; perhaps the light itself causes sufficient deflection of particles in the upper arm to destroy the interference pattern. But, remember that only about half of the particles pass through the upper arm; classical thinking implies that the light sensor should have no influence on particles passing through the lower arm. But in sharp contrast to the classical view, the act of observation of particles in the upper arm somehow changes the behavior of particles passing through both arms. This is a *Renninger negative-result measurement.*

Again we may attempt to fool our " particle waves" into revealing their true nature; this time with the sixth experiment, a *delayed choice experiment.* The lower gate is kept open, and the upper sensor window is closed when each particle enters the interferometer at the left side. From knowledge of particle speed, we are able to determine the time required for the particle to reach the sensor window, which is opened before the expected passage of the particle. In this experiment, the interference pattern is again destroyed! Particles seem to enter the left side of the interferometer "expecting" to act like waves (since the sensor window is then closed) but change their "minds" when the sensor window is opened before they pass the window.

In summary, when both arms of the interferometer are open and no sensor in the arms is turned on, a single particle is somehow represented by two waves, one passing through each arm. But these are not like ordinary physical waves. To see the difference, suppose that a sound wave were to enter a pair of tubes similar to the image in Figure 10–9. The incoming sound wave splits into two waves that can be observed with sensors along either path. By contrast to the interferometer particles, sound waves in each arm remain waves whether or not they are observed. We conclude that one should *not* picture interferometer particles as somehow being "smeared out" and transformed into waves. Rather, the waves provide *statistical information* about the location of particles when they are observed on the sensor screen.

5. WHAT ARE QUANTUM WAVES?

For some readers, quantum ideas may seem too esoteric and far removed from everyday experience to be of general interest, but their consequences are nearly everywhere. Something like a third of the economies of developed countries involves products with components based on quantum principles. Much of modern technology: televisions, cell phones, CD players, computers, automobiles, and other devices rely on modern electronics for which precise understanding of the predictions of quantum mechanics is essential[3]. Furthermore, quantum mechanics provides a deep understanding of natural processes. The disparate properties of different materials, the metals, noble gases, and so forth, may be understood in terms of quantum mechanics, which provides a theoretical framework for the chemical properties of atoms and the periodic table. The amazing paradox is that while quantum mechanics is easily the most successful physical theory in human history, its philosophical interpretation remains murky, controversial, and more than a little strange. The quantum physicist is a bit like some kid who inherited a magic wand from a master magician; the wand works every time, but the kid cannot understand how or why it works.

Quantum mechanics is a theory of the behavior of a mathematical entity called the *quantum wavefunction*, which provides statistical information about the observed behavior of its associated particles. For a single particle moving only in the x direction, the quantum wave amplitude or wavefunction is assigned the Greek letter $\Psi(x, t)$ ("psi"). The information provided by the wavefunction includes the probability density function $|\Psi(x, t)|^2$, which expresses the likelihood of finding the particle at some location x at some time t when a measurement takes place in some experiment, as in the two-slit and interferometer experiments. The interference pattern for the two-slit experiment shown in Figure 10–6 (lower) represents the experimental expression of $|\Psi(x, t)|^2$. The vertical lines around the symbol $\Psi(x, t)$ indicate its magnitude (which is then squared); this notation is needed because $\Psi(x, t)$ is a complex function having real and imaginary parts carrying phase information, the origin of interference phenomena. But just what are quantum waves? Do they have a genuine physical existence analogous to more familiar waves like electromagnetic waves? The usual answer is "no," but this question has been vigorously debated for nearly a century; the question of whether or not quantum waves are real depends partly on just what is meant by the label "real." One can, for example, argue that particles behave *as if* the associated quantum waves are real.

Two traveling *wave packets* (or wave groups) are shown in Figure 10–10; the solid and dashed wave packets in the upper plot move toward the center. These might be short sound wave packets produced by two human voices; in this case, the sound waves carry information between the speakers. When two sound wave packets meet as shown in middle plot; regions of negative pressure cancel regions of positive pressure. The net pressure at each horizontal location is just the sum (*superposition*) of the two sound waves, that is, *wave interference* occurs. The net (summed) pressure at the time of the middle plot is shown in the lower plot. Human voices produce linear waves; as a consequence, the two wave packets pass through each other and emerge undistorted on opposite sides. Thus, several people can talk at the same time and still be understood.

In quantum mechanics, these wave packets were once called *pilot waves*, suggesting that they *guide* their associated particles. Most physicists now avoid notions that quantum waves "guide" particles, although the interpretation by David Bohm and some modern like-minded physicists says just this, as discussed in Chapter 11. Where all physicists do agree is that the waves contain information about particles *observed in later experiments* to have certain

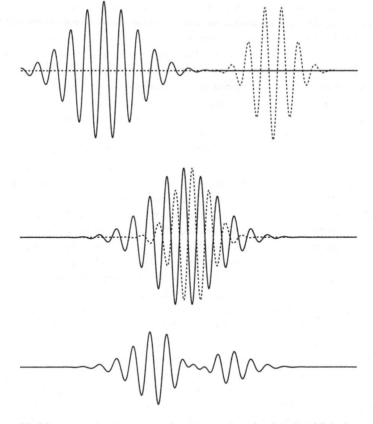

Figure 10–10   (Upper) Two wave packets approach each other. (Middle) The packets collide and interfere. (Lower) The total wave amplitude pattern is the sum of the two packets shown above.

properties like energy E and momentum p. The question of whether a particle can be said to possess these properties before the observation actually occurs has been the subject of intense debate, most notably the early on going exchanges between Bohr and Einstein, but continuing to this day in various contexts.

The motion of each quantum particle is governed by the wave propagation features of its associated wave, which is more safely labeled as a "proxy" wave, a terminology adopted by Nick Herbert.[2] The wave packet moves with a group (packet) velocity that equals the particle velocity. The spatial wavelength λ and angular frequency ω of the waves provide the particle's momentum p and energy E according to

$$p = \frac{h}{\lambda} \tag{10.1}$$

$$E = h\omega \tag{10.2}$$

Planck's constant h is believed to be a fundamental property of the universe, as are the velocity of light and the gravitational constant. The wave frequency f (Hz) is related to angular frequency ω (radians/sec) by the relation $\omega = 2\pi f$. Wavelength (cm) is related to spatial frequency k (radians/cm) by $\lambda = 2\pi/k$.

The wave packets shown in Figure 10–10 represent the motion of unbound (free) particles. By contrast, a bound particle like the electron in a hydrogen atom generally remains part of the atom; such electron is represented by standing waves, several are shown in Figure 10–11. The three gray circles ($n = 1, 2, 3, ...$) represent classical orbital locations of the electron with a nucleus at the center, but electrons don't actually follow classical orbits like planets around the sun. The black lines represent slices (in time and in the plane of the page) of several wavefunctions; the symbol Φ represents only the spatial part of the wavefunction Ψ. The black lines oscillate over time in and out of the gray lines (with nodes at fixed locations) in a manner analogous to guitar strings producing different notes (fundamental and overtones). Since standing waves occur only with discrete frequencies $\omega_n(n = 1, 2, 3, ...)$, the electron's energy is *quantized*, that is, it is allowed to possess only the discrete energies

$$E_n = h\,\omega_n \quad n = 1, 2, 3, \ldots \tag{10.3}$$

Because of the spherical symmetry of the hydrogen atom, these energy levels depend only on the *radial quantum number n*. For example, the part of the

$$\Phi_{nlm}\ (r,\theta,\phi),\ n = 1, 2, 3$$

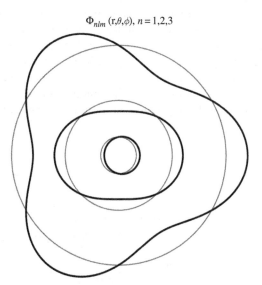

Figure 10–11 Several quantum standing wave functions for an electron in the hydrogen atom are represented by black lines showing departures from average locations (gray lines). The symbol Φ represents spatial parts of the wavefunction Ψ in terms of the three spherical coordinates (r,θ,ϕ) the subscripts are quantum numbers (n, l, m) indicating particular states (energy levels) of the electron.

wavefunction corresponding to the quantum number $n = 3$ has nine associated waves (indicated by the angular quantum numbers l and m) that vary in the two angular directions around the outer sphere. The essential feature determining an element's chemical properties is the statistical spatial distribution of its electrons, mainly the outer shell (valence) electrons, as described by the quantum wavefunction.[4]

The (angular) quantum standing waves are mathematically very similar to the classical Schumann resonances discussed in Chapter 4 (see Fig. 4–12) and the proposed standing brain waves depicted in Figure 7–5. The main difference is that these particular classical waves oscillate only in angular (not radial) directions; their resonant frequencies depend on spatial frequencies (or indexes l and m) over the surface of the Earth or brain. I am *not* suggesting that macroscopic brain waves have any direct connection to quantum mechanics. Rather, the close mathematical similarity occurs because all three systems involve closed shell geometries. Additionally, wave phenomena are found throughout nature, in many physical and biological systems and at multiple hierarchical levels of matter, an illustration of physicist Eugene Wigner's often-quoted "unreasonable success" of mathematics in science.

Several features of quantum mechanics that are quite distinct from classical behavior are illustrated by a system consisting of several particles bouncing about in the bowl shown in Figure 10–12. Suppose these are classical particles, say marbles dropped in your bathroom sink. When the marbles are first dropped, they will have initial potential energies that depend on the heights of their falls into the bowl. The marbles then bounce about in the bowl, transferring energy to the bowl and among each other when they collide. If the initial marble energies are sufficiently small and the bowl sufficiently deep, we can be assured that no marbles will ever escape the sink; the marble system obeys the first law of thermodynamics, the conservation of energy. That is, we can insure that all marbles stay confined by limiting the initial total marble

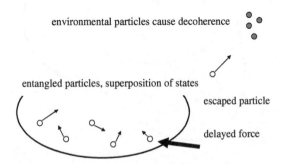

Figure 10–12   Marbles bouncing in a bathroom sink or quantum particles confined by classical forces to a "sink" (perhaps an atom). Unlike classical marbles, an escaped quantum particle remains entangled with sink particles until it interacts with the external environment.

potential energy to a value less than that required for a single particle to escape, accounting for the quite unlikely event that all marble energy gets transferred to a single marble.

With quantum particles, say protons, neutrons, or electrons in an atom, nature's rules are dramatically different. The system of particles is allowed to acquire only discrete energy levels, determined by the size and shape of the bowl and the particle masses, similar to the discrete frequencies given by Equation 10.3. The behavior of the system of particles is described by a single wavefunction $\Psi(x_1, y_1, z_1, x_2, y_2, z_2, ..., t)$ that depends on the simultaneous coordinates (x, y, z) of all the particles, where the numbered subscripts denote particle 1, particle 2, and so forth. In a sense, the particles have lost parts of their individual identities as a result of being confined to the same sink (or atom); in modern quantum terminology, they have become *entangled*. The quantum wavefunction for N particles oscillates in an abstract $3N$ dimensional space, a mathematical generalization of the familiar Euclidean space of three dimensions, called a *Hilbert space*. The entanglement of N particles comes about because of wavefunction phase relationships associated with particle locations.

The probability density function $|\Psi|^2$ provides statistical information about the instantaneous positions and velocities of all the particles. Even when the energy of the system is too low for any particle to escape based on classical thinking, $|\Psi|^2$ tells us that there is always some chance that one or more particles will be found outside the bowl. This uncertainty in particle locations is the basis for many observed properties of nature including *radioactivity*. Many kinds of radioactive decay occur in which atomic nuclei (analogous to our sink) emit various kinds of particles, but it is fundamentally impossible to predict when a particular nucleus will decay. If, however, a mass containing a large number of nuclei is observed in an experiment, $|\Psi|^2$ accurately predicts the expected number of emissions per second from the mass.

The ejected particles can be alpha particles (ionized helium), neutrons, protons, electrons, neutrinos, and so forth. Another example of the non classical behavior of our metaphorical marble—sink system is *quantum tunneling* of electrons through a barrier (analogous to the sink wall) that would be impenetrable according to classical thinking. Such tunneling provides the basis for semiconductors in integrated circuits and other applications, including sensors of the brain's tiny magnetic field (MEG). In the traditional ontological interpretation of quantum mechanics, particles have some chance of being found outside of such confined regions (sinks or *potential wells*) without ever having occupied any location within the barrier (sink wall)! They seem to just appear on one side or the other. In an analogous manner, some of the metaphorical gray balls described in Section 2 will be found outside of the ball machine even when the machine walls lack openings. How do such balls get outside? All we can say is that the balls appear to be magic entities when viewed classically.

Suppose one particle escapes the bowl and flies up toward new particles that are part of the environment in the upper right corner. Just after this escaped particle leaves the bowl, imagine that a force (or potential) is applied to one or more of the remaining particles. If this were a classical system of uncharged particles, say marbles bouncing in a sink, the delayed (after the particle escapes) application of forces to bowl particles would have no effect on the escaped particle. Hit one of the marbles in your the sink with a toothbrush; this action can have no influence on a marble that has already fallen into the toilet. Furthermore, the encounter between the escaped particle and the environmental particles can have no effect on particles remaining in the bowl. But with quantum particles, these common sense classical rules are routinely violated.

The system of particles in the bowl behaves in accordance with its "proxy," the quantum wavefunction $\Psi(x_1, y_1, z_1, x_2, y_2, z_2, ..., t)$. Absent any measurement or other external forces, the system is said to be in a *state of superposition* in which all individual particle locations and velocities are indeterminate as discussed in the following section. The neutrons, protons, and electrons in atoms exist in such a superposition. The wave function yields the probability of finding particles at specific locations when we "look for them" with a specific experimental measurement. A particle escaping the bowl remains entangled to particles remaining in the bowl until such entanglement is lost as the result of interactions (additional entanglement) with the particles that comprise the external environment. If a delayed force is applied to a single bowl particle, this force (Fig. 10–12) alters the behavior of all entangled particles, including the escaped particle. The escaped particle remains entangled with remaining bowl particles until it interacts with environmental particles, but over a (typically) very short time this new entanglement with the macroscopic environment overwhelms entanglement with bowl particles, a process now called *quantum decoherence*. This environmental interaction then alters the behavior of both the escaped particle and the particles remaining in the bowl. Superposition, entanglement, and decoherence are quantum phenomena with no obvious analogs to classical particles.

6. SUPERPOSITION OF STATES: THE COSMIC QUANTUM ORCHESTRA

A basic tenant of traditional quantum mechanics is that individual particles exist in a sort of quantum limbo called a *superposition of states* until an actual measurement is performed. Whereas an atomic electron possesses a definite mass and charge, it occupies an indeterminate location and speed (or momentum) until one of these complementary features is measured. The magic ball experiments (Section 2) and experiments with elementary particles (Sections 3 and 4) demonstrate the general idea, which is quite foreign to intuitive thinking about the classical world of macroscopic objects. While considerable caution should be exercised when classical metaphors are applied to quantum systems, a musical metaphor is quite appropriate for explaining several fundamental features of quantum systems, including superposition and entanglement. The reason that this musical metaphor works so well is that Schrödinger's equation for the particle wavefunction is a linear wave equation,

Individual notes (states)

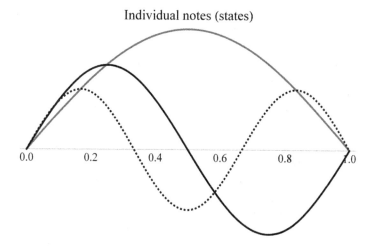

Figure 10–13   A stretched violin string showing its three lowest modes of oscillation with exaggerated amplitudes.

and the sounds produced by musical instruments are governed by very similar wave equations (see the Endnotes for mathematical details[5]). As a result, the dynamic behavior of the quantum wavefunction is nearly identical to the mechanical vibrations of an equivalent part of a musical instrument. Notice, however, that I did *not* say that the quantum particles themselves behave like mechanical vibrations; only the proxy waves behave this way.

Consider the string stretched between fixed supports as shown in Figure 10–13; the spatial shapes of the fundamental and first two overtones are shown with progressively lower amplitudes. These plots represent snapshots in time, but with greatly exaggerated amplitudes for plotting purposes; vertical displacement is very small compared to string length in an actual violin string. This string might be part of any stringed instrument: guitar, violin, piano, and so forth. If a string of length L is plucked at some initial time ($t = 0$), its displacement at all later times $\Psi(x, t)$ may be expressed as a *superposition of states*, that is, a sum (Fourier series) over different temporal frequencies ω_n given by

$$\Psi(x, t) = \sum_{n=1}^{\infty} a_n \cos(\omega_n t) \sin(k_n x) \qquad (10.4)$$

The temporal ω_n and spatial frequencies k_n of string oscillations are related through the string wave *dispersion relation*

$$\omega_n = v k_n = \frac{n \pi v}{L} \quad n = 1, 2, 3, \ldots \qquad (10.5)$$

Thus, each spatial shape (called the *eigenfunction* or characteristic function), shown in Figure 10–13 for a string of length $L = 1$, represents an oscillation with a frequency (musical note) given by Equation (10.5). The dispersion relation originates with the governing wave equation based on Newton's law for the string system. The mechanical string process is very simple: Tension in the string tends to pull it back from displacements about its equilibrium position, and the resulting (horizontal) string wave propagation velocity v depends on the string mass and its tension. The following summary provides some of the general features of standing waves that apply to *both* musical instruments and the wavefunctions of bound elementary particles like electrons in an atom.

- Only discrete musical notes ω_n (frequencies) are produced by the string. Similarly, elementary particles bound to some region have *quantized energy levels* given by $E_n = h\omega_n$, where h is Planck's constant.
- Sounds produced by musical instruments generally consist of multiple notes (frequencies) labeled the fundamental ($n = 1$) and overtones ($n > 1$). In the simple string, all overtones are multiples of the fundamental, that is, harmonics $\omega_n = n\omega_1$, but overtones are generally not harmonics in other oscillating systems. Bound elementary particles exist in a superposition of energy states very similar to Equation (10.4). The lowest allowed energy state ($E_1 = h\omega_1$ or the *zero point energy*) is essentially the fundamental oscillation mode of the quantum wavefunction. A particle with energy equal to exactly zero is not allowed by the uncertainty principle.
- Longer strings produce a lower range of musical notes, as in the bass, cello, and other large-sized members of the violin family. Similarly, a lower *range* of particle energies is allowed in larger quantum systems. Nuclear protons and neutrons, confined by strong nuclear forces to much smaller spaces, have very high energy levels.
- The intensity (loudness) of a particular musical note is equal to the squared coefficients in the superposition (sum over states) expressed in Equation (10.4), that is, a_n^2. The probability that a particle will be found to have energy $E_n = h\omega_n$ when measured by a macroscopic device is also equal to a_n^2, which (unlike the musical note) depends on both the particle itself and the measuring device.
- The two-dimensional version of the string is the square drum membrane with amplitude $\Psi(x, y, t)$ normal to the (x, y) plane. In the case of drum sounds, the single sum in Equation (10.4) is replaced by a double sum (over indices n and m) of spatial waves in the x and y directions; these two-dimensional standing waves oscillate with fundamental and overtone frequencies ω_{nm} similar to one-dimensional waves in a string. Similarly, a single quantum particle moving in two spatial dimensions (or two particles moving in one dimension) is described by the wavefunction $\Psi(x, y, t)$ and has quantized energy levels $E_{nm} = h\omega_{nm}$.
- When the surface of a drum oscillates, separate parts of the membrane displacement are correlated; if you bang a drum at one location, other drum parts are affected. Thus, the drum membrane differs fundamentally from a system consisting of two independent strings; separate parts of the

drum membrane are *entangled*. Similarly, when more than one quantum particle occupies the same region (same atom or sink or *potential well* of some kind), the analogous musical system is *not* two independent strings; rather, it is the drum. The quantum particles are said to be *entangled*.

• The (single electron) hydrogen atom moves in three dimensions and may be described by the wavefunction $\Psi(x, y, z, r, \theta, \varphi, t)$, which depends on the rectangular coordinates of the (proton) nucleus (x, y, z) and the spherical coordinates (r, θ, φ) of the electron with respect to the center of the nucleus. An imagined analogous musical instrument would vibrate in six spatial dimensions. A single wavefunction governs the behaviors of the entangled electron–neutron system; however, because the proton is so much heavier than the electron, an approximate wavefunction governs (approximately) independent electron behavior. The allowed electron energy levels in the atom E_{nlm} involve the three indices or *quantum numbers* (n, l, m) associated with the three spherical coordinates. Several associated standing waves are shown in Figure 10–11.

Table 10–1 lists a number of classical musical analogs to quantum systems. When a guitar or violin is played, we are able to hear multiple notes; our brain

Table 10–1 Musical Analogs of Quantum Waves

Quantum Property	Musical Analogs
Measurements of macroscopic systems	Nonmusical, incoherent sounds
Quantum measurements	Tiny microphones yielding single notes
Wavefunction Ψ providing probability information about particles	Amplitude of mechanical vibration of string, drum, etc., of musical instrument
Particle locations	Locations on string, membrane, etc.
Particle energy state	Musical note (one frequency)
Uncertainty principle. Accurate energy measurements require minimal measurement time t.	Each tone requires a minimum duration t for identification. Musical notes involve both tone and duration.
Quantized energy levels (states) $E_n = \hbar f_n$	Discrete notes, the resonant frequencies of strings, drums, etc.
Superposition of quantum states $\Psi = \sum a_n \psi_n$	Musical chords: multiple tones played simultaneously with relative energies $|a_n|^2$
Lowest energy state	Fundamental frequency of string, membrane, etc.
Excited energy states	Overtones of string, membrane, etc.
Most probable quantum state when measured is the n with largest $|a_n|^2$.	Fundamental or overtone with largest energy
Collapse of the wavefunction	Microphones record only a single note
Wave function interference	Amplitude interference, musical beats
One particle in square well potential	Vibrations of violin string
Two particles in square well potential	Vibrations of square drum membrane

provides the measurements of the intensity and timing of the distinct musical sounds. By contrast, the act of measurement of an electron's energy level mysteriously picks out just one energy level analogous to the weird experience of hearing only a single musical note even though the music contains multiple notes. Complementary features of the particle, for example, its location or momentum, can be picked out from the superposition of states in different experiments (different preparations of the measuring device), subject to the limitations of the uncertainty principle discussed in Chapter 11. If, for example, we set the measuring device to measure particle location with certain accuracy, the particle's momentum will also have some range of indeterminacy dictated by our choice of experimental set-up and the uncertainty principle.

In the traditional interpretation of quantum mechanics, the process by which a single state is identified in an experiment is known as the *collapse of the wavefunction*, suggesting that all but one energy level in the superposition (Eq. 10.4) somehow "vanishes" as a result of the measurement process. It is important to emphasize that this so-called wavefunction "collapse" is an ad hoc addition to the formal mathematics of quantum mechanics, a process roundly challenged by some contemporary physicists. The equivalent outcome in our musical analog would involve some sort of poorly understood (statistically) variable filter measurement system that would allow us to hear only a single note when our system for listening to the sound of a single string is turned on, even though the string actually produces multiple notes simultaneously. The reason that a particular note, say the first overtone, is heard, rather than, say the fundamental or 2nd overtone, is unknown; this is the classical analog of the *quantum measurement problem*. Despite this deep fundamental ignorance, however, one can predict the numbers of occurrence of each observed (heard) note to very high accuracy when the sounds of many identical strings are recorded with identical measuring methods.

Imagine a universe called Oz, apparently consisting of a gigantic ghostly cosmic orchestra with parts of the musical instruments (strings, membranes, air columns, and so forth) representing elementary particles. The inhabitants of Oz are generally unable to hear the music; they hear only the noisy jumble of discordant sounds representing macroscopic objects. However, with careful experiments, they are able to isolate individual parts of musical instruments like a single violin string. But rather than hearing the full complement of the string's sound, only a single note is heard each time their measuring system is switched on. With any single measurement, the observed note cannot be predicted. However, when a large number of experiments are performed on identical strings, the probability of occurrence of each observed note ω_n is found to equal the weighting factor a_n^2 of the sum (Eq. 10.4).

The quantum mechanics represented by Schrödinger's equation is quite separate from the quantum process known as the collapse of the wavefunction. Whereas Schrödinger's equation is well understood and accurately governs the statistical behavior of elementary particles, the mechanism by which specific experiments select a single state (energy level, particle location, and so forth) from the full superposition of states is not understood. If an experiment to find the location of a particle with high accuracy is chosen by the scientist, the particle's velocity (or momentum) will be poorly known as dictated by the uncertainty principle. In other words, nature has apparently erected a fundamental barrier limiting the information accessible to human observers and their scientific instruments. The metaphorical inhabitants of Oz have an excellent model of their ghost orchestra but minimal understanding of the filtering process that forces them to hear only a single note with each measurement; Oz's ignorance is the analog of the *quantum measurement problem*. Some of the ontological issues of quantum mechanics under serious ongoing debate might be boiled down to the following question about our universe: *Is the cosmic ghost orchestra real?*

7. SUMMARY

Quantum mechanics reveals an underlying reality of the world that is foreign to our classical thinking based on everyday experiences with macroscopic systems. To illustrate this point, a metaphorical system is imagined that consists of magic gray balls dropped into the top of a simple ball machine. The balls fall into the machine's body, encounter a fork with two legs, and pass through the legs into two boxes at the bottom. The boxes are then opened and found to contain either the original gray balls or a mysteriously transformed mixture of black and white balls. The mystery deepens when several experiments suggests that such transformations depend on the information available to the observers, who seem to be "joined" to the balls in unexpected ways.

In genuine *quantum two-slit* and *interferometer systems*, an elementary particle like an electron can appear to take two distinct paths at the same time. The metaphorical gray balls and black/white balls are analogous to particle and wave interference patterns, respectively. Particles are shot through a screen containing two slits or alternately through a two-arm device called an interferometer, systems analogous to the magic ball machine. A sensor screen analogous to the ball machine's boxes at the output ends of the quantum systems records the spatial patterns produced when particles hit the screen.

When one particle path (slit or interferometer arm) is blocked, the observed output pattern is the pattern expected of classical particles. However, the first mystery occurs when both paths are open and no sensors along either pathway are active, thereby restricting path information from observers. The observed output at the sensor screen is a wave interference pattern. It may seem at first that each particle is somehow divided into two waves at the slit junction or interferometer fork, each passing through a separate slit or interferometer arm. In this view, the waves would then recombine at the output end to form the interference pattern. But this "obvious" interpretation of wave–particle duality is incorrect; rather, each particle appears to have an associated "proxy" or "information wave" (the quantum wavefunction) that propagates along both open pathways.

The second mysterious outcome occurs when a sensor along one pathway is activated to determine if each particle has passed along its path. This act of gaining information about the particle's path changes the output pattern from the alternating bands characteristic of wave interference to a two-lump pattern characteristic of classical particles passing through two holes or two arms of the interferometer. How can just looking at a particle's path, even when the particle follows the opposite path, change the output pattern?

The third mysterious outcome occurs in the *delayed choice experiment*: the path sensor is turned on only *after* the particle has apparently passed the two-slit wall or fork in the interferometer. Again, the act of turning on the sensor eliminates the interference pattern. This outcome emphasizes that particles do *not* turn into waves at forks in their paths; rather, the wavelike output is eliminated by an action undertaken after the particle or wave (or whatever it is) has passed the fork.

The central practice of quantum mechanics employs a mathematical entity called the *quantum wavefunction*, which provides statistical information about the observed behavior of its associated particles. An isolated particle's energy and momentum is determined by the frequency (or spatial wavelength) of its "proxy" wavefunction. The square of the wavefunction is a probability density function indicating where a particle is most likely to be found in a specified measurement process. Individual particles apparently exist in a quantum limbo called a *superposition of states* until an actual measurement is performed. An atomic electron occupies an indeterminate location and speed (or momentum) until one of these complementary features is observed. Measurement accuracies are limited by the *uncertainty principle*, believed to be a fundamental property of the universe limiting the accessibility of information rather than simply an instrumental limitation.

The wavefunction for any system of particles is governed by Schrödinger's equation, a linear wave equation very similar to the classical equations that govern the mechanical vibrations of musical instruments. As a consequence of this similarity, the dynamic behavior of the quantum wavefunction for a single particle moving in one or two dimensions is nearly identical to the vibrations of a violin string or drum membrane, respectively. The discrete notes produced by musical instruments are closely analogous to the quantized energy states of systems of particles. The system energy state is proportional to the frequency of the wavefunction associated with the full system consisting of all particles. When an individual particle becomes part of a system of particles, it loses aspects of its separate identity to the full system, a process called *quantum entanglement*.

The process by which a single state is picked out from the superposition of states in a quantum experiment is known traditionally as the *collapse of the wavefunction*. This so-called "collapse" is not a property of Schrödinger's equation, but rather an ad hoc addition representing the traditional Copenhagen interpretation of the *quantum measurement problem*. The equivalent outcome in our classical musical analog would involve some sort of measurement system that allows us to hear only a single note from a violin string when our microphone system is turned on, even though the string actually produces multiple notes simultaneously. The probability of hearing any particular note (analogous to the particle's energy level) is accurately predicted by the wavefunction, which may be viewed as a kind of *proxy wave* or *information field* providing statistical information about (measured) properties of particles.

Chapter 11

Ontological Interpretations of Quantum Mechanics

1. THE CLASSICAL MEASUREMENT PROBLEM

Classical experimental science is routinely limited by the act of measurement itself, which can cause an unwanted change in the property being measured. When the temperature of cold water is measured by immersing a room temperature thermometer in the water glass, the water temperature is raised, although the effect is negligible if the heat capacity of the thermometer is much smaller than that of the water. When EEG is recorded from the scalp, tiny scalp currents pass through the EEG amplifiers, but modern amplifiers accept such small currents that the net effect on scalp potentials is negligible.[1]

Consider an example more closely aligned to our discussions of modern physics. Suppose we use a microscope to determine the instantaneous position and speed of an atom, molecule, or other small particle. The particle is illuminated, and the light scattered by the particle is what we (or some instrument) observe while peering through the microscope. The resolving power of the microscope determines the ultimate accuracy of the particle's location, but resolving power is known to increase as the wavelength of scattered light decreases. We are free to choose the light's wavelength for our experiment; with suitable instruments we may even employ electromagnetic radiation outside the visible range as our probe of particle position and velocity. It is known that our particle will experience larger recoil when impacted by light with shorter wavelengths, that is, higher energy (and momentum) photons as given by Equations 10.1 and 10.2. As we shorten the light's wavelength in order to better resolve particle location, we provide a larger "kick" to our particle, thereby forcing a larger, unwanted distortion of the particle's original speed. If, on the other hand, light with longer wavelengths is employed, we obtain better estimates of the particle's speed, but lose information about particle location. If uncertainties in particle location and momentum (the product of mass and velocity) are and Δx, Δp respectively, experimental accuracies are limited by the following version of the *uncertainty principle*

$$\Delta x \, \Delta p \geq \hbar \qquad (11.1)$$

Here $\hbar = h/2\pi$ is Planck's constant, which enters the above analysis because of the known relationship of the momentum p of light quanta (photons) to light wavelength λ given by Equation 10.1. When first reading of this as an undergraduate, my indifferent reaction was "so what?", but it turns out that this simple experiment has profound implications. Rather than the more common label *uncertainty principle*, we might more accurately refer to the *indeterminacy principle* for reasons discussed in the following section.

2. THE UNCERTAINTY PRINCIPLE AND FUNDAMENTAL LIMITS ON INFORMATION

I have purposely placed discussion of the above microscopic particle experiment in a separate section concerned with the classical measurement problem. As implied above, the uncertainty principle at first appears to be just a practical experimental limitation analogous to our experience with classical experiments like measuring water temperature or EEG. The interpretation of Section 1 is essentially classical with just a little quantum flavor; the measurement problem appears to occur only because of technical limitations when measuring small masses. This was the distorted view emphasized in my university classes in the 1960s, but quantum mechanics actually tells us something quite different. Perhaps my professors felt that students required a gentle immersion in quantum thinking before revealing the whole shocking truth. In any case, the big secret that my professors barely mumbled under their breaths is as follows. Quantum mechanics actually says that the uncertainty principle, like the fixed velocity of light, is a fundamental property of our universe and cannot be bypassed with improved technical methods. The uncertainty principle follows from the wavelike behavior of small particles. Particles normally confined to isolated locations sometimes behave *as if* they were guided by quantum waves spread out over large distances.

Consider one critical consequence of the uncertainty principle. Every atom consists of a positively charged nucleus surrounded by negatively charged electrons. Classically, charged particles lose energy when accelerated (as occurs in orbital motion). Why then doesn't the attractive force between charges eventually cause electrons to fall into the nucleus after they have lost speed? The apparent answer is that such action would fix the location of each electron within a very small space, thereby requiring the momentum uncertainty Δp to be very large, implying that electrons would fly out of the atom altogether. But this superficial picture lacks self-consistency; a stable atom actually requires a compromise in which electrons jiggle here and there with moderate uncertainty in both momentum and location within the atom. This emphasizes the central importance of the uncertainty principle even when no experiment occurs. Electrons are evidently *forbidden by nature* to acquire precise locations and speeds at the same time. *If not for the uncertainty principle, stable atoms, molecules, baseballs, and humans would not exist.*

Although quantum mechanics has been fully tested with a myriad of disparate experiments, the results are subject to conflicting ontological interpretations. Quantum mechanical questions may be divided into instrumental questions (expressed in terms of either actual or thought experiments) and purely ontological questions (for which no experimental tests are currently known). Ontological questions, concerning the nature of reality, continue to be argued in both the scientific and general literature, and new experiments may be proposed to move ontological questions into the instrumental category for resolution. I will detail only parts of such discussions here, but the bottom line is that all interpretations of quantum mechanics are weird when considered from our classical, everyday viewpoints. Readers holding classical world views should not expect to find intuitively pleasing explanations of quantum mechanics; scientists much smarter than us have failed in this quest over the past century.

In the traditional (Copenhagen) interpretation of quantum mechanics, an unmeasured particle's properties are, in a certain sense, not real; properties like position and speed are realized only in the act of measurement. Niels Bohr's interpretation is that quantum theory aims to describe certain *connections between human experiences, not* to describe some physical world conceived to exist and have definite properties independently of human observations. An alternate view that some find more satisfying is that while the unmeasured particle is real, its measured properties depend on multiple influences that act over arbitrarily large distances from the measurement site, influences that may be "transmitted" at greater-than-light speed. When we probe a small particle to determine its location, its true location is disturbed by a vast collection of distant events in other parts of the universe. Note that relativity theory prohibits the transmission of signals above light speed, but apparently no such restriction applies to influences that carry no ordinary information useable by observers.

In quantum mechanics, *complementary* measurable properties of particles come in pairs, an idea that follows directly from wave–particle duality. This property is expressed mathematically by the Fourier transform and its inverse. A particle's location and momentum are said to be complementary, as are its energy and the time interval over which the energy measurement is made. The uncertainty principle applies to all complementary pairs of properties of particles and fields. One example is provided by an electric field E with its complementary property equal to the time rate of change of the field $\frac{\partial E}{\partial t}$. If we suppose that the electric field within some region of space at some initial time is exactly zero, the uncertainty principle requires that its time derivative cannot be specified. Such *indeterminacy* then implies that this region of "empty space" is likely to have a non zero electric field an instant later. The implication is that no region of space can remain entirely free of electric field for long; rather, small electric fields continuously pop in and out of existence even with no charge sources present to produce the fields. While this phenomenon seems quite strange, it has been verified by experiments involving pairs of metal plates placed very close together in a vacuum. Quantum theory correctly predicts the force pushing the plates together due to quantum electric field fluctuations. According to quantum mechanics, the vacuum state, which contains no ordinary physical particles, is not truly empty. Rather, it contains fleeting electromagnetic fields and virtual particles that pop in and out of existence. As we found with light speed, so-called "empty" space has some rather unexpected physical properties.

3. SPOOKY INFLUENCES, THE EPR PARADOX, AND BELL'S THEOREM

EPR stands for the scientists Einstein, Podolsky, and Rosen, who introduced a famous thought experiment in 1935 to argue that quantum mechanics is an incomplete physical theory, meaning that particles must have hidden features (*hidden variables*) in addition to the wavefunction that determine their weird behavior. These putative hidden variables might then render the quantum wavefunction analogous to classical statistical measures employed because of the inherent complexity of many interacting elements, as in the example of molecular collisions in a fluid.

One quantum property relevant to this discussion is called *spin*. When a normal object, say a top, spins about some axis, we can imagine the fingers of our right hand pointing in the spin direction. Our thumb is then said to point in the positive spin direction (spin up), a convention is known as the *right hand rule*. Electron or photon spin is sometimes imagined as similar to a spinning baseball or the Earth spinning about the north–south axis, but this picture, like many classical analogs of quantum phenomena, is far too crude. For one thing, the angular speed can only take on discrete (quantized) values. To cite an analogy, the *charge* of an electron is a fundamental property revealed when electrons are exposed to electric fields. Similarly, *spin* is a fundamental property revealed when electrons are exposed to magnetic fields. Thus, the particle properties "charge" and "spin" are defined only by their distinct behaviors in specific experiments.

Electron and photon spin are quantized to single magnitudes but can be either positive (up or counterclockwise) or negative (down or clockwise) *when measured about any axis freely chosen by experimental scientists.* That is, each experimenter chooses some arbitrary direction in space (the chosen axis) and measures the electron spin about that axis; only two results are possible, *spin up* or *spin down*. This experiment tells absolutely nothing about the result that would have occurred had a different axis been chosen. We are concerned here with a particular quantum experiment in which two electrons or photons are emitted by a single source causing them to exist in a state of *quantum entanglement*. In this case, "entanglement" means that if one electron has a positive spin about a certain axis, the electron's twin must have negative spin about the same axis, consistent with the law of angular momentum conservation. But before measurement, it is fundamentally impossible to know which particle spins up and which one spins down about any chosen axis.

The essential ideas of the ERP experiment can be appreciated by the magic dice metaphor indicated in Figure 11–1, in which dice are thrown on different surfaces (analogous to measurements of spin about different axes). That is, the

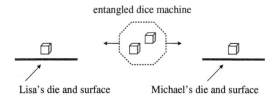

Figure 11–1 Metaphorical dice (containing only 1s and 2s) are first confined to a machine that seems to produce a strange property called *entanglement*. Two scientists each receive a single die at a remote location and toss their die on any one of three (randomly chosen) surfaces. Whenever they happen to choose the same toss surface, their die numbers always match.

dice thrower consciously chooses his surface just as the physicist chooses the axis for the quantum spin measurement as indicated by the analogs in Table 11.1. Each of our imagined die faces exhibits either one or two dots analogous to positive or negative spin. In the case of spin, where there are only two possible outcomes in each measurement, I could have chosen the alternate metaphor of a coin toss yielding either heads or tails. But, I adopt the dice metaphor here because other quantum experiments result in more than just two possible outcomes. The ERP proposal imagines a pair of similar experiments performed at widely separated locations, say by the fanciful pair of physicists Lisa and Michael. Each die number represents a different state of the corresponding particle, but only one realization of these states is observed when the die is tossed on a specific surface. The surfaces used for the dice rolls (spin axes) are independently chosen by Lisa and Michael. Each of our imagined die faces exhibits either one or two dots analogous to positive or negative electron spin about the chosen axis. Our arguments are simplified if we imagine Lisa and Michael's spin sensors to be oriented in *opposite* directions so that a "match" between spins occurs when one electron spins up and the other spins down. Thus, when our metaphorical "entangled dice" are tossed on a surface, the only two possible outcomes are (1, 1) and (2, 2) so that the two die numbers always match when tossed on the same type of surface (no matter how far apart).

Table 11–1 Magic Dice Analog of the Bell-ERP-TypeExperiment

Electron Pair Experiments	Metaphorical Dice Rolls
Particle spin	Upper face of tossed die
Measure particle spin	Act of tossing die
Spin measurement axis	Surface where die is tossed
Spin either positive or negative	Each die shows either a 1 or 2
Local hidden variables	Each die loaded to be correlated with the other
Bell's inequality violated	Dice not loaded
Quantum entanglement	Nonlocal influence between dice

In traditional interpretations of quantum mechanics, the spin of a particular electron or photon is not even "real" until measured. If we measure the spin of one electron as positive (up), any measurement of the spin of the entangled (twin) electron about the same axis must obtain a negative (down) spin. Our dice metaphor gets a little murky at this point as we must imagine some sort of strange connection between the dice forcing a 100% correlation between die numbers observed on each throw, whereas each individual die has only a 50% chance of showing either 1 or 2. When we roll the two separate dice on identical kinds of surfaces, only two outcomes are possible, the dice must exhibit either (1, 1) or (2, 2); the outcomes (1, 2) and (2, 1) are not allowed by quantum theory as verified in many confirming experiments. It then makes absolutely no sense to say that a single die is in the state 1 or 2 before the die is actually cast. Furthermore, the number obtained in the toss depends on both die and toss-surface properties. *The die number is a holistic property of the measuring system and the system being measured.* Perhaps this dice analogy provides us with just a bit more comfort with weird quantum thinking. Our classical roll of a die is analogous to an experiment resulting in the quantum *collapse of the wavefunction.*

Imagine that scientists Lisa and Michael carry out extensive experiments with dice tosses on different surfaces and find that their dice obey classical statistical behavior analogous to that found in quantum mechanics. Their dice theory accurately predicts dice roll probabilities (equal chance of 1 or 2 in the example of unloaded dice), but it cannot predict the outcome of any single die roll. In the quantum system before measurement, each electron is in a state of quantum superposition, consisting of both positive and negative spin, analogous to the state of a die before it is actually tossed. After all, our die faces actually do contain both 1s and 2s, so we might say that the state of the die before tossing is a superposition of states 1 and 2. Collapse of the "die function" (choosing one number) occurs only when the die is tossed.

In the actual quantum experiment, entangled photons or electrons are sent in opposite directions to Lisa's and Michael's detectors at widely separated locations. Suppose Lisa chooses to measure electron spin about, let's say, the vertical axis and finds that her electron has a positive spin. If Michael performs his spin experiment about the same (vertical) axis, quantum mechanics says that, in the absence of information about Lisa's measurement, Michael's spin measurement has an equal 50% chance of being positive (up) or negative (down). But wait! Quantum mechanics also says that once Lisa finds a positive spin for her photon, Michael's electron *must* exhibit a negative spin about the same axis. How can both predictions of quantum mechanics be valid simultaneously?

Our metaphorical dice experiment in Figure 11–1 illustrates the basic idea. Remember that the spin sensors are oriented in opposite directions so that a (1, 1) dice outcome corresponds to electron spins in opposite directions. Suppose Lisa rolls her die on a glass surface and obtains a 1. If Michael throws his die on an identical glass surface in the absence of any information from Lisa's result, according to our dice rules, he has an equal 50% of rolling a 1 or 2. But due to dice entanglement, Lisa's roll of a 1 means that he *must* also roll a 1. How can potentially conflicting rules "control" Michael's die behavior?

A possible classical explanation is that our dice entanglement is much more complicated than we have imagined. Perhaps the dice become loaded during the entanglement process such that Lisa's die is fully predisposed (with 100% chance) to come up 1 and Michael's die is certain to come up 1 when rolled on a glass surfaces; the final states of the dice are actually fixed before they are rolled. Since experiments show that the two possible outcomes of dice rolls are (1, 1) and (2, 2) with equal chance, the next pair of dice may be loaded in either the same or opposite manner. In any roll of a die, there is still only a 50% chance of predicting the outcome, but perhaps this is only because the dice are loaded in a subtle way; they have hidden features that we are unable to observe but behave in agreement with the uncertainty principle.

This "obvious" explanation becomes a bit harder to believe when we realize that the loading of our dice must be very finely tuned to account for rolls on the many different surfaces (spin axes) that Lisa and Michael are free to choose. A second possible explanation involves some sort of "spooky action at a distance," such that Michael's die is informed immediately that Lisa has rolled a 1 with her die. Michael's die then uses this spooky action to determine that it must also show a 1 when rolled.

According to the traditional Copenhagen view of quantum mechanics, nothing is to be gained by such speculations about possible hidden features (or hidden variables). It was argued for at least a full generation that such questions fail to lie within the purview of legitimate science since we cannot settle them with genuine experiments. But, this traditional quantum thinking has been dramatically refuted as a result of a theoretical study by physicist John Bell in 1964, which transformed the ontological issues of the ERP thought experiment into an important issue subject to concrete experiments. Again we recruit our metaphorical magic dice, but this time we allow throws on three different surfaces, say glass, felt, and wood. Bell's theorem (or inequality) is based on experiments with a large number of pairs of entangled electrons or photons (or entangled dice). Our three metaphorical dice surfaces represent particle spin measurements about three different axes oriented 120° apart.

Bell's proposed experiments concern putative hidden features of the entanglement process that may underlie the quantum formalism. In one version of Bell's proposed test, Lisa and Michael receive entangled dice from the central source and agree to perform successive experiments on each die pair. Each die is rolled on one of the three surfaces, chosen at random separately by Lisa and Michael. Suppose that dice entanglement involves local hidden features that may vary for each die pair. Since these putative hidden features must be rather complicated, we may think of them roughly like little computers inside the particles. Say one die is programmed to land on (1, 1, 2) when tossed on glass, felt, and wood, respectively, as indicated in Figure 11–2. Its twin must then also be programmed to land on (1, 1, 2) when tossed on the same three surfaces.

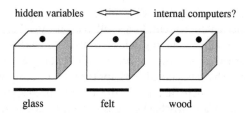

Figure 11–2   An "obvious" explanation for entangled dice behavior is the *local hidden variables* model: Suppose that while together inside the dice machine, each pair somehow becomes "programmed" so that when tossed on, let's say, glass or felt, each die must show a 1, whereas when tossed on wood, each must show a 2. Bell's theorem showed that this hypothesis was subject to experimental tests, and the experiments show that *this local hidden variables explanation is NOT correct.*

Suppose further that subsequent die pairs (emitted later from the magic dice machine) are programmed in a similar manner like (glass, felt, wood) → (2, 1, 2), (2, 2, 1), and so forth.

First consider the case where all dice follow the rule (program) that two surfaces produce the same number (1 or 2), and the third surface produces the opposite number; the conforming example expressed in Table 11–2 is (glass, felt, wood) → (1, 1, 2). Lisa and Michael each have three choices of surfaces for dice tosses; Table 11–2 lists all nine possible combinations. As shown in the third column, Lisa and Michael obtain the same die role in five of the nine cases. All similar combinations generated in the dice machine, (glass, felt, wood) → (2, 1, 2), (2, 2, 1), and so forth, result in the same 5/9 ratio of matches between Lisa and Michael's die. We have neglected the two possible internal programs where dice outcomes are independent of the chosen surface, namely (glass, felt, wood) → (1, 1, 1) or (2, 2, 2). But in these two cases, Lisa and Michael always obtain identical dice outcomes. From this simple analysis, we find the essential

Table 11–2   Nine Possible Outcomes If Magic Dice Are Pre programmed To Yield 1, 1, 2 When Tossed on Glass, Felt, or Wood, Respectively

(1, 1, 2)	Lisa	Michael	Matched Dice?
1	Glass	Glass	Y
2	Glass	Felt	Y
3	Glass	Wood	N
4	Felt	Glass	Y
5	Felt	Felt	Y
6	Felt	Wood	N
7	Wood	Glass	N
8	Wood	Felt	N
9	Wood	Wood	Y

idea of Bell's inequality: If each dice pair is pre-programmed (before being tossed on a surface) to land on a specific number corresponding to each surface, the probability that Lisa and Michael will obtain the same die outcome must be greater than or equal to 5/9.

According to ERP's original argument, each electron or photon entering a detector should have a definite spin about each and every axis even though only spin about one axis at a time can be measured. By the same reasoning, our metaphorical dice should contain features that fix the numbers that occur in any roll of the dice. Bell's theorem shows that even though we can't actually measure electron or photon spin about more than one axis (or obtain a die outcomes on more than one surface at a time), and we are not able to "read" the putative entanglement program, it is still possible to determine if electron spin is fixed ("real") before measurement (or if die outcome is predetermined before the toss).

Quantum experiments based on Bell's theorem have been carried out by several groups and the results appear to be unequivocal.[2] Expressed in terms of the magic dice metaphor, results are as follows:

- When a large number of dice are thrown, the total number of 1s is approximately equal the number of 2s, since each individual die throw has a 50% chance of coming up 1 in agreement with quantum theory as expected.
- The observed correlations between Lisa and Michael's dice throws are significantly lower than the predicted minimum probability of 5/9. We are forced to abandon the local hidden features (or internal computer program) model; the dice cannot have been preloaded to land on a specific number associated with each surface.

We may then be forced to conclude that each electron or photon only acquires a definite spin when measured. In the context of our dice metaphor, this result may, at first, seem not so surprising; the outcome of a throw of an ordinary unloaded die is, in fact, not predetermined by some feature or program hidden within each die; rather, a definite state of the die can only be determined after the die is tossed. But wait! There is more. When Lisa tosses her die and obtains a 1, Michael's toss of the entangled twin die must also yield a 1. Somehow the dice are linked by a strange *nonlocal influence*. Apparently, if Michael tosses first, his die outcome fixes the outcome that Lisa must obtain with a later throw and vice versa.

The influence between magic dice (or electrons or photons) can occur at faster than light speed. Apparently no violation of special relativity need occur, although this issue is subject to some current debate among physicists. Special relativity prohibits any mass from being accelerated to speeds faster than light speed. It also prohibits Lisa from sending a signal to Michael containing ordinary information about her local environment at greater than light speed. She cannot, for example, provide Michael with an instantaneous reading of her local clock; the inevitable delay in such information transfer is central to

Einstein's theory. Imagine that Lisa makes her electron spin measurement just before the twin (entangled) electron arrives at Michael's detector, and Lisa records a positive spin about the vertical axis. The influence of Lisa's measurement is somehow "felt" by the twin electron so that Michael's measurement about the vertical axis must yield a negative spin. Note one additional issue: This description is partly based on classical thinking about time. If relativistic effects occur due to gravitational fields or relative motion, Lisa and Bob do not generally agree on which of their measurements occurred first, thereby confusing the issue of cause and effect.

Experimental tests of Bell's inequality appear to rule out *local realism* once and for all. The *local realism* label applies to particles possessing definite values for certain physical properties like location, speed, spin, energy, and so forth, even though it may be fundamentally impossible to measure complementary properties. Furthermore, in this local interpretation of quantum mechanics, properties cannot change because of spooky actions from distant locations. If our metaphorical dice were locally realistic in this sense, the outcome of each dice roll would be determined in advance by some inner "computer" programmed in the entanglement process but remaining forever hidden from our view.

Experimental rejection of local realism leaves us with two remaining choices; apparently we must either adopt *nonlocal realism* (or *neorealism* described below in Section 5) or abandon realism altogether, meaning that particles do not actually take on certain physical properties until they are measured. In this latter view, particles are suspended in a superposition of states, a quantum limbo, waiting for measurements to bring their attributes into existence. This is essentially the traditional view of quantum mechanics, the view that Einstein vigorously opposed for nearly his entire adult life, famously remarking, "God does not play dice." But, perhaps she does; in one limited sense, this nonrealism interpretation seems quite plausible. Our metaphorical dice are not preprogrammed to fall on fixed numbers, although they may be loaded to prefer some numbers over others. Naturally, we cannot establish the state of a die before it is actually cast. But as far as I can see, this interpretation that abandons realism altogether does not avoid the sticky issue of nonlocality in the quantum entanglement process. When Lisa tosses her die, Michael's die number somehow becomes fixed. How does Michael's die receive its "orders" from Lisa's die?

To summarize, ERP's proposal essentially argued that one of the following must be true

- Lisa's measurements produce instantaneous influences on Michael's measurements at arbitrarily large separations; such *nonlocal* influences can occur at faster than the speed of light. Einstein called this "spooky action at a distance."

  or

- Some parts of Michael's physical reality, as determined by his experiments, cannot be accounted for by quantum mechanics, that is, by the wave function Ψ. Rather, some underlying features or structure of the particles themselves (*local hidden variables*) are required explain observed results.

Experiments based on Bell's theorem eliminate the second option; hidden variables, if they exist at all, must be nonlocal. We may reject *realism* altogether (certain particle properties do not exist before measurement) or adopt *neorealism* (particle properties are determined by *nonlocal* or faster-than-light influences). But, even a full rejection of realism does not appear to avoid the sticky issue of nonlocal influences, which seems to be fundamental to quantum mechanics, as implied by the discussion of quantum particles in the sink shown in Figure 10–12.

4. CAN CONSCIOUSNESS CREATE PARTS OF REALITY?

Several ontological interpretations of quantum theory suggest certain kinds of connections to consciousness, either directly or implied, as discussed in the works of several physicists, including Henry Stapp[3], whose writings include several exchanges with Werner Heisenberg on nuanced versions of the Copenhagen interpretation. Niels Bohr's highly pragmatic version says that the aim of quantum mechanics is merely to describe certain connections between human experiences (experimental observations), rather than to describe a physical world conceived to exist (perhaps erroneously) with definite properties independent of observation. In other words, we are wasting our time by speculating about a putative "reality" that can never be observed. The so-called Copenhagen interpretation is not of a single idea, however, but rather a conceptual framework encompassing a range of related viewpoints. Nevertheless, a common thread is denial of the objective reality of certain aspects of quantum systems in the absence of observation.

Along with Bohr, Heisenberg is the central figure associated with the Copenhagen interpretation; he labeled the macroscopic observed world in terms of "events," with quantum mechanics specifying the "objective tendencies" for such events to occur. In this view, the unmeasured world is just what quantum theory represents it to be: a quantum limbo or superposition of possibilities. In other words, an unmeasured particle is very much like our metaphorical die before it has been tossed on the chosen surface. The act and specific nature of a measurement, involving interaction with a macroscopic system (consciously selected by experimental scientists), brings about a sudden transition in the observed system from the superposition of states to a single realized state. Heisenberg coined the label *collapse of the wavefunction* in 1929 to indicate this transition to the unitary, unambiguous outcomes of such experiments.

Each number on a normal die (with six numbers) represents a single possible state of a particle that has exactly six possible alternative states (a superposition of six quantum states). One number is chosen when a die is tossed on a specific surface picked by the experimenter, this conscious choice of surface is analogous to the design of a quantum experiment aiming for a specific kind of measurement. Heisenberg's interpretation (applied to the dice metaphor) says that quantum mechanics yields only the "propensity" for a die to land on a certain number when tossed on a certain surface.

Heisenberg's expression of the Copenhagen interpretation involves a limited kind of *observer-created reality*, meaning that the experimental scientist consciously chooses in advance to measure, let's say, an electron's location or spin about some axis (metaphorical surface on which to roll the die), but his consciousness does not influence the results of such measurements. Complementary attributes of the particle like the electron's momentum or spin about another axis can have no meaning. Thus, the experimenter's conscious choice of experiment prevents certain features of the particle from becoming actualized; if we never toss a die on the wood surface, its number for the wood surface remains undefined; it has no meaning.

The experimenter does not determine whether a particular attribute (die number) will be acquired or not. That choice is determined by chance, in accordance with the statistical rules spelled out by quantum mechanics, as expressed explicitly by Schrödinger's equation. Note, however, that an electron has a definite charge and mass independent of measurement; evidently, according to this view, only some electron properties (events) are "created" or "actualized" in the measurement process. We consciously choose the surface for a die roll, but our consciousness need have nothing to do with the number obtained when a die roll occurs. If we choose to roll our metaphorical die on a glass surface, the same die's number (property) for a wooden surface roll has no meaning because it is never tossed on wood. We have chosen that part of reality that assigns the die some property (number) for a roll on glass, but have not chosen the number obtained.

When a metaphorical "quantum die" is tossed in accord with Heisenberg's interpretation, there is a collapse of the wavefunction: an event occurs consisting of the selection of exactly one of six possibilities. This outcome depends jointly on the initial quantum state (state of the untossed die) and on which measurement is performed (chosen surface for the die toss). The rules of quantum mechanics yield only the probabilities for each of six possible outcomes, and these are generally not sufficient to specify which particular outcome (die number) actually occurs.

Other ontological interpretations involve more explicit suggestions that consciousness itself creates parts of reality. The mathematical basis for this idea was first developed by the prominent mathematician John von Neumann. He started with the proposition that quantum mechanics provides an accurate picture of the world at all scales. Not only elementary particles, but also the macroscopic devices that measure such particles, are properly represented by quantum wavefunctions (albeit very complicated ones). This view represents a departure from the ideas of Bohr who accorded special status to measuring devices. Between the elementary particles to be measured and the observer's mind, a chain of intermediate devices exists, each represented by its own wavefunction. This chain includes the manmade measuring devices, the peripheral nervous system of an observer, and the observer's brain. In von Neumann's analysis, the quantum measurement problem involves a simple question: Where in this chain does the collapse of the elementary particle's wavefunction occur to yield a single measured state of the particle? Or, in the example of our dice metaphor, where in this chain of devices is a die actually rolled such that the superposition of states (six die faces) reduces to a single state (one die face)? The crux of von Neumann's argument is that the only special place in the chain is the observer's consciousness, which must somehow be responsible for the particle's wavefunction collapse to a specific state.

Einstein was an important early contributor to quantum theory, but a lifelong critic of the Copenhagen interpretation's denial of physical reality in the absence of observation. Einstein famously remarked that he believed that the moon exists even when no one is looking at it. Most physicists agree that macroscopic objects like the moon exist when no one is looking, and also that elementary particles like the electrons bound in atoms actually exist in the absence of observation. Such electrons possess the definitive properties charge and mass, but their atomic locations and velocities (or momentums) are indeterminate. The stability of atoms, as well as their ability to form the chemical bonds required for molecules to exist, depends critically on both parts of this complementary wave–particle duality. Evidently, a fundamental requirement for our universe to contain macroscopic substances is an interchange of ordinary information between the observable and "shadow" realms of existence, the latter identified in various ontological interpretations as the *propensity state, the implicate order*, or the *multiverse*, as discussed in the following section. The "reality" of atoms, molecules, and people apparently demands that the smallest known building blocks, the electrons, be somewhat less than "real," in the sense that the word "real" is employed in normal "macro-speak." I will speculate on shadow realms of existence in the context of *Ultra-Information* in Chapter 12.

5. NEOREALISM AND BOHM MECHANICS

In traditional quantum mechanics, embodied in several nuanced versions of the Copenhagen interpretation, elementary particles cannot be said to have definite properties like location, velocity, or spin until they are actually measured. Like our metaphorical dice that have not yet been cast, these particles are pictured as existing in a quantum limbo (superposition of states) until specific measurements are made. Such measurements involve interactions with macroscopic objects, a process causing *decoherence* in modern parlance, in which a particle's wave properties (energy levels, coherent mode frequencies, interference, and so forth) are lost in the process traditionally labeled as the *collapse of the wavefunction*.

An alternative to the Copenhagen interpretation, now labeled *neorealism*, was originally associated with Louis de Broglie and the idea that the quantum wavefunction consists of "pilot waves" that guide particles. *Neorealism* was more extensively developed in later years by David Bohm (circa 1970–1992). While soundly rejected by most early quantum physicists, this interpretation has recently made a partial comeback, at least to the extent of providing a complementary way of looking at quantum reality that may be useful for some purposes. The re-emergence of Bohm mechanics is partly a result of the ERP-Bell-related experiments revealing unequivocal nonlocal influences between quantum particles. Bohm's interpretation says that particles actually do have definite properties before measurement, but a strange new quantum force (or potential) adds to the usual classical forces.

The new force has the highly unappealing feature (for many physicists) of being *explicitly* nonlocal; it may fail to fall off with distance so that, in theory, distant parts of the universe can provide contributions to forces on local particles. While this may sound unrealistic, it is easily shown (see Endnotes for mathematical outline[4]) that Schrödinger's equation for the motion of a single (non relativistic) particle of mass m may be transformed to obtain the equation

$$m\frac{d\mathbf{v}}{dt} = \mathbf{F}_C + \mathbf{F}_Q \qquad (11.2)$$

This is just Newton's law equating the rate of change of particle's vector velocity $\mathbf{v}$ to the classical vector force $\mathbf{F}_C$, but with the addition of a quantum force $\mathbf{F}_Q$, which is proportional to $\frac{\hbar^2}{2m}$, where $\hbar = h/2\pi$ is Planck's constant. The classical limit of Newton's Law is then approached if the particle mass is sufficiently large of if Planck's constant $\hbar \to 0$.

At first glance, Equation 11.2 might seem like a vast improvement over traditional quantum mechanics. The simple form appears to suggest that elementary particles can be treated semiclassically; all that is required is the addition of a "correction term" $\mathbf{F}_Q$. But on closer inspection of the quantum force $\mathbf{F}_Q$, serious questions quickly become evident. The quantum force $\mathbf{F}_Q$ depends on the quantum wavefunction itself so that experimental predictions, developments in quantum electronics, and so forth still require solution of Schrödinger's equation just like they do in conventional quantum mechanics. Unlike classical forces, the quantum force (or quantum potential) need not add significant energy to the particle but rather provides *information* to guide the particle, rather like a radio signal is used to guide a rocket remotely. This picture seems to imply that particles like electrons have some complicated internal structure (hidden features) that responds to the quantum forces operating at very small scales, hidden variables to be sure, but nonlocal.

The quantum force $\mathbf{F}_Q$ depends on the wavefunction Ψ, but in Bohm's interpretation $|\Psi|^2$ yields the probability that a particle will actually *be* located at a certain location at a certain time, rather than the traditional quantum interpretation in which $|\Psi|^2$ yields the probability of *finding* the particle at a certain location with some measurement. This subtle difference in wording actually pinpoints the major distinction between the Bohm and Copenhagen interpretations: *A Bohm particle actually has a definite location at a certain time even though we can never know its exact location because of uncertainty caused by multiple nonlocal influences.* This is the basis for the label "neorealism." The behavior of a Bohm quantum particle is then somewhat analogous to a classical gas molecule being rapidly bumped unpredictably by other molecules, but with major differences: *(1)* The Bohm quantum particle may be "bumped" (non-locally) by particles at arbitrarily large distances. *(2)* The so-called "bumps" are not random; they occur according to quantum principles and depend critically on the measuring device. *(3)* "Bumps" need not *add* significant energy to the Bohm particle; rather, they guide the manner of energy use, analogous to the role of messenger RNA in protein synthesis in living cells. In philosophical terms, the Copenhagen interpretation focuses more on epistemology (how knowledge is obtained), whereas Bohm's formalism focuses more on ontology (what is actually true).

Since Equation 11.2 was derived directly from Schrödinger's equation, its experimental predictions seem to be identical to those of conventional quantum mechanics. However, a major caveat required for this comparison is that the measurement process itself, associated with wavefunction collapse, involves concepts separate from Schrödinger's equation. Bohm's ontological interpretation, on the underlying nature of quantum reality, differs substantially from conventional quantum mechanics. In traditional quantum mechanics, the uncertainty principle is taken as a fundamental property of the universe; no further explanation is deemed possible. By contrast, Bohm mechanics "explains" the uncertainty principle in terms of unpredictable nonlocal influences, potentially from distant parts of the universe.

The spherical region surrounding the Earth with radius equal to 14 billion light years is the *observable universe*. By contrast, the size of the full universe is unknown; it may be infinite. This raises the possibility of influences on local particles originating at infinite distances! I should emphasize strongly that such nonlocality was *not* introduced by Bohm mechanics. As shown in Section 3, the Bell-ERP-related experiments indicate that nonlocal influences are an integral part of quantum mechanics; Bohm's interpretation just reveals them as too conspicuous to sweep under any mokita-inspired rug.

In Bohm mechanics, there is no strange collapse of the wavefunction caused by measurements. The measuring apparatus and the observed particle participate intimately with each other (become *entangled*), as also occurs in the Copenhagen interpretation. But in Bohm mechanics, the final measured state depends on nonlocal interactions that influence both the observed particle and measuring apparatus. Each particle in the two-slit or interferometer experiments actually follows a definite path; the interference pattern produced by multiple particles striking the sensor screen occurs because individual particles are essentially guided selectively by the (nonlocal) quantum potential. Bohm's labels for the proposed nonlocal property of the universe are *undivided wholeness* and *implicate order* or *enfolded order*, implying that each local part of the universe contains some information about the entire universe. This property is similar to a hologram in which each part of a visual image contains information about the entire image. One may then say that the full image is *enfolded* within each part.

Our metaphorical cosmic quantum orchestra may be employed to demonstrate the general idea of implicate (enfolded) order. The imagined orchestra consists of a nested hierarchy of musical instruments and their substructures: strings (elementary particles), violins (atoms), violin sections (molecules), groups of stringed instruments (small macroscopic particles), and so forth. The metaphorical orchestra needs no conductor or other intelligent agents; the players may be zombies with no music appreciation. Or, instruments may be played in a warm-up period with various groups at different hierarchical levels playing together or playing separately.

Such interactions between distant instruments can occur as a result of *binding by resonance*; for example, if a note produced by one of the flutes matches one of the resonant frequencies of a violin body, the air inside the violin body (and any of its strings with matching resonant frequency) may acquire some tendency to respond selectively at that frequency. For purposes of this metaphor, we neglect sound propagation delays between distant instruments; such resonant binding may then be identified as a nonlocal influence. The allowed (discrete) notes produced by any string, the fundamental and overtones, are analogous to particle energy levels. These are determined by local string properties; however, the selection of a single note in any measurement process is influenced by resonant interactions with distant flutes.

Although I admit the analogy is rather forced, this selection of a single note could occur mechanically as follows. The violin strings themselves produce little sound; sounds are produced mostly by vibrations of the violin body. Thus, we might imagine a resonant coupling between distant flutes and the violin body such that only a single string note tends to be amplified by the body. Furthermore, the distant flutes are imagined to influence our measuring device, perhaps by resonant interaction with a recording microphone's membrane. The selection of one note from the string's "superposition of notes" then results in only a single "observed" note, which might be labeled "collapse of the string overtones." On the other hand, measurements of sounds produced by large groups of instruments (macroscopic systems) employing large numbers of resonant interactions will reveal no such nonlocal influences, an outcome expected if the many nonlocal resonant interactions occur with essentially random phases such that separate oscillations tend to cancel (*decoherence*).

6. THE MULTIVERSE AND MANY WORLDS INTERPRETATIONS OF QUANTUM MECHANICS

One major contender for an ontological interpretation of quantum mechanics involves several versions of the *multiverse*, by definition the whole of physical reality. The putative multiverse may contain many "parallel" universes, and new universes may pop into existence as the result of fundamental quantum processes associated with the uncertainty principle. In one version, particles interact with each other in familiar ways within each universe, and each universe affects the others only weakly through interference phenomena. Thus, a single particle in the two-slit or interferometer experiments produces an interference pattern by interfering with its counterpart in another universe. Such cross-universe interactions may be sufficiently strong to be detectable only between universes that are nearly alike. The multiverse forms the environment for a fanciful story called *Paths to Otherwhere*[5] written by science fiction writer James Hogan and inspired by the writings of physicist David Deutsch. The serial creation of new universes because of fundamental quantum processes is postulated by physicists Lee Smolin, Leonard Susskind, and others as outlined in Chapter 9.

The *many worlds interpretation* of quantum mechanics is one version of the larger *multiverse* category. In the original versions developed by Hugh Everett and later Bryce DeWitt, new universes are constantly branching off when observations occur. Many copies of you and me are imagined to occupy other universes; some are nearly identical, others have substantial differences, but in most universes humans don't exist at all. As far as I am aware, the first account of an imagined world in which all possibilities actually occur was written by famous fiction author Jorge Borges. *The Garden of Forking Paths* was published in 1941, long before such a strange concept entered the physics lexicon.[6] While this view may seem more like science fiction than genuine science, it is taken seriously by more than a few professional physicists, is apparently consistent with all known experiments, and provides a genuine "local" solution to the measurement problem of quantum mechanics. But employing putative influences from other universes seems to me to be a rather expensive price to pay for avoiding the possibility of nonlocal influences in the one universe we know to exist.

One may question whether the multiverse conjecture even fits within the purview of a genuine scientific theory since direct observation of the multiverse requires supernatural or *superuniversal* observers. Proponents of the multiverse might respond to this criticism as follows. Suppose some new theory of quantum gravity, encompassing both general relativity and quantum mechanics in a self-consistent framework, were to be developed. Imagine that the theory enjoys so much success in describing our universe as to apparently qualify as a genuine "theory of everything," perhaps predicting the numerical values of Planck's constant, the gravitational constant, or the velocity of light. If such theory were also to predict the creation of daughter universes, especially if they possessed external features observable in our universe (analogous to the behavior of fields and matter near black holes), the multiverse idea would then achieve substantial scientific acceptance. Even so, tourism to other universes will still be unlikely.

7. SUMMARY

A famous thought experiment (ERP) was proposed by Einstein and colleagues to argue that quantum mechanics is an incomplete physical theory, meaning that particles must possess hidden features (in addition to the wavefunction) that determine their weird behaviors. This hidden variables issue is directly addressed by Bell's theorem and its associated experiments; the ontological implications of the experiments are illustrated here by a magic dice metaphor with each die representing an electron. The surfaces on which the dice are tossed are analogous to the experimenter's choice of electron spin axis measurement, and the number (1 or 2) showing on the toss is analogous to measured spin (up or down). Experimental results inspired by Bell's theorem suggest that we may have no choice but to adopt *neorealism*, meaning that particle properties result partly from instantaneous (nonlocal) influences from distant parts of the universe.

The traditional (Copenhagen) interpretation of quantum mechanics, due mainly to Bohr and Heisenberg, embodies a conceptual framework encompassing several related viewpoints, the common thread being denial of the objective reality of certain aspects of quantum systems in the absence of observation. The unmeasured world is just what quantum theory represents it to be: a quantum limbo or superposition of possibilities. The act and specific nature of a measurement, involving interaction with a macroscopic system, brings about a sudden transition in the observed system from the superposition of states to a single realized state, a process called *collapse of the wavefunction*. Some ontological versions involve limited kinds of *observer-created reality*, for example, scientists consciously choose to measure certain properties of a particle, but such conscious choices do not influence the results of the measurements.

Neorealism is mostly associated with the work of David Bohm, an ontological interpretation that abolishes the traditional collapse of the wavefunction and provides an explicit expression of the inherent nonlocal nature of quantum mechanics. Schrödinger's equation is transformed into a classical-looking form similar to Newton's law except for the appearance of a new quantum force or potential. But unlike classical forces, the quantum force need not add significant energy to particles, but rather provides *information* to guide the particle. Each particle in the two-slit or interferometer experiments actually follows a definite path; the observed interference patterns occur because particles are essentially guided selectively by the (nonlocal) quantum potential. The proposed nonlocal property is called the *implicate order* or *enfolded order*, implying that every part of the universe contains some information about the entire universe.

Another contender for ontological interpretation of quantum mechanics involves several versions of the *multiverse*, defined as the whole of physical reality. The putative multiverse contains many "parallel" universes that may come into existence because of fundamental quantum processes. One universe may influence others weakly by sharing certain kinds of information, accounting for the interference phenomena observed in the two-slit and interferometer experiments. Included in the *multiverse* category is the *many worlds interpretation* of quantum mechanics in which new universes are constantly branching off when observations occur. Many copies of you and me are imagined to occupy other parallel universes; some are nearly identical, others have substantial differences.

In Chapter 12, partial unification of the various ontological interpretations of quantum mechanics will be proposed based on elevating *information* to a more prominent position in the universe (or multiverse). In order to avoid biased interpretations resulting from the varied definitions of the label "information," I will distinguish *ordinary information* from a broader category called *Ultra-Information*. Brain functions clearly involve the processing of ordinary information, but does the existence of *mind* involve more?

Chapter 12

Does the Brain Create the Mind?

1. WHERE HAS OUR JOURNEY TAKEN US AND WHERE ARE WE GOING?

Several aspects of human knowledge have been discussed throughout this book. Epistemological and ontological questions in both the brain and physical sciences were addressed, posing the general question: *What do we know about ourselves and our universe and how do we know it?* Chapters 1–3 advocated complementary models of reality as tools for deepening our understanding of many complex systems including human brains. We also examined appropriate roles for science and religion, considered the graded states of consciousness, suggested that multiple conscious or semi conscious entities can coexist in one brain, and speculated that, in the right circumstances, a single consciousness might even extend beyond brain boundaries.

In Chapters 4–6, human brain anatomy and physiology were outlined, emphasizing that brains consist of many subunits and exhibit intricate nested structures at multiple spatial scales, including cortical minicolumns and macrocolumns interconnected by corticocortical axons. These fibers provide *non-local* interactions, with the hyphen used to distinguish this label from *nonlocal*, meaning influences on quantum systems acting at faster-than-light speed. By contrast, "non-local" brain interactions involve connections that bypass intervening cortical tissue, apparently allowing for much more complex dynamic behaviors than would be possible with only "local" (intracortical, mostly contiguous) interactions. The high relative density of the non-local corticocortical axons in humans compared to lower mammals may be responsible for many of the things that make the human brain "human."

Human brains belong to a broader class of entities called *complex adaptive systems*, which possess the capacity to "learn" from experience and change global behaviors by means of feedback processes. Examples include social systems, ecosystems, and all living systems. Another hallmark of such complex systems is the presence of intricate *fractal-like* dynamic behaviors at multiple scales, meaning the more magnified the observation, the more detailed behavior found. Furthermore, cross-scale interactions are essential features of complex systems in generating multiscale dynamic behaviors. One example is the global human social system characterized by within-scale interactions among persons, corporations, cities, states, and nations, as well as cross-scale interactions between the distinct multiscale entities.

EEG was shown to be a genuine "window on the mind," revealing strong correlations with brain state. A broad range of dynamic signatures or *shadows of thought* have been recorded, each waveform dependent in its own way on time and scalp location. Two of the most promising measures of this dynamics are *coherence* and *covariance*, measures estimating functional interrelationships between network and synaptic field activity recorded at different locations. Consciousness appears to occur in conjunction with large-scale moderately coherent EEG signals, of moderate amplitude and within selected frequency bands observed mostly in the 4 to 13 Hz range in scalp recordings. Unconsciousness in living humans typically occurs with larger EEG amplitudes and frequencies lower than a few Hz. A healthy consciousness may also be associated with a proper "balance" between local, regional, and global mechanisms, perhaps occurring only in states of high dynamic complexity.

Chapter 7 is concerned with dynamic behaviors of cerebral cortex and of several physical systems providing useful analogs. A conceptual framework, embracing the idea of neural networks embedded in global synaptic action fields, is consistent with EEG observations and provides a convenient entry point for the development of a large-scale (global) mathematical model of cortical dynamics. The model provides a number of approximately accurate predictions of the very large-scale dynamic behavior revealed by EEG. The model also directly addresses the so-called *binding problem* of brain science by suggesting top-down resonant interactions between global fields and non overlapping networks. This mechanism may allow brain subsystems to be functionally localized in some frequency bands, but at the same time, functionally integrated in other frequency bands.

Chapter 8 considers the general limits of scientific knowledge and identifies probability as an important measure of human ignorance; scientific predictions are shown to be severely limited in *complex systems*. If artificial consciousness requires accurate simulations of tissue over a wide range of spatial scales, fundamental limits on computer power may preclude creation of artificial consciousness, even if natural brains actually manage to create minds without outside interactions as assumed by most contemporary scientists.

Chapters 9–11 provide an overview of the strange, but experimentally well-established, worldviews based on modern observations of the physical universe. The possibility of deep connections between relativity, quantum mechanics, thermodynamics, and consciousness was labeled *the RQTC conjecture*, independent of the nature of such putative connections. This conjecture is based on several ideas: The study of consciousness is essentially concerned with the nature of reality, and modern physics deals directly with physical reality. Furthermore, modern physical theories may be cast in the form of fundamental information barriers: Relativity, quantum mechanics, and the second law of thermodynamics are all limitations on the speed, quantity, or quality of information transfer.

"Information" is a term with many meanings depending on context; common features involve processing, manipulating, and organizing data in a

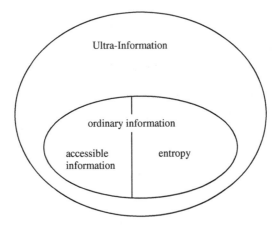

Figure 12-1 Ordinary information consists of accessible ordinary information and ordinary entropy. A broader category, Ultra-Information, is postulated.

way that adds to the knowledge of the person receiving it. But this description is far too narrow for our purposes. In order to bridge the gap between the languages of the physical and mental worlds but, at the same time, avoid some of the hazardous linguistic traps, in this chapter I propose a distinction between normal or *ordinary information* and a broader category called *Ultra-Information*.

The sensory input from the physical world that enters the mind of a human observer involves several kinds of ordinary information transfer and processing, including external physical phenomena like light and sound, as well as internal physiological events like action potentials, cellular integration of synaptic inputs, chemical transmitter actions, and so forth. In this chapter, I address the hard problem of consciousness by posing questions about the possible existence and nature of something beyond ordinary information, that is, *Ultra-Information*, defined broadly to include ordinary information, unknown physical processes, and consciousness as pictured in Figure 12–1. Thus, thoughts, emotions, self-awareness, memory, and the contents of the unconscious are, by definition, categories of Ultra-Information whether or not these mental processes also consist of ordinary information.

In this framework, several basic questions come to mind. Does any separation actually occur between the two ellipses in Figure 12–1 distinguishing ordinary information from Ultra-Information? If so, does any of this space represent conscious processes? We will see that *ordinary entropy* refers to ordinary information that is normally inaccessible but may become accessible with appropriate observations. Does any of the putative Ultra-Information involve a deeper kind of inaccessibility that might be labeled *Ultra-Entropy*? Is all consciousness-related information confined to brain boundaries? What are the material substrates of consciousness encoding? These and several other 64 trillion dollar questions are approached in this chapter.

Here I take seriously the idea that consciousness may be a "fundamental property of the universe." If so, it must be a "fundamental property of the entire universe," which includes everything that exists in our universe. I assume some things exist that lie forever outside the province of our physical observations. Yet such entities might produce indirect observable effects in our physical world, as for example, in the many worlds and several other interpretations of quantum mechanics. The uncertainty principle discussed in Chapters 10 and 11 says that certain physical knowledge is either (1) forever hidden from humans or (2) simply doesn't exist. Can we ever tell the difference between interpretations 1 and 2?

This question has been vigorously debated over the past century and will not be settled here. Nevertheless, physics may have much more to tell as about boundaries between *what is* and *what is not* knowable. Entities that are not knowable but nevertheless exist need not follow established scientific principles; such things themselves need not be part of physics. Here I include one such speculative entity called *Mind* as a sub category of *Ultra-Information*, a category defined so broadly as to include both physical and nonphysical phenomena.

All this discussion about the *existence of the unknowable* may seem rather esoteric; however, we are concerned every day with an unknowable entity that is widely believed to exist; we call this entity *the future*. As discussed in Chapter 8, prediction of future behavior of complex systems is always limited by uncertainty in initial conditions, boundary conditions, and interaction rules. This limitation is fundamental to both classical and quantum systems; it applies to financial markets, humans, climate, and other physical systems. Our predictions of the future must always be of a probabilistic nature even when we hide our ignorance with deterministic language. According to the theory of relativity, even parts of our *past* are fundamentally unknowable. The star Betelgeuse is located 430 light years from Earth. Ordinary information about any event that occurred near this star anytime in the past 430 years is, for humans, hidden by a thick fundamental veil[1]. According to established physics, such events exist but are unknowable.

This chapter involves a number of speculations about possible relationships between entities that may, in actual fact, be unrelated or even fail to exist. I will not apologize for these speculations since I have clearly identified them as such! Figure 12–2 provides a roadmap to Chapter 12 with the solid and dashed lines showing established and speculative connections, respectively. The numbers indicate sections of Chapter 12 most focused on the corresponding entity in each box. Brain and mind clearly depend on ordinary information processing as indicated on the figure's left side; nearly everything else, including *Mind*, is quite speculative. Figure 12–2 represents just one of many possible roadmaps to the study of consciousness; readers are free to offer their own modifications. Some may discount entirely the possible existence of *Mind*; others may insist on placing its box at the top. Still others may add or subtract links and categories. Take your choice.

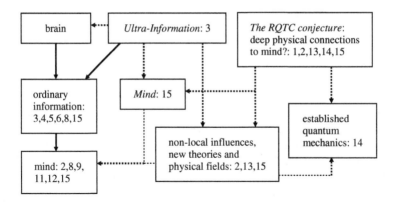

Figure 12–2 A roadmap to Chapter 12 with numbers indicating sections where matching discussion occurs.

2. WHAT IS CONSCIOUSNESS?

Consciousness is often defined as an internal state of awareness of self, thoughts, sensations, and the environment, a circular definition to be sure, but useful as a starting point.[2] Consciousness may be viewed from both the inside and out. The internal experience is fundamentally private; only you can be certain that you are actually conscious. External observers may affirm your consciousness based on language, purposeful behavior, attention to the environment, body language, facial expressions, and so forth. External observers can be quite wrong, however. Discrepancies between internal and external views may occur with dreaming subjects, the nonverbal right hemisphere of a split brain patient, and with the locked-in patents discussed in Chapter 2. Locked-in patients may provide false negative results to external consciousness tests; patients in vegetative states may provide false positives. Neuroimaging methods may be required to sort this out. In addition, neither internal nor external observers may have direct access to the unconscious, which nevertheless receives information from the external world and provides important influences on the brain's conscious entities.

Many neural correlates of consciousness are well known. Brain function changes may be revealed by dynamic measures, as with EEG or fMRI, or by static measures of structural defects caused by injury or disease. Certain EEG patterns are reliably associated with non conscious states like epileptic seizures, deep anesthesia, and deep sleep. fMRI and EEG may provide substantial information about the internal mental world. Widespread damage to both hemispheres of the cerebral cortex results in permanent loss of consciousness. On the other hand, loss of the right cerebral hemisphere or the entire cerebellum typically has only minimal effects on consciousness, at least as judged by (internal) reports from damaged persons as well as most external scientific tests. In patients with damaged or missing right hemisphere, the surviving left hemisphere expresses no sense of loss or even awareness of the absence of his former partner, the right hemisphere. Consciousness seems to arise as a result of the integrated action of large portions of the brain, yet some parts are required much more than others if normal awareness is to occur. Despite all these neural correlates, the genuine nature and origin of consciousness remains a deep mystery.

Some things, especially fundamental entities, are so hard to define that we must settle for circular definitions. For example, electric charge is a fundamental property of elementary particles and can be defined only in terms of its behavior when exposed to external environments consisting of electric fields and other charges. Knowledge of a particle's "charge" provides predictive information about how the particle will behave in certain circumstances. This observed behavior essentially defines "charge." Similarly, an elementary particle's "spin" is defined in terms of its behavior when exposed to magnetic fields; no more fundamental definition of spin is currently available. Since we are unable to define consciousness in terms of more fundamental properties, a plausible working conjecture is that consciousness itself is fundamental.

Energy is another fundamental property but appears in much broader contexts than charge. Chemicals contain stored energy associated with chemical bonds; such energy is released in chemical reactions. Physical objects as well as electromagnetic and gravitational fields possess energy. Gravitational energy is transferred to heavy elements and "stored" as mass in the collapse of super-novae; this stored nuclear energy may be released later in radioactivity and fission bombs. A typical definition of energy is *the amount of work that can be performed by a force*; "work" is the integral of force over distance. "Force" is *the action of one object upon another*, but such action is actually due to interactions of microscopic *electric fields* in the molecular structures. An "electric field" is defined as *the force on a unit charge*. You see the problem; the definitions are circular. We say that charge and energy are "fundamental properties" because, as far as we know, they cannot be reduced to secondary aspects of some more comprehensive entity. The definitions of charge, mass, energy, and electromagnetic field are, in fact, inherently circular, providing only interrelationships between several fundamental entities.

By contrast to energy and charge, the electrical conductivity of a material is not fundamental because it may be explained in terms of interactions of mobile charge carriers (electrons or ions) with the more stationary molecular or atomic structures. Some future generation of scientists may verify the existence of an entity X, perhaps occurring at sub electron scales, and discover that properties like charge and spin are simply different realizations of the more fundamental thing X. String theory (at quantum scales) is one such candidate, suggesting that elementary particle properties result from the vibrations of tiny strings; in this view, different string overtones are manifested as different particles.

To me, consciousness seems more analogous to fundamental physical properties like charge and energy than secondary properties like electrical conductivity, temperature, pressure, strength of chemical bonds, and so forth. Given this argument, I posit that any serious study of consciousness must adopt a conceptual framework that allows for the possibility that consciousness is a fundamental property of the universe. We will not be alone in this view; for example, Max Planck had this to say in 1931:[3] "I regard consciousness as fundamental. I regard matter as derivative from consciousness. We cannot get behind consciousness..." Critics may point to the many known neural correlates of consciousness, those features of brain function that change when some aspect of consciousness changes. My reply is that, yes, science will discover more and more neural correlates, but in the absence of new kinds of fundamental information, will these achievements ever bring us closer to "understanding" the hard problem of consciousness? In the following sections, I pose this basic question in several contexts.

3. THE LANGUAGES OF BRAINS, COMPUTERS, INFORMATION, AND THE UNIVERSE

We are deeply interested here in relationships between the inner world of consciousness and the physical world of brains. Effective discussion of potential links between such seemingly disparate phenomena may be facilitated by adopting language that overlaps both worlds. With this goal in mind, labels like *information, memory, signals, network, knowledge,* and *calculation* are routinely applied in both brain and computer sciences. These common labels indicate useful metaphorical relationships between biological and physical processes having important functional features in common, but they may also differ fundamentally at the core. In *Why the Mind Is Not a Computer*,[4] gerontologist and philosopher Raymond Tallis warns of the pitfalls of such overlapping language. Arguments based on terms like *information*, having so many disguised interpretations, can fool both our conscious and unconscious, hiding logical flaws that fail to stand up in linguistic daylight. As Tallis expresses it, "The deployment of such terms conjures away the barriers between man and machine."

With such warning in mind, I propose here altered definitions for two common entities, *information* (or *ordinary information*) and *computers*, extended here to *Ultra-Information* (Fig. 12–1) and *Ultra-Computers*. Their capitalization serves as a reminder that my usage is much more inclusive than the common interpretations of their lowercase counterparts. Even the ordinary label *information* has multiple meanings depending on context but is typically related to knowledge acquisition, records, patterns, sending and receiving messages, sensory input, and brain processing of this input. Information in "messages" may be transferred from so-called "senders" to "receivers," but none need understand or act on the messages.

The sender may be a distant supernova generating radio waves measured by an antenna (receiver 1) converting radio waves to electric current in a measuring circuit (receiver 2). Next, this electrical information is transformed into a photograph by a transducer (receiver 3); the photograph then provides information to a human retina (receiver 4), followed by a succession of processing steps within a brain (receivers 5, 6, and so forth). All of these steps, including awareness of the photograph in the mind of a human, involve *ordinary information processing*, whether in the external physical systems or in the internal nervous system of the human observer. The internal ordinary information processes include action potentials, integration of cellular synaptic inputs, chemical actions, and so forth. The hard problem may then be expressed in terms of questions about the possible existence of something beyond ordinary information, that is, *Ultra-Information*, and the nature of this new kind of information.

In general, *ordinary information* need not represent actual physical objects or be accurate or even be even related to "truth" in any way. Earthquakes, propaganda, music, art, traffic noise, expressions of emotion, and strangers smiling in restaurants all convey ordinary information, whether or not the events are observed by instruments or living systems. The so-called receivers may be trees, rocks, humans, or just about anything. My goal here is to define "Ultra-Information" broadly to encompass several subcategories: its everyday use as knowledge transfer, its technical interpretation in communication theory, all other ordinary information, and mental processes. Thus, memory, thoughts, emotions, the content of the unconscious, and other aspects of consciousness are, in themselves, categories of Ultra-Information whether or not transference to external receivers occurs. The definition I adopt here is quite broad:

Ultra-Information: That which distinguishes one entity from another.

A familiar definition of *computer* is a machine that manipulates data according to a list of instructions. Included in this category are the usual desktop personal computers, supercomputers, and embedded computers, the small devices used to control other devices like digital cameras, automobile fuel injection, and so forth. But this narrow definition of digital computers ignores analog computers that use physical objects to model phenomena. An electronic analog computer consists of an electric circuit governed by some differential equation matching the identical equation governing a mechanical or other analog system. Once the appropriate analog circuit is constructed, one simply adjusts the circuit control parameters (typically variable resistors), turns on the power, and measures circuit voltages serving as analogs of the desired mechanical variables. But any physical process that models some physical action can be interpreted as an analog computer. Cavemen must have used little pebbles and lines drawn in the sand to plan attacks on other tribes. As kids playing sandlot football, we drew our plays in the dirt: "This pebble stands for that old tire near the big tree; you go out for a pass and I'll hit you just this side of the tire." Someone figured out that little beads on sticks could be adopted for accurate calculations, and the abacus was born, the slide rule followed, and so forth.

Laboratory experiments involve devices with input information chosen by scientists who then observe the outputs; such devices are essentially analog computers. Pour one chemical into a test tube containing another chemical, and measure the results of the reaction; an analog computation has taken place within the test tube. Neuroscientists provide inputs to human brains in the form of requests to perform specific tasks, measuring cognitive outputs like task performance and brain images like EEG and fMRI. The brain is an *Ultra-Computer*; it may even occasionally seem to act like an *ordinary computer*. The universe seems to have started with a quantum fluctuation, followed by the formation of stars that cooked the heavy elements required for complex structures like life and brains to emerge; the universe is an Ultra-Computer. In Section 6, we see that the universe is actually a quantum Ultra-Computer that has both analog and digital features. Given this background, my inclusive definition is:

Ultra-Computer: Any system that processes *Ultra-Information*.

As we have defined Ultra-Information quite broadly, the Ultra-Computer definition covers just about any physical or biological system and more; one may rightly question whether this definition is far too broad to be useful. *But here is my main point*: If more restrictive definitions of Ultra-Information or Ultra-Computer were chosen, we would be faced with the difficult decision of where to draw the line distinguishing entities that fall within the more restrictive category from those that belong outside. This would seem to be an arbitrary choice. Thus, I propose broad categories here that, by definition, include both the physical and mental worlds.

This approach to questions about consciousness and information may be viewed as somewhat analogous to historic arguments about the existence and nature of God. Following 18th century philosopher Immanuel Kant, one may define God in sufficiently broad terms such that we can all agree that he (or she or it) *exists*. Our arguments may then be confined to questions concerning the *nature* of God. Similarly, rather than argue whether or not consciousness involves any kind of information processing or if brains are similar to computers or other dynamic physical systems, I here define "Ultra-Information" and "Ultra-Computer" in terms broad enough to include mind. Thus, our approach to the hard problem of consciousness reduces, in part, to questions about the nature of Ultra-Information and its processing by the matching category of Ultra-Computer. As far as I can see, the only legitimate objections to this linguistic trick concern its usefulness or lack thereof.

4. ARE BASEBALLS REAL?

Our everyday experiences with material objects provide us with strongly biased, mechanical views of the structure of reality. Only in the face of overwhelming evidence and with great reluctance did early 20th century physicists abandon their overly mechanical views of the physical world. This section offers a little warm-up exercise to introduce non mechanical concepts and subsequent arguments in Section 6, where information (or Ultra-Information) is afforded a lofty status, well above that given to material objects.

A baseball consists of a cork center wound with layers of string and covered with a stitched leather covering. When a baseball flies through the air, light is reflected from the ball's leather cover and enters the observer's retina where photoreceptor cells containing a special protein absorb photons. Photons (the electromagnetic field) carry energy and information causing changes in membrane potentials, essentially providing signals to receptor cells. Substantial preprocessing of information, involving action potentials and other physiological events, occurs at the retina stage such that the 130 million receptor cells converge on the 1.2 million axons forming the optic nerve, carrying information (mostly) to the thalamus, which then relays information to primary visual cortex by means of action potentials. This transformed (ordinary) information is then relayed to secondary areas of visual cortex, also by means of action potentials, and integrated with memory and emotional content, perhaps initiating a motor response such as swinging a bat.

Multiple feedback processes in the brain between cortical and sub cortical regions are responsible for conscious perception of the baseball. The processes linking the "real" physical baseball to the baseball image in observer brains and minds involve a sequence of complex steps in which both energy and information are transformed in various ways. Note that I have associated "ordinary information" processing with known physical events like action potential propagation, integration of inputs to cells, and so forth. A wide range of neuroscience data suggests that memory retrieval and emotional content also involve ordinary information processing; the open question is whether these and other aspects of consciousness involve something more, that is, some category of Ultra-Information that exists outside the ordinary information subset of Figure 12–1.

Two observers, say a cricket player and a baseball player, might experience different perceptions of the same baseball even when their retinas receive identical information. Furthermore, an alien would likely experience an entirely different baseball reality or perhaps not even be aware of the baseball's existence. Unfortunately I have no close alien friends on which to test this idea, but my golden retriever (Savannah) can serve as a substitute. We often walk in a wildlife area bordering an athletic park containing several Little League baseball fields. Using her superior olfactory "intellect," she nearly always manages to find at least one lost baseball within the leaves and bushes. Other than noting her apparent fondness for baseballs, I can't say much about her baseball perceptions, except that they seem to differ substantially from mine.

Despite disparate internal perceptions, we say that baseballs are "real" because they possess certain physical properties that we can all agree on; properties that exist even when they are not observed. An approximate macroscopic description of a moving baseball might consist of its size, shape, mass, location, and velocity. More detailed information is needed to predict its trajectory, however, including its spin about three axes and the condition of its surface. Spin provides the pitcher with an effective weapon, the curveball, against the batter. Before 1920, the spitball was also legal; earlier pitchers tried many ways to alter baseball surfaces, scuffing using foreign objects, spit, and even tobacco juice, thereby adding to trajectory uncertainty, both real and imagined by batters. The macroscopic state of a moving baseball might be described in great detail, including the surface coordinates of its raised stitches contributing to its trajectory, by perhaps 20 variables with, let's say, four-digit precision or roughly 18 bits of information.

If matter behaved classically and was continuous down to arbitrarily small scales, a physical object like a baseball would contain an infinite amount of information. The amount of information in any *finite* description would then depend on the precision assigned to, let's say, the locations and velocities of each small piece of the baseball. By contrast, in quantum theory, material objects are believed to contain finite rather than infinite information because of the fundamental limitations on precision dictated by the uncertainty principle. A complete microscopic description of a baseball in terms of the locations and velocities of its elementary particles would consist of something like 10^{26} bits of information. Most of this information is inaccessible to observation, and such *inaccessible information* is identified as *entropy* in Sections 5 and 6. According to quantum mechanics, it is fundamentally impossible to add precision or information beyond 10^{26} bits to this description of a baseball. If any additional baseball information exists, it is *unknowable* according to current science. This label is meant to be taken literally: "Unknowable" means absolutely and forever unknowable; "inaccessible" means not easily known.

If some new theory, more fundamental than quantum mechanics, should be discovered, a new kind of information, some category of Ultra-Information, would be implied. For example, according to current physical theory, there exists a minimum length scale, called the Planck length, at which the structure of space-time itself becomes dominated by quantum effects. In several theories, space-time takes on a sort of foamy structure at very small scales. The ratio of the smallest physical scale that can currently be studied (10^{-16} cm) to the Planck length (10^{-33} cm) is 10^{17}, about equal to the ratio of the Earth–sun separation to the size of a living cell. This huge range allows plenty of room for all kinds of sub electron structure, perhaps even arranged in a nested hierarchy. Such structure might contain Ultra-Information of many kinds and be related to or interact with *nonlocal hidden variables, the implicate order, the propensity state,* or the *multiverse* as discussed in Chapter 11. Here is still another wild speculation: It might even have some connection with consciousness.

5. VERY BASIC INFORMATION THEORY

This section represents a short detour from our journey to the more central layers of our metaphorical "onion" of consciousness. Ultra-Information is defined quite broadly but includes ordinary information as a subcategory as indicated in Figure 12–1. Ordinary information is itself divided into *accessible ordinary information* and *inaccessible ordinary information* or *entropy*. This detour section has two goals:

- To quantify ordinary information so that we may consider the *amount* of ordinary information processing taking place in various complex systems. The question of whether it is even possible to quantify other kinds of Ultra-Information is left unanswered.
- To provide a simple description of inaccessible ordinary information (entropy). Later I will speculate about the possible existence of a deeper kind of inaccessibility, *Ultra-Entropy*, which may be fundamentally unknowable.

Even the restricted label *ordinary information* can have quite a few meanings depending on context but is typically related to concepts like records, patterns, sending and receiving messages, sensory input, and processing of this input by the brain. In this section, we focus on specific kinds of ordinary information from the field of *information theory* as adopted in physics, computer science, and communications engineering, although our discussion overlaps ordinary "information" as used in other fields.

The basic unit of information in a message is the *bit*, shorthand for *binary digit*. A bit is either 0 or 1; bits might be used to represent a written language or the state of some physical device like the local magnetic field direction stored in a computer memory. Bits might also represent the spin direction of an elementary particle in a quantum computer. A string of bits can represent any symbol; all possible 3-bit numbers are (000, 001, 010, 011, 100, 101, 110, 111) normally representing the base-10 numbers 0 through 7. Larger base-10 numbers and other symbols require longer bit strings. The standard computer code ASCII consists of 7-bit numbers, for example, the letter "g" is (1100111). A 7-bit number (sequence) can represent $2^7 = 128$ symbols.

Communication engineers are concerned with finding the most efficient way to encode messages. Suppose a message consists of 1000 random bits; say I toss a coin 1000 times, and send you the sequence, H, H, T, H, and so forth. The information content of my message is 1000 bits; the fact that this "information" is of no use to either of us is not yet an issue in our discussion. Consider a collection of messages consisting of bit sequences of equal length; the information content will generally vary from message to message. Perhaps counter intuitively, the random (and useless) bit sequences contain the maximum amount of "information," as defined in this context.

Suppose I replace coin tosses with tosses of a six-faced fair die and send the sequence of results; the probability of any particular number showing on a single toss is 1/6. Representing the die numbers 1 through 6 in my message requires a sequence of 3-bit numbers; thus, I could relay the entire sequence of 1000 die tosses using a string of 3000 bits. But, it turns out that this is not the most efficient encoding; I can relay the same information with shorter bit strings.

One improved strategy is to lump the die tosses in groups of three; the number of possible (base-10) die outcomes like (1, 2, 1), (3, 6, 2), and so forth in each group is then $6^3 = 216$. With 8-bit sequences, I can send all of these cases by encoding any number between 1 and $2^8 = 256$. In the original inefficient scheme, the base-10 outcome (1, 2, 1) would be encoded as the three 3-bit sequences (001, 010, 001), whereas the same lumped group of three tosses might be more efficiently represented by the single 8-bit sequence (00000110), representing a reduction from 9 to 8 bits for each group of three die tosses. The total number of bits required to transfer the same information is then reduced from 3000 to $(8/9) \times (3000)$ or 2667.

While it might appear that finding the most efficient coding scheme requires a lot of trial and error, information theory provides a simple equation applicable to messages consisting of bit strings when the probability of each event leading to a bit string is known. The most efficient possible encoding of the sequence defines the information content of each bit transmitted in the message and is given by

$$\text{bits/action} = -\sum_x p(x)\log_2[p(x)] \tag{12.1}$$

Here the sum is over all possible actionable outcomes, each having probability $p(x)$. Note that the logarithmic operation on the function $p(x) \leq 1$ yields either 0 or a negative number so the number of bits per action is always 0 or positive. In our die example, x is the die number occurring with probability $p(x) = 1/6$ in each die toss (action), and the sum is over the six possible outcomes. The transmitted information expressed in minimum bits per die toss as obtained from Equation 12.1 is then 2.585; thus, the minimal number bits required to transmit the desired information produced by 1000 die tosses is 2585 rather than the values 2667 or 3000 bits required by the less efficient encoding schemes. In the case of a coin toss with $p(x) = 1/2$, the sum of two outcomes (heads and tails) in Equation 12.1 yields 1 bit per coin toss as expected.

Equation 12.1 has an important alternate interpretation as the entropy $H(p)$ of a generally unknown system. Suppose the probability $p(x)$ of outcomes x is unknown; our six-sided die may be loaded, for example. If we have absolutely no knowledge about the die, $p(x) = 1/6$ as a result of this ignorance, and the entropy $H(p)$ attains its maximum possible value of 2.585. On the other hand, suppose we take a close look at the die and find that two of the faces are printed with 1s but no face is printed with a 6. If the die is otherwise fair, we conclude that $p(1) = 1/3$ and $p(6) = 0$, Equation 12.1 then yields $H(p) = 2.252$. *We have gained important information about the die system; as a result, its entropy has decreased.* In the extreme case of perfect knowledge of die outcomes, say because all faces are printed with 1s, $p(1) = 1$ and the entropy $H(p) = 0$. Entropy is often said to be a measure of system *disorder*, here interpreted to mean that increased entropy occurs as our ignorance of the likelihood of die outcomes increases. For purposes of our interest in information and consciousness, our essential conclusion is this: *Entropy is information inaccessible because of ignorance, a basic measure of observer ignorance.*

6. UNIVERSAL ORDINARY INFORMATION

As discussed in Chapters 9–11, the three fundamental theories of the universe, relativity, quantum mechanics, and the second law of thermodynamics all involve limitations on the transfer, accessibility, quantity, or usefulness of information. Relativity prohibits the transfer of messages (ordinary information) or particles at faster-than-light speed; the uncertainty principle prohibits quantum particles from having definite speeds and locations at the same time. The second law of thermodynamics fundamentally limits our ability to use energy and information. Perhaps then, we should consider information itself as a fundamental property of the universe, promoting information to a status equal to or perhaps even greater than that afforded energy and its relativistic equivalent, mass.

This idea of treating information as a fundamental property is not proposed simply as a metaphor; rather, it is a view adopted by number of smart physicists who even appear to be quite sane. In order to summarize the framework supporting this view, I have borrowed much of the material in this section from the writings of MIT professor and quantum computer scientist Seth Lloyd[5]. For purposes of discussion in this section, ordinary information and Ultra-Information are treated as identical; that is, the inner ellipse in Figure 12–1 is assumed to fill the outer ellipse consistent with treatment of quantum mechanics as a complete theory, discounting possible contributions from any extraordinary (Ultra-) information.

Table 12–1 lists short descriptions for a number of ordinary information-related entities from Lloyd's perspective; these should be interpreted as complementary rather than conflicting with the more conventional descriptions from traditional physics and engineering. The amount of information contained in a physical system equals the number of atoms in the system multiplied by the

Table 12–1   Seth Lloyd's Information Jargon

Total (ordinary) information	The sum of accessible information and inaccessible information. Total information never decreases and exists independent of observation.
Accessible information	Directs physical action; messages received and acted on.
Inaccessible information	Also called *entropy* (see below). Decreased locally by observations causing known information to increase (local decrease of ignorance).
Computer	Any system that processes information.
Quantum computer	Operations based on superposition of states; a bit can be 0 and 1 at the same time (superposition). No distinction between analog and digital computation.

(*continued*)

Table 12–1 (Continued)

Observable universe	Spherical region with radius equal to 14 billion light years with earth at the center. The largest known machine that processes information. Energy and information have equal status. A quantum computer that "computes" its own behavior by registering and transferring information. Has performed no more than 10^{122} operations since the universe began with the big bang.
Universe	Cosmic computer of unknown size; might be infinite. A quantum system with many of its parts entangled; entanglement is responsible for the generation of new information.
Energy	An entity that causes objects to perform physical action.
Entropy	The information required to specify the motions of atoms, molecules, and so forth, information generally inaccessible to humans. A measure of the disorder of small particles; a measure of ignorance. Limits the efficiency of heat engines.
Fields, waves	Information and energy organized in specific ways.
Mass, particles	Information and energy organized in specific ways.
First law	Energy is conserved.
Second law	Total information never decreases; the laws of physics preserve information. Arises from the interplay between accessible information and inaccessible information (entropy).
Space	Paths along which information flows; essentially the "wires" of the universe connecting "quantum logic gates."
Bit	Basic unit of information; a byte is 8 bits.
ASCII code	Sequences of bits (binary numbers) representing computer keyboard letters, symbols, etc.
Chaos	Infection of macroscopic bits by microscopic bits.
Effective complexity	The amount of information required to describe a system's *regular features*, the properties essential for successful operation.
Flipping a bit	Operation of replacing 1 by 0 or 0 by 1. May be accomplished in quantum computation by resonant interaction between laser and atom. Occurs through continuous intermediate sequences of superpositions.
FLOPS, ops	Standard measure of computer speed, floating point operations per second, or basic operations per second (ops)
Free energy	Energy with a small amount of entropy. The amount of work (or useful energy) that can be extracted from a system.
Temperature	Energy per bit.

number of bits registered by each atom; that is, the total number of bits required to describe the positions and velocities of all atoms at the smallest possible scale. If matter were continuous "all the way down" to arbitrarily small scales, the "information" contained in any system would be infinite by this definition. But quantum mechanics defines the precision (smallest scale) to which an atom's position and velocity can be specified. As a result, each atom registers only something like 20 bits, and physical systems possess finite information content. Any one kilogram mass, if fully converted to energy, would produce 10^{17} joules of energy, enough energy to run one million 400 horsepower engines for 100 hours. However, there is a big difference between 1 kg of mud and 1 kg of enriched uranium; only the uranium can be converted to energy with current technology. The difference between uranium and mud can be attributed to differences in their informational structures.

Based on the number of atoms and the atomic precision dictated by quantum mechanics, the total information in the physical structure of this book is about 10^{26} bits. By contrast, the verbal information content represented by the 100,000 or so printed words is about 10^6 bits, and the images of the book's pages printed at, let's say, 300 dots per inch total about 10^9 bits. Thus, several kinds of information are potentially available to observers with different interests and armed with different measuring devices. Nevertheless, total (ordinary) information is independent of observation and may be expressed as the sum of accessible and inaccessible information, the latter assigned the label *entropy*. For a book that is read in the normal manner, the information accessible to an unaided human observer is 10^6 bits and the entropy is $10^{26}-10^6$ $\approx 10^{26}$ bits. Special instruments, a microscope and so forth, can be employed to convert entropy to accessible information, say by finding the locations of all pixels on the printed pages. Such a detailed observation would reduce book entropy, but this reduction must be compensated for by an increase in observer entropy. The second law of thermodynamics says that total information and entropy can never decrease; the laws of physics create ordinary information. The *second law of thermodynamics* arises from the interplay between accessible ordinary information and ordinary entropy.

7. COMPLEX SYSTEMS

Complex systems generally consist of multiple interacting parts such that a system taken as a whole exhibits emergent properties not obvious in any single part: airplanes, hurricanes, living cells, ant colonies, economies, and human social systems are common examples. But what makes one system more or less complex than another? Can we establish a useful definition of complexity? A number of semi quantitative definitions have been advanced; in particular, Seth Lloyd has proposed more than 30 different definitions of complexity. His proposal (with Murray Gell-Mann) for a quantity labeled *effective complexity* is outlined in the following paragraphs.[6]

Every physical system has total (ordinary) information determined at the atomic level; part describes the *random* aspects, and part describes the *regular* aspects. In an engineering system like an airplane, the "effective complexity" is essentially the length of the airplane's blueprint, the amount of information required to construct the airplane. The blueprint specifies the wing shape and the chemical content for the metal alloy used to construct the wing. But the blueprint does not specify just where each atom is located; these are not needed for the airplane to fly. Good design attempts to minimize the effective complexity of an engineered system while maintaining the system's ability to function properly. As the old engineering adage goes, *keep it simple, stupid* (KISS), but not too simple.

Lloyd defines effective complexity as the amount of information required to describe a system's *regular features*. But what are these so-called "regular features" of the system? They are the properties essential for successful operation. A simple thought experiment might distinguish information associated with regular from that of random features: Flip any bit in the system (for example, transform one of the 0s to a 1); a bit flip that affects the ability of the system to attain its purpose contributes to the system's regular features and effective complexity. This test makes sense for manmade systems, but what are the "purposes" and successful operations of living systems? Living systems are apparently "successful" when they consume energy and reproduce efficiently, but at least some of us seem to have other things to do in addition to just eating and engaging in sex.

Another problem with this definition of effective complexity concerns the spatial and temporal scales at which the description of the system's "regular" features is to be truncated. Again consider an airplane blueprint. One important component of the airplane shell is aluminum, an abundant element in the Earth's crust, but too chemically reactive to occur naturally as a free metal; it must be separated from bauxite ore. Furthermore, aluminum is typically alloyed with the element titanium to enhance its physical properties. Should these alloy production processes be included in the blueprint, thereby adding to effective complexity? What about instructions for mining the titanium and bauxite ore, including perhaps political information about the third world country where the ore is obtained? If these are made part of the blueprint, perhaps one should also include the following instructions for creating aluminum and titanium: *Go ye forth into the universe and use gravitational attraction to attract clumps of hydrogen. Wait a few billion years or so for a star to form and produce the required metals by nuclear fusion, then wait awhile longer for the star to end its life in a supernova and expel the desired metals.* But perhaps these instructions are still not enough; maybe we require our blueprint to include instructions to create the universe in the first place. With these arguments about the meaning of "complexity" in mind, I consider multiscale contributions to brain complexity and information coding in the following sections and their possible links to consciousness. But unfortunately finding good definitions for "complexity" is not a simple task; it is, in fact, rather complex.[6]

8. BRAINS, INTEGRATED INFORMATION, AND PATTERNS IN NESTED HIERARCHIES

Giulio Tononi, Professor of Psychiatry at the University of Wisconsin, has proposed the concept of *integrated information*, defined as the information generated by a "complex" of interacting elements over and above the information generated by all elements acting in isolation.[7] Giulio notes that everyday consciousness involves brains making fine discriminations between large classes of alternative choices. Furthermore, consciousness is not an all-or-nothing phenomenon. Rather, consciousness is graded as evidenced by the drowsy transition periods between waking and sleeping, light anesthesia, alcohol intoxication, multiple stages of Alzheimer's disease, the active unconscious, and the other varied conscious states indicated in Figure 3–1. Based partly on this general notion, Giulio suggests that integrated information generated by "complexes" of neural elements may provide a plausible quantitative measure of consciousness. This picture may also account for a number of puzzling observations: Consciousness is associated with cortical-thalamic neural assemblies but not obviously with the cerebellum, and unconscious functions evidently occur in many cortical and sub cortical networks. The concept of integrated information in neural complexes overlaps and serves to extend our discussion of graphs (or networks) in Chapter 7 if "complexes" are identified with multiscale neural networks.

Interactions might occur between individual neurons, cortical columns, or other neural structures at arbitrary spatial scales as indicated in Figures 3–6 and 4–8. For integrated information (defined at a particular scale) to be high, the system must be interconnected such that the informational effect of interactions among its basic elements dominates the effect of interactions inside individual elements. In this manner, integrated information can be much larger than that which would be produced by the same collection of isolated elements. As emphasized in Chapters 4 and 7, a hallmark of complex adaptive systems is the presence of distinct dynamic behavior at multiple scales and important interactions across scales. Evidently, such cross-scale interactions can add substantially to integrated information, which might also be labeled *emergent information*, matching the concept of *emergent behavior* typically attributed to a broad class of complex adaptive systems.

Top-down and bottom-up hierarchical interactions across spatial scales occur in many systems; such phenomena are a hallmark of complex systems. Complex dynamic phenomena have been studied in physical, biological, social, and financial systems. Small-scale events cause new events to occur at larger scales, which in turn influence both smaller and even larger scales in the system's nested hierarchy, a general process termed *circular causality*. Take the human global social system as an example: Families, corporations, cities, and nations form nested hierarchies and interact with each other, at the same scales and across scales, as discussed in several contexts in earlier chapters (see Figs. 3–6 and 4–8). Even the highest ranking national leaders act as small-scale units, but they may exert strong bottom-up influences on humans worldwide; such influences can be felt at several larger scales. At the same time, the actions of such leaders are influenced top-down by larger scales, including global events like world wars and financial crises as well as mesoscopic (intermediate scale) events like corporate bankruptcies or political action at state levels. Cross-scale interactions appear to be essential to brain function, including its dynamic behavior and, as I conjecture throughout this book, consciousness itself.

Complex systems often exhibit *fractal-like* dynamic behavior. The word "fractal" (derived from "fractional dimension") indicates geometric shapes that exhibit fine structure at arbitrarily small scales. Magnify an image of a coastline, mountain range, or brain tissue, and you find more intricate structural patterns as the magnification is increased. Technically, "fractals" are supposed to possess a mathematical property called *statistical self-similarity*, roughly meaning cross-scale "similarity" (in some sense) of spatial shapes. But in order to avoid over restrictive definition, I adopt the label "fractal-like" to refer to both geometrical features like the (static) multiscale columnar structure of cerebral cortex and the (dynamic) electrical behavior recorded with electrodes of different sizes. In both the static and dynamic cases, the closer we look, the more detail we expect to find. Weather systems are famous for exhibiting fractal-like dynamic behavior: Global systems contain hurricanes at the scale of hundreds of miles. The hurricanes may contain 100 meter-scale tornados and water spouts, which themselves contain progressively smaller vortices, all the way down to very small scales where matter no longer behaves as a fluid. Still more intricate dynamic behaviors await any "incredible shrinking observer," including semi classical molecular interactions and full quantum behavior at electron scales.

Metaphors like weather or the human global social system are useful for providing an introduction to the dynamics of complex systems, but more realistic models are needed in genuine brain science. Artificial neural networks can be useful in this regard as they can exhibit relatively complex dynamics while processing input information in ways that appear to mimic aspects of human performance, albeit quite limited ones. Artificial networks can learn to classify patterns as in practical tasks like speech or text recognition; for example, networks analogous to the graphs shown in Figures 7–1 and 7–2 can be constructed with distinct processing stages and interaction rules. Despite their ability to perform simple tasks, artificial networks consisting of a few hundred or a few thousand nodes provide only very hollow representations of genuine brains consisting of 100 billion neurons arranged in a nested hierarchy of structure: minicolumns, macrocolumns, and so forth. By analogy, we would expect even a perfectly accurate social model of an isolated tribe living in the Amazon rain forest to be inadequate as a model of the human global system.

To overcome some of the formidable modeling limitations, my colleague Lester Ingber developed a statistical mechanical theory of neocortical interactions in the early 1980s based on new mathematical developments first applied in statistical and quantum mechanics in the 1970s.[8] Macroscopic variables like EEG and large-scale neural firing patterns are indentified through a chain of interactions across spatial scales ranging from single neurons to minicolumns to macrocolumns. One might loosely term this approach "crossing the fractal divide." The theory's outcomes are statistical predictions of spatial-temporal patterns of action potential firings. Lester's theory predicts that cerebral cortex should possess something like 5 to 10 *dynamic memories* consisting of propensities to generate specific firing patterns, which typically persist for several hundreds of milliseconds based on actual physiological parameters; no free parameters (or fudge factors) are introduced in the theory.

To illustrate what is meant by a "dynamic memory," consider an ordinary deck of cards used to produce multiple hands in some card game. Three or four normal human shuffles will typically fail to randomize the deck. As a result, each new round of hands is dealt from a deck with statistical memories created in earlier hands. In the poker game *five-card draw*, the chances of higher cards being dealt close together will be greater than in a random deck, and this pattern will be more pronounced for the aces and face cards than for lower cards. This memory is created because players in earlier hands with a pair of aces in the first betting round will have discarded three cards, keeping their aces together, even after receiving three new cards. Similarly, in the game of *bridge*, an enhanced tendency for cards of the same suit to occur in bunches will occur. A deck of cards can hold several distinct kinds of memory simultaneously.

One important outcome of Lester's theory is the prediction of neural firing patterns persisting for several hundred milliseconds; these patterns are the dynamic memories of whatever activity produced the patterns in the first place. If several firing patterns can exist simultaneously, then several memories can be stored simultaneously. Thus, the dynamic memories predicted by theory are candidates to represent genuine human short-term memory, which occurs on roughly the same timescale and has a reported capacity of about 7 ± 2 items. This capacity apparently is approximately valid even for exceptional memory performers whose achievements are based on a mental strategy of grouping larger patterns into single items. As short-term memory is an important feature of consciousness, this theory provides a link between one aspect of awareness and the brain dynamic behavior predicted by genuine physiology and anatomy.

9. CONSCIOUSNESS ENCODING AT VERY LARGE OR VERY SMALL SCALES?

Can information associated with consciousness be encoded at the very large scales (greater than several centimeters) at which the EEG is recorded? In Chapter 7, I proposed a convenient strategy to view the large-scale dynamics generating EEG: The sources of this dynamics may be pictured as neural networks *embedded* in synaptic action fields, the latter defined as the numbers of active excitatory and inhibitory synapses per unit volume of cortical tissue. The synaptic fields, which may appear as large-scale standing or traveling waves or other global dynamic behavior, are distinct from the electric fields that they generate. Highly asynchronous synaptic fields may fail to produce any measureable extra cranial electric field at all, for example.

In this picture, neural network (or cell assembly) and synaptic field descriptions constitute complementary models of cortical reality, with the label "network" indicating dynamics over a range of mesoscopic (millimeter to centimeter) scales and "synaptic fields" indicating the largest-scale brain dynamics. The network and field descriptions overlap at intermediate (several centimeter) scales, as in the case of regional networks interconnecting cerebral lobes. Neural networks may be viewed as embedded in cortical synaptic fields in a manner analogous to social networks embedded in human cultures. Thus, important top-down and bottom-up interactions across spatial scales are anticipated. For example, networks embedded in an exceptionally excitatory global field environment may be more likely to become active or spread their actions to other networks. In extreme cases, *epilepsy* is expected as the observable outcome. Or, remote, non overlapping networks may become correlated as a result of immersion in a common global field, perhaps oscillating in a narrow frequency band. This latter process, called *binding by resonance*, was discussed in Chapter 7. The coexistence of network and global synaptic field activity constitutes one kind of *fractal-like dynamic behavior*.

Hermann Haken, the well-known founder of the field of *synergetics* (the science of cooperation), and his former student, physicist-turned-neuroscientist, Viktor Jirsa, have advanced the idea of complementary local and global processes by showing that local network models and my global EEG model discussed in Chapter 7 are naturally compatible in both the mathematical and physiological senses.[9] Hermann and Viktor showed mathematically that the brain may act similar to a parallel computer at small scales by means of local or regional neural networks, while simultaneously producing the global field patterns that I have advocated at macroscopic scales, that is, fractal-like dynamics. In one experimental test, their local-global model was able to predict important aspects of MEG dynamics recorded during a motor task.[10]

Conjectures concerning possible material substrates underlying consciousness are not limited to neurons, their larger scale complexes like cortical columns, or global synaptic fields. Information (or Ultra-Information) associated with consciousness might also be stored at very small scales. Herms Romijn of the Netherlands Institute for Brain Research has published a highly speculative paper proposing that the fleeting, ordered three-dimensional patterns of electric and magnetic fields surrounding the dendritic trees of neural networks might encode conscious experiences.[11] These microfields can exhibit a rich dynamic behavior at millisecond and micrometer time and space scales, providing for much finer-grained spatial details than patterns occurring at neuron and larger scales. In this view, consciousness did not actually "emerge" during evolution; rather, the germs of rudimentary consciousness have long existed as a fundamental property of the universe, manifested in its omnipresent electric and magnetic fields. Perhaps an absence of the appropriate kind of detailed spatial-temporal structure needed to support fine-grained fields prevented genuine awareness from emerging before familiar life forms evolved. Neural networks may then be viewed as contributing to consciousness by the generation of highly ordered complex field patterns, thereby allowing for subjective experiences to emerge in the localized informational spaces we now know as "brains." While I view this specific idea as a real long shot, it does suggest possible future arguments in the context of unknown physical fields or other entities.

11. CONSTRUCTION OF AN ARTIFICIAL BRAIN: A PROVOCATIVE THOUGHT EXPERIMENT

Consider a thought experiment where one attempts to create a *conscious entity* (a class of Ultra-Computer) using a blueprint, perhaps supplied by the fanciful alien Moses introduced in earlier chapters. The central question addressed here concerns the *effective complexity* of this blueprint, that is, the amount of regular information and the limiting precision or smallest scale of the blueprint, issues similar to those considered for the airplane blueprint in Section 6. Proponents of the idea that artificial consciousness can be created in the near future have envisioned construction of artificial networks of, let's say, 10^8 to 10^{10} interacting units representing minicolumns or individual neurons, respectively, with each unit obeying simple input-output rules. But genuine neurons are complicated dynamic systems in and of themselves, and accurate simulation of even single cells down to molecular scales is well beyond current computer technology. Furthermore, the molecules themselves exhibit their own complex nested hierarchies. So our basic question is this: Can artificial neurons or columns with simple input-output rules adequately replace real neural structures if the ultimate goal is to create genuine awareness? The answer seems to hinge, at least in part, on the scale at which the information (or Ultra-Information) associated with consciousness is encoded. If, for example, Romijn's model were to be valid and (quasi static) micro electric and micro magnetic fields encode information critical to consciousness, interacting simple units representing neurons, even in very large complexes, would seem to remain forever free of awareness, irrespective of their proficiency with human tasks or ability to pass Turing tests.

Complex systems like spin glasses (magnets with certain complex properties), lasers, chemical mixes, weather, ecology, and so forth typically generate *multiscale* dynamic behaviors that bridge gaps between microscopic and macroscopic scales. In fact, many physical systems exhibit intricate dynamic behaviors at multiple scales in the absence of fixed multiscale structures. The simultaneous production of hurricanes, tornadoes, and smaller multiscale vortices provides a common example from fluid mechanics. Neocortex is especially interesting in this context because of the presence of fixed mesoscopic tissue scales, both anatomically (multiscale columnar structures) and physiologically (scale-dependent inhibitory and excitatory interactions). This multiscale structure would appear to encourage greatly the production of attendant multiscale dynamic behaviors. In this regard, neuroscientist Walter Freeman has long studied the dynamic behaviors of multiscale neural structures that he labels "K-sets." Walter identifies neural KO sets through KV sets, representing different scales, types of interconnections, and input-output characteristics, and suggests their possible selective contributions to various aspects of conscious experience.[12]

Another way to address these issues is to employ our analog global social system shown in Figure 4–8 and pose the following question: Which substrate (or scale) codes the information required to describe human social activity?

Perhaps the best answer is individual humans, but on reflection, the answer is not quite so obvious. For one thing, we have argued that each human consciousness emerges from interactions of multiple unconscious and quasi conscious subsystems, suggesting the importance of smaller-scale substrates for the social system. On the other hand, families, cities, and nations display emergent dynamic properties resulting from interactions at smaller scales; as such they become candidates for larger-scale substrates. Adopting Giulio Tononi's language, the larger human structures process *integrated information*, which exceeds the sum of informational processing of isolated humans inside the human "complexes," or in Walter Freeman's parlance, "K sets."

Based on the arguments of this chapter, I see no compelling reason to focus on any single scale as *the* foundational substrate of consciousness. As each spatial scale is crossed through interactions, new (integrated) information is evidently created together with the attending emergent properties in the larger systems. The information (or Ultra-Information) of consciousness can apparently exist and be processed at multiple scales simultaneously. I am reminded of the well-known passage by neuroscientist Vernon Mountcastle, discoverer of the columnar organization of cerebral cortex in the 1950s: "...the brain is a complex of widely and reciprocally interconnected systems and the dynamic interplay between these systems is the very essence of brain function."[13] To this "essence" I suggest adding interactions across scales and fractal-like dynamic behaviors at multiple scales; these are hallmarks of a wide variety of complex systems, and my guess is that they are also critical in the pre-eminent complex systems the we call "brains."

If these conjectures about the critical importance of cross scale interactions are correct, we are then faced with the following fundamental question: *Where do we make the small-scale cut-off below which physical structures may be treated simply?* Or said another way: *Where does the fractal-like character of the nervous system stop?* Whereas many neuroscientists implicitly or explicitly choose the single neuron scale for this barrier, I see no obvious support for this assumption. In the following section, I will address similar issues in the context of different kinds of memory storage.

12. INFORMATION STORAGE AND MEMORY

The word "memory" refers to a very familiar but, nevertheless, strange collection of phenomena, some closely aligned with awareness. We remember genuine past experiences, thus memory differs both from *imagination* and *perception*, the awareness of current sensory information. Recalling dramatic events like those of September 11, 2001 can elicit vivid visual memories of the people and objects located nearby on such occasions. I can clearly picture a fellow student's animated face and body language as he excitedly approached me on November 22, 1963, shouting, "The president's been shot!" One may pose two distinct questions about memory: Where are various kinds of memory stored? And,

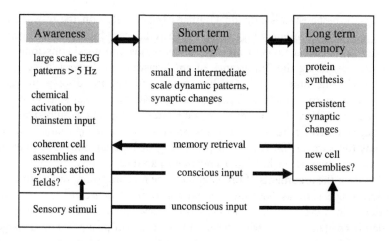

Figure 12–3   An overview of memory systems.

what are the physical representations of memory, the means of memory information storage called *memory traces* or *engrams*?

Cognitive scientists make relatively sharp distinctions between *short-* and
long-term memory, but long-term memory consists of several sub categories
including: *episodic memory* (of specific past events), *semantic memory* (knowledge
about the external world), *procedural memory* (use of objects or body movements), and *emotional memory*. Long-term memory is thought to be widely
distributed throughout the brain, but different memory categories seem to be
preferentially located in the regions most involved with the original experiences.
The *cerebellum* and *limbic system* (an extensive collection of interconnected sub
cortical structures) are, for example, linked to procedural and emotional
memories, respectively. At least some aspects of memory appear to be essential
for the presence of genuine consciousness.

Figure 12–3 provides a highly oversimplified overview that includes long-
term memory storage resulting from sensory input that fails to register in the
conscious mind. Examples of "unconscious storage" include patients under
general anesthesia, subliminal messages hidden in very brief visual or auditory
input embedded in other signals, and *blindsight*, involving persons perceptually
blind in certain areas of their visual fields. Subjects in these experiments may
have no awareness of the target stimuli but are able to predict various aspects of
the targets at levels significantly above chance by being forced to guess between
alternatives.

Short-term memory is associated with both dynamic spatial patterns and
modifications of synaptic strengths. Long-term memory is known to involve
construction of new proteins within cell bodies as well as new synaptic pathways
reinforcing the strengths of neuron-neuron connections.[14] Such a general outline, however, provides almost no detail about how vast amounts of memory

information (or Ultra-Information), seemingly required for normal human functions, are stored and retrieved. The physical representations of memory, the *engrams*, are largely unknown. Is it plausible that all of the vast information content of the long-term memory of an adult human could be stored in new cell assembly (network) formation, especially given that many of these same cells apparently participate in perception and processing of current events? If so, are different kinds of memory stored in networks simultaneously operating at different spatial scales? Is it possible that important aspects of memory are stored at smaller scales, say in protein molecules or even at still smaller scales?

Small-scale memory storage associated with awareness may not seem so farfetched if we recall that several other kinds of "memory" are stored at single-cell and molecular scales. The success of vaccinations against disease is based on *immunological memory* in which vertebrate immune systems exposed to pathogens store this contact information in "memory cells" able to mount chemical responses to new exposures. *Antibodies* are protein molecules produced in these cells that identify and neutralize foreign bodies. *Genetic memory* in the form of species-specific genes is passed between generations as DNA molecules.[15] DNA contains the information needed to construct specific protein molecules making up the cells of the offspring, essentially providing the blueprint for the construction of all parts of the new living creature. DNA also carries the information determining when and where in the body different genes turn on and off.

In summary, short-term, long-term, immunological, and genetic memories all require information storage, but on progressively longer time scales. Short-term memory is associated with dynamic patterns and cell assembly formation; immunologic and genetic memories are stored at smaller spatial scales including cellular and large molecular scales. The usual sharp distinction between short- and long-term memories makes for convenient discussion, but apparently masks a continuum of processes involving cross-scale interactions. I am unaware of any evidence for memory storage at sub molecular scales, but such storage does not appear to violate physical laws.

13. ULTRA-INFORMATION CANDIDATES

Mankind's understanding of the universe has progressed slowly over the past four hundred years or so, but with greatly accelerated knowledge development in the past century. These periods represent only about 0.00001% of the history of life on Earth and 0.1% of the time of Homo sapiens' existence. Given our very short history of scientific literacy, we must wonder about unimagined new phenomena that await discovery. One of the most useful of scientific concepts developed in the past hundred years or so is that of the *field*, a mathematical function that assigns some quantity to each point in space and time. The nature and existence of "fields" is determined by the observed effects they produce on the various entities that "match" the appropriate field. Place a charged particle in an electromagnetic field or a massive object in a gravitational field, and they will behave in a predictable manner. The existence of specific kinds of fields is revealed only when the behavior of the matching "antenna" (charge or mass) is observed. This raises the genuine possibility that so called "empty" space may contain many kinds of fields that are currently unknown. Nonlocal influences evidenced by the Bell-ERP-inspired experiments and the nonlocal Bohm quantum potential are possible candidates for fields that may fall in the Ultra-Information category. Furthermore, who knows what strange phenomena may lurk in the shadows of sub electron scales or rolled up in the extra space dimensions proposed by string theory?

Unknown fields may also act on macroscopic objects. *Dark matter* is hypothetical mass whose existence is inferred from the observed motion of stars and galaxies. Such inference is analogous to the theoretical prediction of the existence and location of the planet Neptune based on unexpected orbital behavior of Uranus. In addition to dark matter, some sort of *dark energy* appears to permeate space as it provides an explanation for the observed accelerated expansion of the universe. Surprisingly, dark energy plus dark matter appear to make up 96% of the mass-energy of the observable universe, with visible matter like stars and intergalactic gas accounting only for the remaining 4%. If dark energy and dark matter have genuine physical properties, associated *dark information* must also exist. I am *not* claiming that such dark information has anything to do with consciousness. Rather, the apparent discovery of these strange new fields serves to remind us that still more fields, as yet unknown, may be found; some might even have links to consciousness. I offer no support for this conjecture, only the glib (and not altogether convincing) retort, *absence of evidence is not evidence of absence.*

14. DUALISM AND QUANTUM MECHANICS

René Descartes, famous 17th century philosopher, scientist, and mathematician, proposed *Cartesian* (or *substance*) *dualism*, in which the body (and brain) are essentially machines following physical laws, but the mind is a separate nonmaterial entity that occupies an independent realm of existence outside of the physical world. This position is essentially Plato's view and matches many of today's religions if "mind" is identified with "soul." Cartesian dualism runs counter to much modern thinking in the brain sciences as many, if not most, scientists believe that mind emerges as a direct result of neural interactions within the brain. This modern view is based on a wealth of data showing strong correlations between observed brain dynamic patterns (revealed with EEG, FMRI, and so forth) or structural deficits (due to injury or disease) and conscious experience. The mind clearly relies on brain anatomy and physiology to operate normally as discussed in Chapters 5 and 6. These data from brain studies may seem to some to essentially prove that the brain creates the mind; consciousness appears to be an emergent property of neural interactions, a view known as *property dualism* in the philosophy of mind.

While some battles between science and religion originate with an apparent conflict between Cartesian and property dualism, scientific bases for nuanced versions of Cartesian dualism have been advanced. Philosopher David Chalmers has proposed a thought experiment, perhaps inspired by the movie *The Matrix*, in which Cartesian dualism appears consistent with science: A computer simulation is created in which the bodies of the simulated beings are controlled by their minds, but their minds remain external to the simulation. The simulated beings perform sophisticated experiments, but discovering the origins of their minds appears to be fundamentally impossible, as their minds reside outside of their observable universe. One may say that these beings live in a universe containing information that is fundamentally more inaccessible than ordinary entropy; in my proposed terminology, this is *Ultra-Entropy*. There is at least a metaphorical link between this Cartesian dualism and the established *physical dualism* of quantum mechanics discussed in Chapter 11 and in the following paragraphs. One may take this idea a little further and question if the link may be more than simply metaphorical.

Each of the ontological interpretations of quantum mechanics outlined in Chapter 11 can be interpreted as a *physical dualism* (just within the physical world itself), irrespective of the status afforded to mind by each ontology. Quantum mechanics divides the universe into two parts corresponding to wavelike and particle-like features of nature. Heisenberg describes this separation of reality into (wavelike) *propensity states* consisting of "objective tendencies" or statistical weights for certain observable (particle-like) "events" to occur. In Bohm's language, reality is divided into the *enfolded* (or *implicate*) *order* and the *explicate order*, in which observable events occur. In the many worlds interpretation, events observed by the inhabitants of one universe are influenced by events in other universes. In each of these interpretations, the universe is divided into observable and non observable parts, with the latter providing subtle influences on events in the former. We might then say that limited kinds of Ultra-Information pass between the separate realms of reality. In the Heisenberg-von Neumann interpretations, at least, interactions between the separate realms are not strictly limited to the atomic level. Rather, macroscopic events like reading a measuring device by an observer are viewed as holistic outcomes of interactions between the quantum world and the measuring system. Our cosmic quantum orchestra of Chapter 11 might be adopted as crude metaphor for this non observable realm of existence, which might be labeled *the propensity state, the implicate order, the multiverse, the Platonic world, the world of Ultra-Information*, and so forth.

The physical dualism implied by quantum mechanics may or may not be directly related to the hard problem of consciousness. If nothing else, however, the general notion that physical dualism is a fundamental property of the physical universe should perhaps cause us to be quite skeptical of narrow materialistic views based on classical physics, in which the challenge of consciousness is trivialized or even banished as an illusion. In the late 19th century, the famous biologist Thomas Huxley labeled the conscious mind an *epiphenomenon,* an accidental byproduct of the physical brain. Paradoxically, this very classical-mechanistic view was expressed just before the dawn of the new era of quantum mechanics in which the classical world view was over-thrown. For some prominent physicists, notably Roger Penrose[16] and Henry Stapp,[17] much of today's brain science and philosophy remains mired in outdated 19th century classical thinking when addressing the hard problem of consciousness.

15. CONCLUDING REMARKS: DOES THE BRAIN CREATE THE MIND?

With today's science, fundamental entities like charge and energy cannot be defined without relying on circular arguments. Similarly, science is currently unable to explain consciousness in terms of more fundamental processes. Given such deep ignorance, I have argued that we must allow for the possibility that consciousness itself is fundamental. I offer a choice between two possibilities: *(1)* Consciousness emerges from complex dynamic interactions confined to the brain. In other words, the brain creates the mind, the mainstream scientific view. *(2)* Consciousness is a fundamental entity that exists at least partly in space-time, and each brain acts like an "antenna" interacting with this entity.

In either of these views, a wealth of modern scientific data point to brain tissue as something very special, whether actually creating consciousness or selectively interacting with some external consciousness-producing entity. But just what is so special about these little blobs of tissue called brains, distinguishing them from other complex systems? One proposal is that, in some sense, brains are much more complex even than kidneys or hearts or even the Amazon rain forest, for example.[16] This is an attractive idea, but in what sense are brains more complex? Unambiguous quantitative measures of "complexity" are hard to come by. It was suggested in Chapters 4 and 6 that brain dynamic complexity may maximize in states intermediate between global coherence and extreme functional localization. Healthy brains may require the proper dynamic balance. Some have also emphasized various measures of information processing in brain tissue, but, again, "information" can have multiple interpretations.

This book has repeatedly emphasized the dynamic complexity resulting from multiscale interactions. Cerebral cortical tissue is structured in a nested hierarchy consisting neurons, columns of various sizes, and lobes. Such multiscale structure encourages fractal-like dynamic behavior and interactions across spatial scales, both top-down and bottom-up, a *circular causality* with common analogs in complex physical systems. This multiscaled structure together with the (non-local) corticocortical interactions evidently provides a highly effective anatomical-physiological substrate for complex dynamic behavior. Furthermore, different parts of the brain can do different things, providing functional isolation at some scales, in some frequency bands, or both. At the same time, the brain may remain functionally integrated at the largest scales, in other frequency bands, or both. Is this anatomical-physiological substrate, of itself, sufficient for consciousness to emerge from brain dynamic processes?

Or does the substrate and attendant dynamic complexity merely produce a functioning antenna?

In order to facilitate our discussion, I have proposed a choice of language designed to avoid the linguistic traps that may blur genuine distinctions between man and machine. To this end, the common label *information* is replaced by *ordinary information*, and a broader category, *Ultra-Information*, is defined, perhaps provocatively, as *that which distinguishes one entity from another*. This definition is meant to encompass ordinary information, conscious processes, and putative physical phenomena that might not qualify as ordinary information, perhaps encompassing nonlocal influences (occurring at faster-than-light speed), as in the Bell-ERP experiments outlined in Chapter 11. Thoughts, emotions, self-awareness, memory, contents of the unconscious, and other aspects of consciousness are, by definition, considered here to be categories of Ultra-Information whether or not these mental processes consist exclusively of ordinary information. Ultra-Information might be located both inside and outside of brains.[18]

Starting with the prevailing assumption that consciousness emerges from brain dynamics, several additional questions were raised in this chapter. What are the physical and biological entities that store the information (or Ultra-Information) of consciousness; that is, what are the material substrates of mind? How is the information stored and retrieved? Which spatial scales are involved in consciousness-related information storage and processing? I have argued that consciousness substrates need not be limited to neurons. Brains belong to a class of dynamic entities called *complex adaptive systems*. Interactions across scales and fractal-like dynamic behaviors at multiple scales are the hallmarks of many such systems. Given that cross-scale interactions and distinct dynamic behaviors are critical to complex dynamic systems, one may reasonably conjecture the critical importance of such general phenomena to brain function. Thus, the information associated with various aspects of conscious experience may be stored and processed at multiple spatial scales, ranging from synaptic fields encompassing most or all of neocortex to regional cell assemblies (several centimeters) to columnar scale (millimeter) assemblies to molecular or even sub electron scales.

The electric fields produced by valence (outer shell) electrons are essentially the "glue" that holds atoms together to form molecules; every chemical reaction involves interactions between intricate, small-scale electric field patterns. We readily accept that genetic memory is stored in DNA molecules. Could other molecules hold other kinds of memory or selected aspects of consciousness? If information is stored "in molecules," can we just as easily say that this information is stored in the corresponding microscale electric field patterns holding molecular structures together?

To expand on this last question, note that many biological processes involve microelectric fields acting on brain chemicals: for example, absorption of photons by retinal cells, opening of voltage-gated ion channels, initiation of action potentials in cell membranes, release of chemical neurotransmitters on the arrival of action potentials at synapses, and the actions of these neurotransmitters on postsynaptic cells. We describe transmembrane voltages as "changing molecular structure," as in opening voltage-gated ion channels. But more detailed descriptions of the same processes would depict the intricate interactions of the membrane's internal electric field with the smaller-scale atomic field patterns within the protein molecules forming the ion channels.

At which scale can we say that the fractal-like character of the nervous system stops? In other words, how much detail (*effective complexity*) is required in a brain blueprint? Is it possible that still more storage and processing of "conscious information" (or Ultra-Information) occurs at atomic or even sub atomic scales? If so, direct influences from quantum processes would be implied, thereby supporting the *RQTC conjecture*.

Where is the ordinary information or Ultra-Information of consciousness stored? Many scientists will claim no need for a new information category; ordinary information and today's established physics may be all that is required for consciousness, a view apparently enjoying majority support from contemporary neuroscientists. Known neural correlates suggest that memory and other consciousness-related information are widely distributed throughout various parts of the brain even though their substrates remain mostly unknown. Yet even the most extensive and robust neural correlates cannot insure that *all* of consciousness is actually confined to brain boundaries.

A recent book, *Irreducible Mind*,[19] provides an extensive overview of empirical data collected over the past century, beginning with the classic works of William James and F. W. H. Myers and addressing well-established phenomena of mind such as unconscious processes, extreme forms of psychophysical influence (hypnotic blisters, stigmata, and so forth), hypnosis, multiple personality, and memory. The book goes further, offering a generally positive view of the possibility that, at least in special circumstances such as occurring under conditions of deep general anesthesia and/or cardiac arrest, consciousness need not be confined to brain. While much of this latter material is highly controversial,[20] the book offers systematic entry to unconventional studies of consciousness and possible new experiments that might test some of the ideas outlined here.

If a consciousness-causing external entity were actually to exist, how would it interact with brains? Recall our analogy with electron charge and spin, the fundamental physical properties that act as "antennas" revealing the presence of electric and magnetic fields. At a larger scale, the photoreceptive cells of the retina are neurons acting as antenna systems sensitive to electromagnetic fields in the very narrow frequency band called *light*. With such analogs in mind, I have speculated in this chapter on the possible existence of some undiscovered physical field or even a nonphysical entity, a subcategory of Ultra-Information, which interacts with brains in some unknown manner.[21] In this highly speculative picture, whole brains or special parts of brains might behave like antenna systems sensitive to an unknown physical field or other entity that, for want of a better name, may be called *Mind* as indicated in Figure 12–2. This interaction could, for example, occur at sub molecular or even sub electron scales, allowing "absorption" of very small-scale Ultra-Information that would later work its way "up the hierarchical stairway" to the large scales of brain dynamics by cross-scale interactions. Delays incurred in crossing small scales could easily be short, say small fractions of a millisecond. Since consciousness of external stimuli takes several hundred milliseconds to develop, the micro delays could be negligible.

I am unable to offer supporting evidence for this "crazy" conjecture; rather, I suggest that, given man's ultra short scientific history and profound ignorance of the origin of consciousness, the possible existence of *Mind* cannot be dismissed out of hand. I offer no definitive experiments to test this speculation, but perhaps clever scientists will think of some in the future. Does the brain create the mind? Or do brain and *Mind* act as partners to create the mind? Your guess is as good as mine.

Endnotes

Chapter 1

1. Parts of his book are concerned with professional philosophy; a convenient and up-to-date online general reference is E. N. Zalta (Ed.), *The Stanford Encyclopedia of Philosophy* [URL http://plato.stanford.edu/]. Books aimed specifically at the philosophy of mind include:
   P. S. Churchland, *Neurophilosophy*, Cambridge, MA: MIT Press, 1986.
   D. C. Dennett, *Consciousness Explained*, Boston: Little Brown & Company, 1991.
   J. Searle, *The Rediscovery of the Mind*, Cambridge, MA: MIT Press, 1992.
2. Cal Thomas, Consensus or censorship, *Tribune Media Services*, March 26, 2009.
3. V. Braitenberg, *Vehicles. Experiments in Synthetic Psychology*, Cambridge, MA: MIT Press, 1984.
4. J. Hogan, *Code of the Lifemaker*, Ballantine Books, 1983.
5. The current casino-like banking system in the United States, seemingly designed to funnel money to the finance and insurance industries, began to emerge after 1980 during the presidency of Ronald Reagan. One of the first major consequences is described in Martin Mayer, *The Greatest-Ever Bank Robbery: The Collapse of the Savings and Loan Industry*, 1990. Unfortunately, such lessons of extreme deregulation were not well absorbed as evidenced by the much greater taxpayer robberies surfacing in 2008–2009. Two Nobel Prize–winning economists, Joseph Stiglitz and Paul Krugman, have written of how politicians with close ties to the banking industry formed unholy alliances to prevent adoption of good government policies. The banking villains were not by any means limited to Republicans. As many, including journalist Robert Scheer, have observed, the huge expansion in collateralized mortgage debt was the direct result of enabling deregulatory legislation that occurred during the Clinton presidency due largely to the efforts of then Treasury Secretaries Robert Rubin and Lawrence Summers. They essentially partnered with then Fed Chairman Alan Greenspan and congressional leaders James Leach and Phil Gramm to facilitate unrestricted gambling by the banking industry. Reaganomics has had a dramatic effect on the 0.01% wealthiest Americans, whose incomes rose by a factor of seven between 1980 and 2007 while the median income rose by only about 20%. See also T. Philippon and A. Reshef, Wages and human capital in the US financial industry, 1909–2006, *NBER Working Paper* 14644, January, 2009 [URL http://www.nber.org] and J. R. Talbott, *Contagion*, Hoboken, NJ: Wiley, 2009.

6. Many think of missile defense as originating with Ronald Reagan's Strategic Defense Initiative (SDI) in 1983, commonly known as "Star Wars." But defense scientists were thinking about defensive missiles by the early 1950s. An official government program was initiated in 1963, and I performed scientific work in this area in 1969–1971 just after receiving my PhD. Shortly thereafter I switched fields to neuroscience, partly in reaction to U.S. involvement in Vietnam. One of the many problems with missile defense is its destabilizing effect; the easiest and cheapest response to an enemy's defensive system is typically to increase your own offensive capability. Thus, when the Soviet Union deployed a defensive system around Moscow, a natural U.S. response was to "MIRV" its offensive missiles, meaning the placement of multiple (individually targeted) nuclear weapons on each missile. As a net result of deploying the defensive system, Moscow apparently became much *less* safe.

   The catalyst for Reagan's SDI was his interaction with Edward Teller, the so-called "father" of the H bomb (My PhD advisor, Sinai Rand, was one of Teller's students; Teller was one of Heisenberg's students). Reagan, seemingly ignorant of the limitations of missile defense, instituted an "end run" around sound scientific advice to create the expensive new research program SDI. Because both the United States and USSR had finally come to appreciate the destabilizing influence of missile defense in 1972, they then had then signed the Anti-Ballistic Missile Treaty prohibiting new ABM deployments. SDI in 1983 was officially a research program, so it did not violate the existing treaty. But in December, 2001 the Bush administration withdrew from the treaty opening the door for actual deployment and raising the following question: Just *who* is missile defense to be deployed against? The putative enemy must be sufficiently advanced to develop both a reliable intercontinental ballistic missile system and compact, sophisticated nuclear warheads appropriate for this system (hard problems), but at the same time, so technically backward that they cannot implement effective measures to counter a U.S. defensive system (a relatively easy problem). In essence, this imagined enemy must be technically smart and dumb at the same time, an interesting combination to say the least. See also note 6 under Chapter 3 regarding Teller's autobiography.

   In 1984, scientists seeking SDI funding were invited to a meeting held in a large conference room overlooking the Pacific Ocean in La Jolla. I attended even though I had no intention of seeking SDI funds; I simply wanted to witness the historic feeding frenzy, a sort of "mini-Woodstock" based on financial profit rather than music, peace, and love. I was not disappointed; government bureaucrats communicated the following (barely disguised) message to excited defense contractors in attendance: *We are required to spend all this new money on SDI but have little idea of how we can possibly spend so much so fast; please help us get rid of this stuff!*

7. A number of excellent books have been written about the Iraq and Vietnam wars. For Iraq, see T. E. Ricks, *Fiasco*, London: Penguin Books, 2006. Absurd claims that the Vietnam War had to do with "freedom for the Vietnamese" provide an excellent example of George Orwell's prescription, "He who controls the present controls the past and he who controls the past controls the future." Such revisionist history makes future military action, including the Iraq invasion, far more palatable to the public. For a partial history of the Vietnam War see N. Sheehan, *A Bright and Shining Lie*, New York: Vintage Books, 1988, and *The Pentagon Papers. Gravel Edition, Boston: Beacon Press*, 1971 (the *top secret* history commissioned by U.S. Secretary of Defense Robert Strange McNamara in 1967, officially titled *United States–Vietnam Relations, 1945–1967: A Study Prepared*

by the Department of Defense). Here is what McNamara said in an interview with journalist Robert Scheer in 1995:

> Look, we dropped three to four times the tonnage on that tiny little area as were dropped by the Allies in all of the theaters in World War II over a period of five years. It was unbelievable. We killed—there were killed—3,200,000 Vietnamese, excluding the South Vietnamese military. My God! The killing, the tonnage—it was fantastic. The problem was that we were trying to do something that was militarily impossible—we were trying to break the will; I don't think we can break the will by bombing short of genocide [URL http://www.truthdig.com].

So the war did, in fact, result in a kind of "freedom" for a million or so Vietnamese (including countless civilians living in small villages) and the 58,000 American soldiers who returned in body bags.

8. U.S.-backed overt and covert military actions in Central and South America often used the Cold War as an excuse, but in most cases, the main motivations were clearly economic, that is, protecting the interests of U.S. corporations and investors, not to mention a pathological fear that left-leaning governments might become successful, thereby setting a 'bad" example for the U.S. See, for example, N. Chomsky, *Hegemony or Survival. America's Quest for Global Dominance*, New York: Henry Holt and Company, 2003.

9. The free-market model also fails when management compensation is misaligned with the interests of corporate shareholders. Bonuses and stock options, in particular, provide management with incentives to grab quick profits at the expense of the long-term health of their firms. In scientific parlance, management and shareholders attempt to maximize their benefits on different time scales.

10. A common fallacy is that insider trading is illegal. In the United States, trades made by corporate insiders in their company's stock are considered fraudulent only if based on "material nonpublic information." However, as soon as the corporate report is issued to the public, insider trades based on information (perhaps well hidden) in the report are perfectly legal. Given the creative accounting tricks that have surfaced in recent years, it appears that the intent of the law is easily circumvented. Furthermore, the passage of subtle but critical information between insiders and cronies, say by raising an eyebrow or a smile or frown at the appropriate time, also cannot be controlled, resulting in even more positive feedback to make the rich even richer.

Chapter 2

1. R. Dawkins, *The Blind Watchmaker*, New York: WW Norton & Co, 1996.
2. R. W. Sperry, Lateral specialization in the surgically separated hemispheres, In F. O. Schmitt and F. G. Worden (Eds.), *The Neurosciences 3rd Study Program*, Cambridge, MA: MIT Press, pp. 5–19, 1974 (the famous work that led to Sperry's Nobel Prize). Figures 2–1 and 2–3 reproduced with permission from this article.
3. F. S. Collins, *The Language of God*, New York: Free Press, 2006.
4. J. Bauby, *The Diving Bell and the Butterfly*, New York: Alfred A. Knopf, 1997.
5. *The Medical Durable Power of Attorney* designates an agent to make decisions in case of incapacity and can give written guidance for end-of-life decisions. This feature differs from other legal instruments that may require interpretation by physicians or

court-appointed guardians. *The Medical Durable Power of Attorney* takes the job of interpretation out of the hands of strangers and gives it to a person trusted by the patient. Such instructions to designated agents or family members should consider religious beliefs, age, financial capacity, the law's limitations, and so forth. In the case of locked-in patients, the anguish of being trapped in the "diving bell" or "buried alive" should also be considered. Each person must choose his own instructions to his agent. Some may agree with me and find that the following example statements fit their wishes; others may opt to prolong their lives in the face of severe adversity: *(1)* I have executed *The Medical Durable Power of Attorney* so that my wife, in consultation with my children, is free to make decisions about my fate if I am unable to communicate my wish to either live or die. I designate my wife as my agent for this purpose. *(2)* If in the opinion of qualified medical staff, I am in an irreversible unconscious or semiconscious state lacking the ability for unequivocal communication, I choose to die in the quickest and most painless manner feasible. If this cannot be accomplished locally because of state law, I wish to be transported to a location (perhaps Oregon) where my life can be ended without placing my agent or medical staff in legal jeopardy. *(3)* If I am in a semi-locked-in state with the ability to communicate at least one letter of the alphabet, I wish to be asked at least once per day whether I wish to live or die. If I answer with the letter *L*, it means I wish to live at least one more day. If I answer with the letter *D* three times in a row, it means I wish to die as quickly as possible under the conditions of #2 above. *(4)* If I am in a fully locked-in condition so that I am unable to communicate my wishes, I choose to die under these same conditions. I also favor #4 in the case of late-stage (zombie-like) Alzheimer's disease, but this may pose difficult legal problems.

Chapter 3

1. For an easy-to-read overview, see: S. Pinker, *How the Mind Works*, New York: W. W. Norton & Company, 1997. For excellent descriptions of how perceptions of reality are altered by brain disease or trauma see: V. S. Ramachandran and S. Blakeslee, *Phantoms in the Brain*, New York: Harper, 1998 (which could be subtitled *The Man Who Mistook His Foot for a Penis*). Todd Feinberg, a clinical neurologist, also provides interesting clinical accounts of unusual conscious states. Todd further emphasizes the critical importance of the brain's nested hierarchical structure in producing consciousness, a view in agreement with many ideas expressed in this book. See T. E. Feinberg, *Altered Egos*, New York: Oxford University Press, 2001, and *From Axons to Identity: Neurological Explorations of the Nature of the Self*, New York: Norton, 2009.
2. Figure 3–1 was inspired by a similar figure in the chapter: N. D. Schiff, Large-scale brain dynamics and connectivity in the minimally conscious state. In V .K. Jirsa and A. R. McIntosh (Eds.), *Handbook of Brain Connectivity*, Berlin, Germany: Springer, pp. 505–520, 2007.
3. B. Libet, *Mind Time*, Cambridge, MA: Harvard University Press, 2004.
4. F. Hoyle, *The Black Cloud*, New York: The New American Library, 1957.
5. F. Hoyle, *Home Is Where the Wind Blows*, Mill Valley, California: University Science Books, 1994 (autobiography).
6. Evidently, one of the favorite recreations of many mid–20th century physicists (especially those working on the Manhattan project) was poker with friends and colleagues. John von Neumann, one of history's most talented mathematicians and

theoreticians, consistently lost at poker throughout his life, a point often emphasized by his friends after publication of his classic book on game theory: J. von Neumann and O. Morgenstern, *Theory of Games and Economic Behavior*, Princeton, NJ: Princeton University Press, 1944. For more detailed descriptions of physicists and poker, ballistic missile defense, and other scientific and political issues, see E. Teller, *Memoirs*, Cambridge, MA: Perseus Publishing, 2002. I strongly disagree with Teller on many issues, but I am reminded of an old Buddhist saying, "Your enemy is your best teacher." His autobiography provides a unique perspective on an especially critical period of history by someone who played a major role in shaping this history—the good, the bad, and the ugly.

7. The goal of professional poker players is to maximize their winnings against opponents of varying abilities. Thus, the professional's optimum strategy is much more directed toward weaker players. By analogy, the most successful lion is especially good at identifying the weakest wildebeest and efficiently catching it; strong wildebeests are to be avoided as they are quite capable of injuring lions. Similarly, the most successful poker player is not necessarily the best player judged by head-to-head competition against other professionals (or computer). For an interesting test of computer program versus Texas Hold'em players of varying ability, see D. Billings, N. Burch, A. Davidson, R. Holte, J. Schaeffer, T. Schauenberg, and D. Szafron, Approximating game-theoretic optimal strategies for full-scale poker, *International Joint Conference on Artificial Intelligence*, 2003.

8. A. H. Maslow, *Toward a Psychology of Being*, New York: Van Nostrand Reinhold Company, 1968.

Chapter 4

1. A general reference on the nervous system with plenty of nice pictures is M. F. Bear, B. W. Connors, and M. A. Paradiso, *Neuroscience: Exploring the Brain*, Baltimore: Williams & Wilkins, 1996.

2. Technical issues faced in EEG and related neurophysiology are addressed in P. L. Nunez and R. Srinivasan, *Electric Fields of the Brain: The Neurophysics of EEG*, 2nd edition, Oxford University Press, 2006 (Figure 4–1 was reproduced from this source with permission).

   Dynamic issues in cerebral cortex and analog physical systems are treated in P. L. Nunez, *Neocortical Dynamics and Human EEG Rhythms*. New York: Oxford University Press, 1995 (Figures 4–4, 4–5, 4–8, and 4–14 were reproduced from this source with permission).

   The title of this chapter matches a short overview of similar topics: P. L. Nunez and R. Srinivasan, Hearts don't love and brains don't pump: Neocortical dynamic correlates of conscious experience, *Journal of Consciousness Studies* 14:20–34, 2007.

3. V. B. Mountcastle, An organizing principle for cerebral function: The unit module and the distributed system. In F. O. Schmitt and F. G. Worden (Eds.), *The Neurosciences 4th Study Program*, Cambridge, MA: MIT Press, 1979 (a classic chapter on the columnar structure of cerebral cortex).

4. M. E. Scheibel and A. B. Scheibel, Elementary processes in selected thalamic and cortical subsystems–the neural substrates, In F. O. Schmitt and F. G. Worden (Eds.), *The Neurosciences 2nd Study Program*, Cambridge, MA: MIT Press, pp. 443–457, 1970.

5. V. Braitenberg, Comparison of different cortices as a basis for speculation on their function. In H. Petsche and M. A. B. Brazier (Eds.), *Synchronization of EEG Activity in Epilepsies*, New York: Springer-Verlag, pp. 47–63, 1972.

6. Krieg, W. J. S., *Connections of the Cerebral Cortex*, Evanston, IL: Brain Books, 1963. Figure 4–9 was reproduced from this book with permission.

   Krieg, W. J. S. *Architectronics of Human Cerebral Fiber System*, Evanston, IL: Brain Books, 1973.

7. Here is a sample of Walter Freeman's work at UC Berkeley:

   W. J. Freeman, *Mass Action in the Nervous System*, New York: Academic Press, 1975.

   W. J. Freeman and C. A. Skarda, *Brain Research Reviews*, 10:147–175, 1985.

   W. J. Freeman and C. A. Skarda, John Searle and his critics, In E. Lepore and R. van Gulick (Eds.), *Mind/Brain Science: Neuroscience on Philosophy of Mind*, Oxford, UK: Blackwell, pp. 115–127, 1990.

   W. J. Freeman, Scale-free neocortical dynamics, E. Izhikevich (Ed.), *Encyclopedia for Computational Neuroscience*, 2007 [URL http://www.scholarpedia.org/article/Scale-free_neocortical_dynamics].

   W. J. Freeman, Intentionality, In E. Izhikevich, Entry for Encyclopedia for Computational Neuroscience, 2007 [URL http://www.scholarpedia.org/article/Intentionality].

   W. J. Freeman, H. Erwin, Freeman K-set. Scholarpedia 3:3238, 2008 [URL http://www.scholarpedia.org/article/Freeman_K-set].

8. Lester Ingber is a Karate expert (8th Dan Black Belt), physicist, theoretical neuroscientist, and contributor to several other disparate fields [URL http://www.ingber.com]. A sample of publications most relevant to this book follows:

   L. Ingber, Statistical mechanics of neocortical interactions. Dynamics of synaptic modification, *Physical Review A* 28:395–416, 1983 [URL http://www.ingber.com/smni83_dynamics.pdf].

   L. Ingber, Statistical mechanics of neocortical interactions: Stability and duration of the 7 ± 2 rule of short-term memory capacity, *Physical Review A* 31:1183–1186, 1985 [URL http://www.ingber.com/smni85_stm.pdf].

   L. Ingber, Statistical mechanics of multiple scales of neocortical interactions, In P. L. Nunez (Author), *Neocortical Dynamics and Human EEG Rhythms*, New York: Oxford University Press, pp. 628–681, 1995 [URL http://www.ingber.com/smni95_scales.pdf].

   L. Ingber and P. Nunez, Statistical mechanics of neocortical interactions: High resolution path-integral calculation of short-term memory, *Physical Review E* 51:5074–5083, 1995 [URL http://www.ingber.com/smni95_stm.pdf].

   L. Ingber, AI and ideas by statistical mechanics (ISM), In *Encyclopedia of Artificial Intelligence*, J. R. Rabual, J. Dorado, and A. P. Pazos (Eds.), New York: Information Science Reference, pp. 58–64, 2008.

9. P. L. Nunez, The brain wave equation: A model for the EEG, *Mathematical Biosciences* 21:279–297, 1974. This model was originally presented at the American EEG Society Meeting, Houston, TX, August, 1972 and submitted to the *Biophysical Journal* about the same time. The journal held the paper for more than 7 months before rejecting it. One reviewer said that it was *obvious* that brain waves were actually waves, therefore the paper had no point. The second reviewer said just the opposite; brain waves were clearly *not* really waves so the analysis must be wrong.

10. The first four Schumann resonances (Hz) are: theoretical (10.6, 18.3, 25.8, 33.3) and experimental (8, 14, 20, 26). The experimental fundamental and overtone frequencies are accurately predicted by multiplying the theoretical frequencies by the constant factor 0.78, a correction required because the simplified theory idealizes the boundaries as perfectly conducting. The near matching of the fundamental Schumann resonance to the alpha rhythm is apparently a coincidence. One might wonder if some sort of coupling of ambient electromagnetic fields to evolving brains might have occurred. But this conjecture doesn't seem consistent with data indicating that the alpha band does not clearly enjoy special status in mammalian brains other than humans and (evidently) dolphins. As far as I am aware, no one has attempted to record EEG from the larger brains of elephants and whales.

Chapter 5

1. Magnetoencephalography (MEG), developed around 1980, has long been promoted by a combination of legitimate scientific arguments and scientifically unjustified commercial pressures. While it is often claimed that MEG spatial resolution is superior to EEG, this claim is largely false as shown in *Electric Fields of the Brain* (#2 below). The essential reason is as follows: While tissue is transparent to magnetic fields, providing an advantage to MEG, this advantage is essentially cancelled by the increased distance of MEG sensors from brain sources. EEG electrodes sit on the scalp approximately 1 cm from the dominant cortical sources in unfolded (gyral) cortex, whereas MEG coils are typically located 2 to 3 cm above the scalp or about 3 to 7 cm from its dominant cortical sources. The larger end of this estimate takes into account the selective sensitivity of MEG to sources tangent to its sensor coils. Such sources are more likely to occur in cortical folds, which occur deeper (1–3 cm) than sources in unfolded cortex. MEG's advantage in recording sources in cortical folds is apparently due to its *insensitivity* to sources in the crowns of cortical gyri, which often dominate EEG recordings. In other words, if for some reason one is interested mainly in localized sources in a cortical fold (perhaps an epileptic focus), the widely distributed sources in unfolded cortex may be viewed as "noise." Ignoring this "noise" by choosing MEG over EEG then reinforces the localized source model. In summary, EEG and MEG mostly record dipole sources oriented perpendicular and parallel to the scalp surface, respectively; they are selectively sensitive and complementary measures of brain dynamics.

2. Several sources for electroencephalography (EEG) information are:

B. J. Fisch, *Fisch & Spehlmann's EEG Primer, 3rd Edition*, Amsterdam, The Netherlands: Elsevier, 1999.

P. L. Nunez, *EEG*, In V. S. Ramachandran (Eds.), *Encyclopedia of the Human Brain*, *Vol. 2*, La Jolla, CA: Academic Press, pp. 169–179, 2002.

J. C. Shaw, *The Brain's Alpha Rhythms and the Mind*, Amsterdam, The Netherlands: Elsevier, 2003.

P. L. Nunez, Electroencephalography and neural sources, In G. Adelman and B. H. Smith (Eds.), *Encyclopedia of Neuroscience, 3rd Edition*, New York: Elsevier, 2004 [URL http://www.elsevier.com/locate/encneu].

P. L. Nunez and R. Srinivasan, *Electric Fields of the Brain: The Neurophysics of EEG*, *2nd Edition*, Oxford University Press, 2006 (Figures 5–1, 5–6 through 5–12 were reproduced from this book with permission; Figure 5–8 is a simplified version of Figure 8–7 from this book).

P. L. Nunez and R. Srinivasan, *Electroencephalogram*, Scholarpedia, 2007 [URL: http://www.scholarpedia.org/article/Electroencephalogram]

G. Buzsaki, *Rhythms of the Brain*, New York: Oxford University Press, 2006.

3. P. L. Nunez, L. Reid and R. G. Bickford, The relationship of head size to alpha frequency with implications to a brain wave model, *Electroencephalography and Clinical Neurophysiology* 44:344–352, 1978. Our study attempted to select subjects based on extreme head sizes to improve statistical power. In our resulting pool of approximately 150 subjects, significant negative correlations between head size and alpha frequency were found ($r = -0.21$ or -0.23; $p = 0.02$ or 0.01, depending on our definition of alpha peak frequency). As far as I am aware, only one other published study looked for a possible correlation between head (or brain) size and peak alpha frequency: D. Posthuma, M. C. Neale, D. I. Boomsma, and E. J. C. de Geus, Are smarter brains running faster? Heritability of alpha peak frequency, IQ, and their interrelation, *Behavior Genetics* 31:567–579, 2001. This project first addressed the possibility of a correlation between IQ score and alpha frequency. But because IQ is apparently positively correlated with head size and alpha frequency is apparently negatively correlated with head size (based on my earlier paper), the Posthuma et al. study adopted an appropriate correction. But even with this correction, no significant correlation between IQ and alpha frequency was found in the population of the 631 subjects (chosen with no attempt to find extreme head sizes). However, this study did confirm both the expected positive correlation between head size and IQ ($r = 0.15$ to 0.23 depending on test; $p < 0.001$) and the expected negative correlation between head size and alpha frequency ($r = -0.12$; $p = 0.003$). In other studies, the Cuban Human Brain Mapping Project is looking for a possible relation between alpha frequency and cortical surface (using MRI) as well as other issues involving EEG dynamics. Based on the standing wave theory, the predicted negative correlation is actually between the average cortico-cortical fiber length (or global delay time) and peak frequency, so there are some subtle issues to consider in the experiments.

4. W. Penfield and H. Jasper, *Epilepsy and the Functional Anatomy of the Human Brain*, Boston: Little Brown, 1954 (Classic book with intracranial data perhaps not so easily duplicated in modern studies because of changing ethical standards and the condition of modern epilepsy patients with possibly drug-altered EEGs). Figure 5–4 was reproduced from this book with permission.

5. The spatial distribution of potential over the scalp is generally influenced by the choice of reference electrode location. The EEG recordings shown in Figures 5–9 through 5–12 were obtained using the common average reference, which usually provides the closest approximation to a reference-free recording when large electrode arrays are employed. Very similar spatial properties, including robust frontal alpha rhythms, are obtained with neck or ear references as discussed in *Electric Fields of the Brain* (#2 above). The high-resolution estimates, obtained with the New Orleans (surface) spline-Laplacian algorithm, are entirely reference independent. The alternate choice for high-resolution algorithm discussed in *Electric Fields of the Brain* is Melbourne dura imaging (developed by Peter Cadusch and Richard Silberstein), which yields estimates of cortical surface potential patterns that are nearly identical to the New Orleans estimates when applied with high-density electrode arrays, say more than 100 scalp electrodes.

Chapter 6

1. P. L. Nunez, B. M. Wingeier, and R. B. Silberstein, Spatial-temporal structure of human alpha rhythms: Theory, microcurrent sources, multiscale measurements, and global binding of local networks, *Human Brain Mapping* 13:125–164, 2001.

   B. M. Wingeier, *A High-Resolution Study of Large-Scale Dynamic Properties of Human EEG*, PhD Dissertation, Tulane University, April, 2004 (Figures 6–2 and 6–3 were reproduced with permission from this document).

2. M. N. Livanov, *Spatial Organization of Cerebral Processes*, New York: John Wiley & Sons, 1977 (classic work translated from Russian).

3. Alan Gevins is head and founder of The San Francisco Brain Research Institute and Sam Technology Inc. [URL http://www.eeg.com]. Figure 6-7 was obtained by personal communication from Gevins to Nunez. Here are some of Alan's sample EEG papers:

   A. S. Gevins and M. E. Smith, EEG in Neuroergonomics, In R. Parasuraman and M. Rizzo, (Eds.) *Neuroergonomics: The Brain at Work,* New York: Oxford University Press, pp. 15–31, 2008.

   A. S. Gevins, Electrophysiological imaging of brain function, In A. W. Toga and J. C. Mazzioto (Eds.), *Brain Mapping: Methods*, San Diego, CA: Academic Press, pp. 175–188, 2002.

   A. S. Gevins, M. E. Smith, and L. K. McEvoy, Tracking the cognitive pharmacodynamics of psychoactive substances with combinations of behavioral and neurophysiological measures, *Neuropsychopharmacology* 26:27–39, 2002.

   A. S. Gevins, M. E. Smith, L. McEvoy, and D. Yu, High resolution EEG mapping of cortical activation related to working memory: Effects of task difficulty, type of processing, and practice, *Cerebral Cortex* 7:374–385, 1997.

   A. S. Gevins, N. H. Morgan, S. L. Bressler, B. A. Cutillo, R. M. White, J. Illes, D. S. Greer, J. C. Doyle, and G. M. Zeitlin, Human neuroelectric patterns predict performance accuracy, *Science* 235:580–585, 1987.

   A. S. Gevins, R. E. Schaffer, J. C. Doyle, B. A. Cutillo, R. L. Tannehill, and S. L. Bressler, Shadows of thought: Shifting lateralization of human brain electrical patterns during brief visuomotor task, *Science* 220:97–99, 1983.

4. D. Regan, *Human Brain Electrophysiology: Evoked Potentials and Evoked Magnetic Fields in Science and Medicine*, New York: Elsevier, 1989.

5. Richard Silberstein is founder of the Brain Sciences Institute of Swinburne University in Melbourne, Australia, where he remains a professor. In 2005, he started *Neuro-Insight*, a market research company as a means to support his scientific interests [URL http://www.neuro-insight.com.au]. A few of his relevant publications follow; others are listed under Nunez references:

   R. B. Silberstein and G. E. Nield, Brain activity correlates of consumer brand choice shift associated with television advertising, *International Journal of Advertising* 27:359–380, 2008.

   R. B. Silberstein, J. Song, P. L. Nunez, and W. Park, Dynamic sculpting of brain functional connectivity is correlated with performance, *Brain Topography* 16:240–254, 2004.

   R. B. Silberstein, F. Danieli, and P. L. Nunez, Fronto-parietal evoked potential synchronization is increased during mental rotation, *NeuroReport* 14:67–71, 2003.

   R. B. Silberstein, P. L. Nunez, A. Pipingas, P. Harris, and F. Danieli, Steady state visually evoked potential (SSVEP) topography in a graded working memory task. *International Journal of Psychophysiology* 42:219–232, 2001.

R. B. Silberstein, Steady-state visually evoked potentials, brain resonances, and cognitive processes, In P. L. Nunez (Author), *Neocortical Dynamics and Human EEG Rhythms*, Oxford University Press, pp. 272–303, 1995.

R. B. Silberstein, Neuromodulation of neocortical dynamics, In P. L. Nunez (Author), *Neocortical Dynamics and Human EEG Rhythms*, Oxford University Press, pp. 591–627, 1995. This is a discussion of the possible roles of neurotransmitters acting selectively at different cortical depths to move the dynamic behavior between more *hypocoupled* and more *hypercoupled* states. In more recent cognitive EEG studies not ready in time to include in this book, Richard has verified that the neurotransmitter dopamine does indeed reduce functional coupling (coherence). Such selective decoupling appears to be as important as specific coupling for cognitive functions.

6. G. M. Edelman and G. Tononi, *A Universe of Consciousness*, New York: Basic Books, 2000 (a nice little book on the author's works including contributions by Ramesh Srinivasan on frequency tagging experiments).

7. Ramesh Srinivasan holds a joint faculty appointment in Cognitive Science and Biomedical Engineering at the University of California at Irvine and runs the EEG laboratory. A few of his relevant publications follow; others are listed under Nunez references:

R. Srinivasan, D. P. Russell, G. M. Edelman, and G. Tononi, Frequency tagging competing stimuli in binocular rivalry reveals increased synchronization of neuromagnetic responses during conscious perception, *Journal of Neuroscience* 19: 5435–5448, 1999.

R. Srinivasan, W. R. Winter, J. Ding, and P. L. Nunez, EEG and MEG coherence: Measures of functional connectivity at distinct spatial scales of neocortical dynamics, *Journal of Neuroscience Methods* 166:41–52, 2007.

R. Srinivasan, W. Winter, and P. L. Nunez, Source analysis of EEG oscillations using high resolution EEG and MEG, In C. Neuper and W. Klimesch (Eds), *Progress in Brain Research*, Amsterdam, The Netherlands: Elsevier, 2007.

8. P. L. Nunez and R. Srinivasan, *Electric Fields of the Brain: The Neurophysics of EEG*, *2nd Edition*, Oxford University Press, 2006.

9. MEG issues. See note #1 under Chapter 5.

10. J. R. Wolpaw, N. Birbaumer, D. J. McFarlanda, G. Pfurtschellere, and T. M. Vaughan, Brain–computer interfaces for communication and control, *Clinical Neurophysiology* 113:767–791, 2002.

11. The following figures were generated by the software package Mathematica (Wolfram Research Inc.): 5–2, 5–3, 6–1, 7–2, 7–5, 7–7, 8–1, and 8–2.

Chapter 7

1. D. J. Watts, *Small Worlds*, Princeton, NJ: Princeton University Press, 1999.

2. A. N. Wilson, *The Casino Gamblers Guide*, New York: Harper & Row, 1965.

3. A mechanical example of compression of normal mode frequencies due to increased connectivity may be found in Nunez, 1995 (note #6 below, pp. 452–456).

4. F. C. Hoppensteadt and E. M. Izhikevich, Thalamo-cortical interactions modeled by weakly connected oscillators: Could brain use FM radio principles? *Biosystems* 48:85–92, 1998.

E. M. Izhikevich, Weakly connected quasi-periodic oscillators, FM interactions, and multiplexing in the brain, *SIAM Journal on Applied Mathematics* 59:2193–2223, 1999.

The Izhikevich-Hoppensteadt oscillators are pairwise weakly connected to themselves and to a so-called "central" oscillator $\mathbf{X}_0$. While these mathematicians imagined $\mathbf{X}_0$ to be located in the thalamus, I have suggested that $\mathbf{X}_0$ might just as easily represent the global field. The entire coupled system of N oscillators is described by the vectors $\mathbf{X}_n(t) = \{x_{n1}(t), x_{n2}(t), ..., x_{nK(n)}(t)\}$ indicating $K(n)$ scalar dynamic variables for each weakly coupled oscillator n. The coupled equations are of the form

$$\frac{d\mathbf{X}_n}{dt} = \mathbf{F}_n(\mathbf{X}_n) + \varepsilon \sum_{j=1}^{N} \mathbf{G}_{nj}(\mathbf{X}_n, \mathbf{X}_j, \mathbf{X}_0, \varepsilon) \quad n = 1, N$$

Here the vector functions $\mathbf{F}_n$ and $\mathbf{G}_{nj}$ are largely arbitrary. The main point is that the oscillators only substantially interact (that is, interact on a time scale of $1/\varepsilon$) when certain resonant relations exist between the autonomous oscillators.

5. Figure 7–4 was generated by a computer algorithm that progressively inflates each brain hemisphere and transforms them into spheres. The figure was kindly generated for me by Armin Fuchs of Florida Atlantic University based on computer methods described in A. M. Dale, B. Fischl, and M. I. Sereno, Cortical surface-based analysis I: Segmentation and surface reconstruction, *NeuroImage* 9:179–194, 1999; and B. Fischl, M. I. Sereno, and A. M. Dale, Cortical surface-based analysis II: Inflation, flattening, a surface-based coordinate system, *NeuroImage* 9:195–207, 1999.

6. A short overview of global (holistic) brain field theory follows. The label *global theory* is used here to indicate mathematical models in which delays in the (non-local) corticocortical fibers forming most of the white matter in humans provide the underlying time scale for the large-scale EEG dynamics. Periodic boundary conditions are generally essential to global theories because the cortical–white matter system of each hemisphere is topologically close to a spherical shell. This is in marked contrast to *local theory*, which refers to mathematical models of cortical or thalamocortical interactions for which corticocortical propagation delays are neglected. The underlying time scales in local theories are typically postsynaptic potential rise and decay times due to membrane capacitive-resistive properties. Thalamocortical networks are also "local" from the viewpoint of a surface electrode, which cannot distinguish purely cortical from thalamocortical networks. These theories are also "local" in the sense of being independent of global boundary conditions. The following "stripped down" version of global theory proposes equations for two field variables:

$\delta\Psi_e(\mathbf{r}, t) \equiv \Psi(\mathbf{r}, t)$ modulation of excitatory synaptic action density
$\delta\Theta(\mathbf{r}, t)$ modulation of action potential density

The excitatory synaptic action density $\Psi_e(\mathbf{r}, t)$ is defined as the number of active excitatory synapses per unit area of cortical surface in the two-dimensional version of the theory or number per unit length of a cortical strip in the one-dimensional version. The modulation of the cortical synaptic field $\delta\Psi_e(\mathbf{r}, t)$ due to modulation of action potential input $\delta\Theta(\mathbf{r}, t)$ is considered first. Here we treat the inhibitory synaptic action density as a parameter (influencing background cortical excitability) to keep this presentation simple.

In the linear version of the theory, a dynamic transfer function (or its inverse, the dispersion function) is obtained from a basic integral equation relating these two variables as indicated below. The dispersion relation is determined by the poles of the transfer function in the usual manner of linear systems analysis. An equivalent linear differential equation in the variable $\delta\Psi_e(\mathbf{r}, t) \equiv \Psi(\mathbf{r}, t)$ follows directly from the dispersion relation. Nonlinear versions of this equation are developed based on plausible physiological arguments, especially the postulate that instability is prevented in healthy brains by recruitment of additional inhibitory mechanisms (negative feedback) from thalamus or contiguous cortex (lateral inhibition).

Dispersion relation for an idealized cortical medium: The excitatory synaptic action at cortical location $\mathbf{r}$ may be expressed in terms of an inner integral over the cortical surface $S(\mathbf{r}_1)$ and outer integral over distributed axon propagation speeds v_1 as

$$\delta\Psi_e(\mathbf{r}, t) = \delta\Psi_0(\mathbf{r}, t) + \int_0^\infty dv_1 \int\int_{S(\mathbf{r}_1)} \Gamma(\mathbf{r}, \mathbf{r}_1, v_1)\delta\Theta\left(\mathbf{r}_1, t - \frac{|\mathbf{r} - \mathbf{r}_1|}{v_1}\right) dS(\mathbf{r}_1)$$

(7.a)

The corticocortical and thalamocortical fibers are believed to be exclusively excitatory (or nearly so). Thus, Equation 7.a is based on the simple, noncontroversial idea that excitatory synaptic action at cortical location $\mathbf{r}$ is due to excitatory subcortical input $\delta\Psi_0(\mathbf{r}, t)$ plus excitatory action potential density $\delta\Theta(\mathbf{r}, t)$ integrated over the entire neocortex. Action potentials at location $\mathbf{r}_1$ produce synaptic activity at location $\mathbf{r}$ only after a delay that is proportional to cortical separation distance and inversely proportional to axon speed v_1. Distances are defined on an equivalent smooth cortex (see Fig. 7–4). All the complications of white matter (corticocortical) fiber tracts (after smoothing) are included in the kernel or distribution function $\Gamma(\mathbf{r}, \mathbf{r}_1, v_1)$. The outer integral is generally distributed over corticocortical propagation velocities v_1. This is a *linear integral equation*, but it must be combined with a second (generally nonlinear) equation to be solved.

In the simplest *one-dimensional version* of the global theory, axons are assumed to run only in the anterior–posterior direction of each hemisphere (see Fig. 7-5). The corticocortical axons are parceled into M fiber systems with connection densities that fall off exponentially with separation distance $|x - x_1|$. But here we keep only the system with the longest fibers and assume a single axon velocity such that $f(v_1) = \delta(v_1 - v)$. By expanding an assumed sigmoid relationship between action potential density and synaptic action, the required second equation is obtained

$$\rho\delta\Theta(x, t) = 2\beta\delta\Psi(x, t) - \alpha\delta\Psi(x, t)^3$$

(7.b)

where ρ is the number of synapses per long axon. In the linear limiting case ($\alpha \to 0$), the complex frequency is given in terms of real and imaginary parts by

$$\omega(k) = \omega_R(k) + j\gamma(k)$$

(7.c)

This yields the *dispersion relation* in terms of real and imaginary frequencies

$$\omega_R(k) = v\sqrt{k^2 - \beta^2\lambda^2}$$
$$\gamma = v\lambda(\beta - 1)$$

(7.d)

The first of Equations 7.d is identical to Equation 7.3 with the substitution $\omega_R = 2\pi f$ and $k = \frac{2n\pi}{L}$ (standing waves in a closed cortical loop of circumference L). The parameter λ refers to the characteristic exponential fall-off in number density in the longest fiber system. The frequency of each mode decreases as the background excitability of the cortex β increases, suggesting EEG changes associated with sleep and anesthesia. These oversimplified linear waves become unstable when $\beta > 1$, but nonlinear theory suggests several physiological mechanisms in healthy brains that limit growth in wave amplitudes. More physiologically realistic distributed axon velocities yield $\beta = \beta(k)$. Ron Katznelson's solution for standing waves in a spherical shell yields qualitatively similar results (see below). Various versions of the global (holistic) field theory of large-scale dynamics in cerebral cortex and related papers have been published over a 34-year period; a partial list follows:

P. L. Nunez, The brain wave equation: A model for the EEG, *Mathematical Biosciences* 21:279–297, 1974 (originally presented at the American EEG Society Meeting, Houston, TX, August, 1972).

H. R. Wilson and J. D. Cowan, A mathematical theory of the functional dynamics of cortical and thalamic nervous tissue, *Kybernetik* 13:55-80, 1973 (the classic paper on strictly local theory).

P. L. Nunez, Wave-like properties of the alpha rhythm. *IEEE Transactions on Biomedical Engineering* 21:473-482, 1974 (early frequency-wavenumber spectral study suggesting the existence of an EEG dispersion relation).

R. D. Katznelson, *Deterministic and Stochastic Field Theoretic Models in the Neurophysics of EEG*, PhD Dissertation. La Jolla, CA: The University of California at San Diego, 1982 (Solution obtained in a spherical shell; also presented in Chapter 11 of Nunez, 1981, *Electric Fields of the Brain* (1st edition) and the appendix of Nunez, 1995, listed below).

P. L. Nunez, Generation of human EEG by a combination of long and short range neocortical interactions, *Brain Topography* 1:199-215, 1989 (an early "marriage" of global to a local theory published by Ab van Rotterdam and Fernando Lopes da Silva).

P. L. Nunez, *Neocortical Dynamics and Human EEG Rhythms*, Oxford University Press, 1995.

V. K. Jirsa and H. Haken, A derivation of a macroscopic field theory of the brain from the quasi-microscopic neural dynamics, *Physica D* 99:503–526, 1997 (a comprehensive "marriage" of Nunez global theory to the local theory of Wilson and Cowan).

H. Haken, What can synergetics contribute to the understanding of brain functioning? In *Analysis of Neurophysiological Brain Functioning*, C. Uhl (Ed.) Berlin, Germany: Springer-Verlag, pp. 7–40, 1999.

P. L. Nunez, Toward a quantitative description of large scale neocortical dynamic function and EEG. *Behavioral and Brain Sciences* 23:371-437, 2000 (invited target article).

P. L. Nunez, Neocortical dynamic theory should be as simple as possible, but not simpler, *Behavioral and Brain Sciences* 23:415–437, 2000 (response to 18 commentaries on above target article by various neuroscientists).

B. M. Wingeier, P. L. Nunez, and R. B. Silberstein, Spherical harmonic decomposition applied to spatial-temporal analysis of human high-density electroencephalogram. *Physical Review E* 64:051916-1 to 9, 2001 (one of the experimental verifications of EEG wave behavior; a more extensive coverage is provided in Chapters 10 and 11 of the following Nunez & Srinivasan book).

B. M. Wingeier, *A High-Resolution Study of Large-Scale Dynamic Properties of Human EEG*, PhD Dissertation, Tulane University, April, 2004 (contains strong evidence for the existence of an alpha wave dispersion relation as well as estimates of phase and group velocities; summarized in *Electric Fields of the Brain*, below).

P. L. Nunez and R. Srinivasan, *Electric Fields of the Brain: The Neurophysics of EEG*, 2nd edition, Oxford University Press, 2006 (first edition authored by P. L. Nunez, 1981).

P. L. Nunez and R. Srinivasan, A theoretical basis for standing and traveling brain waves measured with human EEG with implications for an integrated consciousness,

Clinical Neurophysiology 117:2424–2435, 2006 (non mathematical summary of global theory and related experiments).

7. This note looks at several issues that may require consideration when making comparisons between mathematical models of cortical dynamics and experimental EEG (or other) data. Global boundary conditions (including system size), noise, and recording methods are all potentially important factors influencing genuine (observable) dynamics in complex nonlinear systems. Such influences may not be well appreciated when complex systems are reduced to simple ordinary differential equations like the famous Lorenz system. By contrast, genuine complex systems possess boundary conditions that may impose spatial structure that inhibits temporal chaos. Another potential influence of boundary conditions is to facilitate spatial coherence even when the temporal behavior of individual modes becomes chaotic (see the Tabor book and Bishop et al. paper in list below). Chaotic effects can also become "lost" in noise so that experimental observations are unable to distinguish between stochastic and chaotic behaviors (Ingber et al.). Finally, spatial filtering (as in scalp-recorded EEG) can easily influence observed temporal dynamics (Nunez et al.). This short look at fluid convection introduces several of these issues.

The original explosion of interest in chaos was based on work in the papers by Saltzman and Lorenz listed below. If these were proverbial "shots heard around the world," it required about 15–20 years for most scientists to hear them. The fluid convection system under study is governed by a pair of complicated nonlinear partial differential equations in two dependent variables: the stream function $\Psi(\mathbf{r}, t)$ and the temperature perturbation $T(\mathbf{r}, t)$ with respect to the case of no convection. The stream function yields the fluid velocity by means of the curl operation, $\mathbf{v} = \nabla \times \Psi$. Saltzman and Lorenz sought solutions in two dimensions (x, z) of the form:

$$\Psi_y(x, z, t) = \sum_{m=1}^{\infty} \sum_{n=1}^{\infty} A_{mn}(t) \sin\left(\frac{m\pi a x}{h}\right) \sin\left(\frac{n\pi z}{h}\right) \qquad (7.\mathrm{e})$$

$$T(x, z, t) = \sum_{m=0}^{\infty} \sum_{n=1}^{\infty} B_{mn}(t) \cos\left(\frac{m\pi a x}{h}\right) \sin\left(\frac{n\pi z}{h}\right) \qquad (7.\mathrm{f})$$

This system is roughly equivalent to a rectangular "tank" of depth h, width h/a, and infinite in the 3rd dimension. Lorenz instituted an extreme truncation by keeping only three terms in the expansions (A_{11}, B_{02}, B_{11}) based on numerical work by Saltzman. These are the three dependent variables of the famous Lorenz equations that led to the modern fuss about chaos. The independent variable is a nondimensional time τ that applies to the full expansion of the partial differential equations as well as the simple, truncated Lorenz system; the time variable is

$$\tau = \frac{\pi^2 (1 + a^2) \kappa t}{h^2} \qquad (7.\mathrm{g})$$

where κ is the fluid thermal conductivity. In order to show the isolated effect of tank depth h on spectra obtained for a wide range of dynamic behavior, I simply chose κ to be a uniformly distributed random variable (over a factor of 10), kept a (the ratio of depth to width) constant, and let the depth vary over $1 < h < 3$. The "central" oscillation frequency is then simply $f = \tau^{-1}$, which applies to chaotic and well as periodic solutions of the set (7.e) and (7.f). In other words, I "cheated" by never solving the actual system. *Here is the point of this little exercise*: an imagined fluid experimentalist with no access to theory would only have the experimental data showing the behavior in Figure 7-7, making him somewhat analogous to today's brain scientists. This suggests that system size and other boundary conditions can generally be expected to make important contributions to the dynamic behavior of complex systems, including brains.

B. Saltzman, Finite amplitude free convection as an initial value problem-I, *Journal of Atmospheric Sciences* 19:329–341, 1962.

E. N. Lorenz, *Deterministic nonperiodic flow, Journal of Atmospheric Sciences* 20:*130–141, 1963.*

A. R. Bishop, K. Fesser, P. S. Lomdahl, and S. E. Trullinger, Influence of solitons in the initial state or chaos in the driven, damped sine-Gordon system. *Physica* 7D:259-279, 1983.

M. Tabor, *Chaos and Integrability in Nonlinear Dynamics,* New York: Wiley, 1989.

P. L. Nunez and R. Srinivasan, Implications of recording strategy for estimates of neocortical dynamics using EEG. *Chaos: An Interdisciplinary Journal of Nonlinear Science* 3:257–266, 1993.

L. Ingber, R. Srinivasan, and P. L. Nunez, Path-integral evolution of chaos embedded in noise: Duffing neocortical analog, *Mathematical and Computer Modelling* 23:43–53, 1996 [URL http://www.ingber.com/path96_duffing.pdf].

8. P. L. Nunez, Modeling inflation in an idealized fictitious society with implications for the U.S. economy, to be submitted sometime.

Chapter 8

1. L. Mlodinow, *The Drunkard's Walk,* New York: Pantheon Books, 2008.
2. N. N. Taleb, *Fooled by Randomness,* New York: Random House, 2005.
   N. N. Taleb, *The Black Swan,* New York: Random House, 2007.
3. T. A. Bass, *The Eudemonic Pie. Or Why Would Anyone Play Roulette Without a Computer in His Shoe?* Boston: Houghton Mifflin, 1985.
4. R. Feynman, *Lectures on Physics,* Vol. 2, Palo Alto, CA: Addison-Wesley, 1963.
5. E. N. Lorenz, *Predictability: Does the Flap of a Butterfly's Wings in Brazil set off a Tornado in Texas?* Presented at the meeting of the American Association for the Advancement of Science in Washington, DC, 1972.
6. A. Scott, *Stairway to the Mind.* New York: Springer-Verlag, 1995.
7. Papers by Lester Ingber are listed for Chapter 4, note #8.
8. J. R. Searle, *The Rediscovery of the Mind,* Cambridge, MA: MIT Press, 1992.
   J. R. Searle, *The Mystery of Consciousness,* New York: The New York Review of Books, 1997.
9. E. F. Kelly and E. W. Kelly, *Irreducible Mind,* Lanham, MD: Rowman & Littlefield, 2007.
10. See Chapter 6, note #11.

Chapter 9

1. Skepticism about a possible deep role for quantum mechanics in consciousness is summarized in a letter by neuroscientist Christof Koch and physicist Klaus Hepp, Quantum mechanics in the brain, *Nature* 440, 611–612, 2006. K & H focus on coherent quantum states that most physicists agree cannot survive in brains, stating "...brains

obey quantum mechanics, but do not seem to exploit any of its special features." But, do not chemical reactions "exploit" "special" quantum features like entanglement? In Chapter 12, I argue that elementary particle systems, molecules, cells, brains, and the universe can be viewed as "quantum Ultra-Computers" operating in a grand nested hierarchy. These "computers" follow instructions called the laws of physics. Unlike the primitive man made quantum computers cited by K & H, nature's "computers" use *both* entanglement and decoherence to their advantage. Some of the open questions about putative quantum connections to consciousness may be expressed in the context of the following thought experiment: What level of hierarchical complexity in a "blueprint" would be required to build a conscious brain? Could, for example, classical chemical models provide adequate substitutes for full quantum instructions? Web-published criticisms of K & H include a tendency to equate neural correlates with consciousness itself (B. Alan Wallace, Illusions of knowledge, Response to "Quantum mechanics and the brain" by Christof Koch and Klaus Hepp [URL http://www.sbin-stitute.com/KHresponse.pdf] and discounting possible macroscopic quantum effects that might not be suppressed by environmental decoherence (Henry P. Stapp, Quantum mechanics in the brain [URL www-physics.lbl.gov/~stapp/koch-hepp.doc]).

2. H. P. Stapp, *Mind, Matter, and Quantum Mechanics*. Berlin, Germany: Springer, 1994.

   H. P. Stapp, *Mindful Universe*. Berlin, Germany: Springer, 2007.

3. P. Davies, *God and the New Physics*, New York: Simon & Schuster, 1983.

   P. Davies, *About Time*, New York: Simon & Schuster, 1995.

   P. Davies, *The Fifth Miracle*, New York: Simon & Schuster, 1999.

   P. Davies, *The Goldilocks Enigma*, New York: First Mariner Books, 2006.

   S. Hawking, *A Brief History of Time*, New York: Random House (Bantam Books), 1988.

4. B. Green, *The Fabric of the Cosmos*, New York: Vintage Books, 2004 (includes user-friendly descriptions of Bell-ERP related experiments similar to my description in Chapter 11).

   L. Smolin, *Three Roads to Quantum Gravity*, New York: Basic Books, 2001.

5. J. Barrow and F. Tipler, *The Anthropic Cosmological Principle*, New York: Oxford University Press, 1986.

6. L. Smolin, *The Life of the Cosmos*, New York: Oxford University Press, 1997.

7. L. Susskind, *The Cosmic Landscape*, New York: Little, Brown, and Company, 2006.

Chapter 10

1. A similar analog system is described in B. Rosenblum and F. Kuttner, *Quantum Enigma*, New York: Oxford University Press, 2006.

2. R. Feynman, *Lectures on Physics*, Vol. 3, Palo Alto, CA: Addison-Wesley, 1963 (a core reference for the two slit experiment as well as many technical issues).

   N. Herbert, *Quantum Reality*, New York: Anchor Books, 1985.

   D. Deutsch, *The Fabric of Reality*, New York: Penguin Books, 1997.

   J. Al-Khalili, *Quantum. A Guide for the Perplexed*, London: Weidenfeld & Nicolson, 2003 (includes many color pictures and provides a nice updated summary of different ontological interpretations; I found this book especially well written and useful).

3. T. Hey and P. Walters, *The Quantum Universe*, London: Cambridge University Press, 1987 (practical applications in quantum mechanics with many color pictures).

4. L. Pauling and E. B. Wilson, Jr., *Introduction to Quantum Mechanics*, New York: Dover Publications, 1935 (I cite this old book to emphasize that the basic mathematics of quantum mechanics remains largely unchanged after 70+ years).

5. The close analogy between the mechanical vibrations of musical instruments and the quantum wavefunction is outlined here. Note that quantum physicists typically adopt symbolic shorthand known as Dirac notation, which is strictly avoided here in order to emphasize links to the classical analog. The classical wave equation for the displacement $\Psi(\mathbf{r}, t)$ of a mechanical medium with propagation speed c (say a vibrating string or membrane) with an added inhomogeneous "stiffness" influence $V(\mathbf{r})$ is given by the partial differential equation

$$\frac{\partial^2 \Psi}{\partial t^2} = c^2 \nabla^2 \Psi - V\Psi \tag{10.a}$$

The solution in one spatial dimension may be expressed as a sum over terms having different oscillatory frequencies ω_n, that is

$$\Psi(x, t) = \sum_{n=0}^{\infty} (a_n \cos \omega_n t + b_n \sin \omega_n t)\psi_n(x) \tag{10.b}$$

The spatial *eigenfunctions* $\psi_n(x)$ are solutions of the ordinary differential equation

$$c^2 \psi_n''(x) + \left[\omega_n^2 - V(x)\right]\psi_n(x) = 0 \tag{10.c}$$

To take one example, a stretched string fixed at both ends with a system of distributed attached springs of constant natural frequency ω_0 yields $V(x) = \omega_0^2$ and the dispersion relation

$$\omega_n^2 = \omega_0^2 + c^2 k_n^2 \tag{10.d}$$

The same dispersion relation is obtained in several other classical systems, for example, electrical transmission lines and hot plasmas. When the stiffness (spring) parameter $\omega_0 = 0$, the usual *nondispersive waves* (which propagate without changing shape) are obtained, that is, $\omega_n = ck_n$, where the $k_n = \frac{n\pi}{L}$ are the spatial frequencies allowed by the (fixed-ends) boundary conditions in a string of length L. In this case, the solution (10.b) may be expressed

$$\Psi(x, t) = \sum_{n=0}^{\infty} (a_n \cos \omega_n t + b_n \sin \omega_n t)\sin k_n x \tag{10.e}$$

Note that the solution (10.e) involves two sets of arbitrary constants that must be evaluated from the initial conditions, $\Psi(x, 0)$ and $(\partial \Psi/\partial t)_{t=0}$, consistent with the fact that Equation 10.a is second order in the time variable.

Schrödinger's equation for a wavefunction Ψ of a single non relativistic particle of mass m subject to a classical potential $V(\mathbf{r})$ is

$$j\hbar \frac{\partial \Psi}{\partial t} = -\frac{\hbar^2}{2m} \nabla^2 \Psi + V\Psi \tag{10.f}$$

The solution to Equation 10.f in one spatial dimension is similar to 10.b except that, unlike the classical wave amplitude, the quantum wavefunction is complex. Also in contrast to the classical wave equation, Schrödinger's equation is first order in time, so a unique solution involves only one set of constants evaluated from $\Psi(x, 0)$. The spatial part of the solution is given by the same ordinary differential equation (10.c) as the classical system

$$\frac{\hbar^2}{2m}\psi_n''(x) + [\hbar\omega_n - V(x)]\psi_n(x) = 0 \qquad (10.g)$$

If a particle is placed in a one-dimensional *infinite square well potential* of length L (essentially a trough with very thick walls), the classical potential $V(x)$ is zero inside the well and infinite at well walls. The boundary conditions on the wavefunction, $\Psi(0,t) = \Psi(L,t) = 0$, are identical to those of a string with both ends fixed. In this case, the quantum dispersion relation analogous to the classical dispersion relation (10.d) is

$$E_n = \hbar\omega_n = \frac{n^2\pi^2\hbar^2}{2mL^2} \qquad (10.h)$$

The particle in the trough is *forbidden by nature from acquiring arbitrary energies*; the only allowed energies are given by the discrete values E_n, $n = 1, 2, 3, \ldots$ The solution for the quantum wavefunction is very similar to the classical solution (10.e), that is

$$\Psi(x,t) = \sum_{n=1}^{\infty} A_n e^{-j\omega_n t}\sin k_n x \qquad (10.i)$$

where $e^{-j\omega_n t} \equiv \cos\omega_n t - j\sin\omega_n t$. If the well walls have finite thickness such that $V(x)$ is finite for $x < 0$ and/or $x > L$, the quantum system is analogous to a classical string with flexible end supports. The wavefunction $\Psi(x,t)$ is no longer zero at well walls and "leaks" into the external world, demonstrating quantum tunneling, a case where the particle has some chance of escaping the (classically inescapable) well by quantum "magic."

Chapter 11

1. One notable case of measurement-created distortion in EEG is thus: Psychologists doing evoked potential research in the 1970s and 1980s linked (conductively) the subject's ears or mastoids to form the so-called *linked ears reference*. This approach changed the natural potential distribution over the scalp (noted early on by my colleague, Ron Katznelson). The second, more serious, problem was that it produced an essentially random reference electrode location depending on electrode contact impedances. See the following:

    P. L. Nunez, Comments on the paper by Miller, Lutzenberger, and Elbert, *Journal of Psychophysiology* 5:279–280, 1991.

    P. L. Nunez and R. Srinivasan, *Electric Fields of the Brain: The Neurophysics of EEG*, 2nd Edition, Oxford University Press, 2006.

2. A. Aspect, Bell's inequality test: More ideal than ever, *Nature* 398:189, 1999.

3. Henry Stapp's references are listed in Chapter 9, notes 1 and 2. See also [URL www-physics.lbl.gov/~stapp].

4. Bohm mechanics is outlined as follows: Schrödinger's equation for a single non relativistic particle of mass m subject to a classical potential V is

$$j\hbar\frac{\partial\Psi}{\partial t} = -\frac{\hbar^2}{2m}\nabla^2\Psi + V\Psi \qquad (11.a)$$

Express the wavefunction in polar form in terms of the new variables (R, S)

$$\Psi = R e^{(jS/\hbar)} \tag{11.b}$$

to yield separate equations for the two new variables R and S

$$\frac{\partial S}{\partial t} + \frac{(\nabla S)^2}{2m} + V - \frac{\hbar^2}{2m}\frac{\nabla^2 R}{R} = 0 \tag{11.c}$$

$$\frac{\partial R^2}{\partial t} + \nabla\bullet\left(R^2\frac{\nabla S}{m}\right) = 0 \tag{11.d}$$

Note that $R^2 = |\Psi|^2$ is the probability density function yielding the probability of finding the particle between $\mathbf{r}$ and $\mathbf{r} + \Delta\mathbf{r}$ at time t. R is unitless, and from Equation 11.b, S has the units of erg sec, so the term $\frac{\nabla S}{m}$ has units of velocity. Equation 11.d may then be seen as identical to the basic conservation equation (8.2), in this case indicating that probability density is conserved. Essentially, this means only that an *observed* particle must be found *somewhere*. When $\hbar \to 0$, Equation 11.c takes the form of the standard Hamilton-Jacobi equation governing motion of a classical particle when subjected to a classical potential V. This formalism represents an alternate expression of Newton's law of motion in which the particle velocity is given by $\frac{\nabla S}{m}$. From Equation 11.c we conclude that a quantum particle subjected to a classical potential V behaves *as if* it is a classical particle subjected to the total potential $V + Q$, where the (new) *quantum potential* and *quantum force* are given by

$$Q = -\frac{\hbar^2}{2m}\frac{\nabla^2 R}{R} \quad \text{and} \quad \mathbf{F}_Q = \frac{\hbar^2}{2m}\nabla\left(\frac{\nabla^2 R}{R}\right) \tag{11.e}$$

The implied equation motion for the non relativistic quantum particle exposed to a classical force $\mathbf{F}_C = -\nabla V$ is then

$$m\frac{d\mathbf{v}}{dt} = \mathbf{F}_C + \mathbf{F}_Q \tag{11.2}$$

Note that the quantum force in Equation 11.e is not affected when the wavefunction Ψ is multiplied by a constant. That is, the quantum force is independent of the intensity of Ψ, but rather depends on its three-dimensional form in space. The quantum force does not generally fall off with distance; it is *explicitly nonlocal*. In the Bohm interpretation, the quantum force $\mathbf{F}_Q$ acts to *guide* the particle along what might be quite an intricate path, perhaps through one of the two slits or interferometer arms shown in Figures 10–5 to 10–9 or perhaps through a classically impenetrable barrier.

D. Bohm and B. J. Hiley, *The Undivided Universe*, New York: Routledge, 1993.
5. J. P. Hogan, *Paths to Otherwhere*, Riverdale, NY: Baen Publishing Enterprises, 1996.
6. Seth Lloyd has described his "many worlds encounter" with Borges (Chapter 12, note #5).

Chapter 12

1. I have neglected the possibility of speculative structures like *wormholes* connecting distance regions of space-time that might or might not allow the passage of ordinary information.

2. A modern overview may be found in S. Laureys and G. Tononi (Eds.), *The Neurology of Consciousness: Cognitive Neuroscience and Neuropathology*. Amsterdam, The Netherlands: Elsevier, 2009.

3. Quoted by C. E. M. Joad in *Guide to Modern Thought*, London: Faber & Farber, pp. 94–94, 1933, from an interview with one J. W. N. Sullivan in *The Observer*, January 25, 1931.

4. R. Tallis, *Why the Mind Is Not a Computer*, Charlottesville, VA: Imprint Academic, 2004 (first published in 1994).

5. S. Lloyd, *Programming the Universe*, New York: Random House (Vintage Books), 2007.

6. For a quick overview of complexity, see: O. Sporns, *Complexity*, Scholarpedia, 2007 [URL http://www.scholarpedia.org/article/Complexity]. See also M. Gell-Mann and S. Lloyd, Information measures, effective complexity, and total information, *Complexity* 2:44–52, 1996.

   Effective complexity is one plausible category, but we typically describe the relative complexity of living systems in terms of their potential range of behavior. Human brains, for example, are able to build tools that greatly extend the capacity of human minds and bodies. One might describe such behaviors as motion in multi-dimensional spaces, the higher the dimensionality in which the system can move, the more complex the system. *Complexity would then be the amount of freedom to explore Hilbert space.* Just saying this is one thing, expressing it in some useful mathematical context is quite another.

7. K. J. Friston, G. Tononi, O. Sporns, and G. M. Edelman, Characterizing the complexity of neuronal interactions, *Human Brain Mapping* 3:302–314, 1995.

   G. Tononi, Consciousness as integrated information: A provisional manifesto, *Biological Bulletin* 215:216–242, 2008.

8. Lester Ingber references are listed under note Chapter 4, note #8.

9. H. Haken, *Synergetics. An Introduction*, 3rd edition, Berlin, Germany: Springer-Verlag, 1983.

   H. Haken, What can synergetics contribute to the understanding of brain functioning? In *Analysis of Neurophysiological Brain Functioning*, C. Uhl (Ed.) Berlin, Germany: Springer-Verlag, pp. 7–40, 1999.

   V. K. Jirsa and H. Haken, A derivation of a macroscopic field theory of the brain from the quasi-microscopic neural dynamics, *Physica D* 99:503–526, 1997.

10. C. Uhl (Ed.), *Analysis of Neurophysiological Brain Functioning*, Berlin, Germany: Springer-Verlag, 1999.

11. Herms Romijn, Are virtual photons the elementary carriers of consciousness? *Journal of Consciousness Studies* 9:61–81, 2002.

12. Walter Freeman's references are listed under Chapter 4, note #7.

13. V. B. Mountcastle, An organizing principle for cerebral function: The unit module and the distributed system. In F. O. Schmitt and F. G. Worden (Eds.), *The Neurosciences 4th Study Program*. Cambridge, MA: MIT Press, 1979.

14. E. R. Kandel, *In Search of Memory*, New York: WW Norton & Company, 2006.

15. J. D. Watson, *DNA. The Secret of Life*, New York: Alfred A. Knopf, 2004.

16. R. Penrose, *The Emperor's New Mind*, Oxford, UK: Oxford University Press, 1989.

    R. Penrose, *The Large, the Small and the Human Mind*. Cambridge, UK: Cambridge University Press, 1997.

17. Henry Stapp's references are listed in notes #1 and #2 for Chapter 9.

18. In 1989 Roger Penrose published his famous book *The Emperor's New Mind*, implying that some new theory of quantum gravity (encompassing both quantum

mechanics and general relativity) may be the key to unlocking the secrets of consciousness. This conjecture was strongly criticized by many neuroscientists and physicists, for example, by open peer commentary in *Behavioral and Brain Sciences* (13:643–706, 1990). My personal response to the Penrose position at that time was something like, "this idea is absurd." But, I have since taken Penrose's general idea more seriously even though his postulated neuro quantum mechanisms appear to me to be real long shots. Here are some reasons why I have come to take his *general* idea seriously. The worldview due to Isaac Newton was dramatically altered in two distinct directions by quantum mechanics and general relativity. Quantum mechanics altered the relationship between observer and observed such that observer becomes an active participant. But quantum mechanics kept the old Newtonian view in which space and time act as the passive stage on which events unfold. By contrast, general relativity did just the opposite; it retained the Newtonian observer–observed relationship but elevated space-time from a passive stage to an active participant in the action. Physicist Lee Smolin and others suggest that any successful theory of quantum gravity must have purged both "parochial" Newtonian views so as to conform to both quantum mechanics and general relativity in appropriate limiting cases. The imagined new theory must be analogous to a play in which the ever-expanding stage and props are dynamically influenced by the actors. Furthermore, the play's outcome may evolve partly as a result of audience–actor interactions. I am reminded of one of the small experimental playhouses in San Diego in the 1970s, where the audience was always limited to 12 "jury members" who voted on the guilt or innocence of the defendant played by an actor. On some nights he was found guilty, other nights innocent. This theater analogy is way overstated because the universe evolved for 14 billion years before human consciousness appeared. Yet it is still possible that some kind of fundamental informational structure has existed from the beginning and underlies both the physical and mental worlds. The two leading contenders for a full theory of quantum gravity are string theory, with its roots in quantum mechanics, and loop quantum gravity, which stems from general relativity. Both approaches describe physics on very small scales, roughly the Planck length of 10^{-33} cm. Can these disparate approaches be made compatible? Smolin (one of the originators of loop quantum gravity) suggests a possible picture in which space is actually "woven" from a network of strings like cloth woven from a network of threads. Regardless of whether this picture has any approximate validity, he suggests that the universe must be just *an evolving network of relationships* and any correct theory of *quantum cosmology must be a theory of the information exchanged between subsystems of the universe.* As an example of the possible fundamental role of information, Israeli physicists Vigdop and Fouxon (2009) propose that the universe may consist of a complex information web made up of entities interacting by resonance principles. This web does not exist within space-time, rather spatial-temporal physical laws (classical and quantum mechanics, general relativity, etc.) and space-time itself emerge from web interactions. These "informational resonances" between web entities are independent of physical distances. The web extends the familiar spatial-temporal links between objects, possibly accounting for the structure of classical chaos and the nonlocal influences of quantum mechanics. The postulated informational web appears to have properties in common with David Bohm's implicate order and the Ultra-Information that I posit in Chapter 12.

L. Smolin, *Three Roads to Quantum Gravity*, New York: Basic Books, 2001.

A. J. Vidgop and I. Fouxon, Web as a fundamental universal system [URL http:// arxiv.org/pdf/0907.0471v2].

19. E. F. Kelly and E. W. Kelly, *Irreducible Mind*, Lanham, MD: Rowman & Littlefield, 2007.

20. Legitimate scientists participating in psi experiments face severe and unusual risks, including becoming fraud victims. My personal view, as one unfamiliar with psi literature, is unavoidably colored by the ubiquitous psi fraud of supermarket ilk, although I note several intriguing reports in *Irreducible Mind* (note 19). But even if robust psi-positive data are available, my guess is that general scientific acceptance would require, at minimum, active participation of an interdisciplinary team of highly prestigious scientists. The team might design and carry out an experimental program aiming to verify or refute earlier positive psi reports. In my view, such team would require an independent "sheriff" to insure that no participant (including the lead scientists running the study) engage in fraud or self delusion. The reason for such extreme measures is that any report of positive psi results would be viewed with great suspicion, even of the scientists enjoying impeccable reputations before the study is carried out. Recruitment of such a "dream team" and its "sheriff" would be quite difficult and add substantially to the cost but might be possible if the earlier, controversial results were deemed sufficiently compelling and private funding could be obtained. But, don't hold your breath.

21. My brief summaries of relativity, quantum mechanics, and thermodynamics in the context of the RQTC conjecture provide only an introduction to modern physics. Non physicists might well question if more comprehensive treatments provide solutions to the cited mysteries. But as far as I can tell, the ontological issues introduced here appear just as deep and perplexing when advanced physics is employed. For a comprehensive overview, see R. Penrose, *The Road to Reality. A Complete Guide to the Laws of the Universe*, New York: Vintage Books, 2007 (first published in 2004), a very clearly written, but nevertheless formidable, tome (1099 pages with plenty of mathematics). Penrose introduces the label *quanglement* to indicate quantum information or (nonlocal) quantum influences. Quanglement may be considered a sub category of Ultra-Information.

Index

Note: A *t* or *f* following a page number indicates tabular or figure material.